The Complete Home Healer

ABOUT THE AUTHOR

ANGELA SMYTH is a medical journalist and author who has written extensively for health and science publications in the United Kingdom and the United States. She is a frequent contributor to the *Independent* and the *Guardian,* as well as to *Here's Health* and *BBC Good Health.* She is the author of *S.A.D.: Winter Depression.*

Consultant editor Dr. Hilary Jones is British television's best-known doctor. He contributes to a number of publications and is also a practicing general practitioner.

CONTRIBUTORS

Leon Chaitow, N.D., D.O. (naturopathy)

Robert Bridge, R.S. Hom. (homeopathy)

Kathryn Marsden (diet)

Helena Bridge, D.O. (osteopathy/massage)

Shirley Price (aromatherapy)

Dr. Julian Kenyon (acupressure)

Anthony Attenborough (Bates Method)

The Complete
Home Healer

YOUR GUIDE TO
EVERY TREATMENT AVAILABLE
FOR OVER 300 OF THE MOST
COMMON HEALTH PROBLEMS

ANGELA SMYTH

FOREWORD BY ELSON M. HAAS, M.D.

PREFACE BY HILARY JONES, M.D.

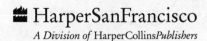
HarperSanFrancisco
A Division of HarperCollins*Publishers*

THE COMPLETE HOME HEALER: *Your Guide to Every Treatment Available for Over 300 of the Most Common Health Problems.* Copyright © 1994 by Angela Smyth. Printed in the United States of America. All rights reserved. No part of this book may be used or reproduced in any manner whatsoever without written permission except in the case of brief quotations embodied in critical articles and reviews. For information address HarperCollins Publishers, 10 East 53rd Street, New York, NY 10022.

The Author hereby asserts the Author's right to be identified as the author of the Work.

FIRST EDITION

Library of Congress Cataloging-in-Publication Data

Smyth, Angela.
    The complete home healer : your guide to every treatment available for over
    300 of the most common health problems / Angela Smyth : consultant editor,
    Hilary Jones. — 1st ed.
        p. cm.
    Includes index.
    ISBN 0-06-250844-x (hdcvr : acid-free paper)
    1. Medicine, Popular—Encyclopedias. 2. Alternative medicine—Encyclopedias.
    3. Self-care, Health—Encyclopedias. I. Title.
    RC81.A2S67 1994
    616.024'03—dc20   93–40025
                                                                              CIP

94 95 96 97 98 CWI 10 9 8 7 6 5 4 3 2 1

This editon is printed on acid-free paper that meets the American National Standards Institute Z39.48 Standard.

///////// Contents

///////// *Note to the Reader*

FOREWORD

I HAVE BEEN WAITING FOR A PUBLICATION like HarperCollins's *The Complete Home Healer* for quite some time. This extensive book will be a valuable resource for my practice and for my patients. People now will be able to assess their therapeutic options by having this book at their fingertips rather than just accepting their doctor's prescription, which may be based only on one (limited) set of theories/beliefs and one therapeutic approach.

Western medicine, i.e. allopathic medicine, does not work for many of the problems it attempts to treat. Its strength is in acute and crisis care, diagnostic evaluations, and technical surgeries. Its weakness is clearly in the treatment and management of chronic disease, the generation of which I believe it contributes to as much as it helps by the regular use or overuse of strong medicines and chemicals. There is clearly a need for "alternative" treatments.

Integrated medicine, i.e. complementary medicine as it is referred to by Ms. Smyth, blends together conventional (orthodox) practice with traditional (alternative) medical approaches. In my opinion, a more integrated medical path is clearly the answer to the health care crisis and the personal long-term well-being of our people.

It is important and imperative that medical practitioners understand and utilize a larger approach to health care. The managing physician must be able to suggest the safest, most effective therapy for the individual patient, avoiding over treatment, side effects, and excessive costs—all so inherent in our medical system's treatment of both crisis and chronic conditions. Furthermore, Western medicine alone most often does not correct the common chronic conditions, such as hypertension and cardiovascular diseases, diabetes, and cancer, because it does not really address the causes, which are most often found in our lifestyle and exposures to chemicals and toxic agents. Clearly, the more wisdom we gain in how to live will help us prevent some of these chronic conditions, a much more valuable outcome.

A more integrated way to look at health and illness suggests that our body—our physical functions, energy levels, vitality, mental and emotional balance—is a by-product of our life. Our basic constitution and upbringing, our past problems and how we treated them, our diet, stress levels, relationships, the level of joy in our work or service, and more—all contribute to our overall health.

An integrated approach utilizes multiple systems of healing to allow the best choice to be applied to each specific concern. For simpler and transient problems, milder and subtler forms of treatment that support the body's healing mechanisms are appropriate, whereas for really serious or intense symptoms or illnesses, stronger interventions that kill germs or suppress overactive systems may be required. And most significantly, an integrated approach interacts with personal illness from a different perspective, whereby your initial question moves from "How can I get rid of this?" (the attack and conquer approach) to more revealing questions, such as "Why do I have this now? Body, what are you telling me? and What can I do to heal?"

The Complete Home Healer takes a multi-disciplinary approach to everything. I love it! The application of dietary changes and nutritional supplements, herbs, Chinese medicine and acupuncture, Osteopathy and cranio-sacral therapy, and homeopathy to name a few of the treatment modalities—I have found very useful in helping people resolve many conditions. Each treatment has its strengths and weaknesses, and *The Complete Home Healer* helps you apply the most useful therapies per condition.

For example, the reduction of *allergies* is often greatly aided by nutritional supplements, herbs, homeopathic remedies, and/or acupuncture, as well as some anti-allergy dietary changes where appropriate. Ms. Smyth's multidisciplinary approach to *back pains* works, as experienced by many patients at my medical center. The hands-on treatment by osteopathic physicians and physical therapists, along with relaxation and exercise/stretching, and some Western medicines or herbs/homeopathics constitute a very effective healing regimen in most cases.

The Complete Home Healer also takes a preventive approach to many chronic and advanced conditions, such as *hypertension and cardiovascular disease,* which can even be helpful with those people who are prone to or just beginning these life-limiting problems. I also find useful the common sense preventive approach for many acute problems as well, such as *viral illnesses, bronchitis, colds,* and *flus.* For acute problems, you have the Western conventional treatment plus the homeopathics and herbs useful for such problems as *diarrhea* and *dysentery,* and for chronic concerns, you have a focus on prevention and slow non-toxic interventions. Even the problems that require primarily a Western drug or surgical approach like *acute appendicitis* or *bone fractures,* also have other supportive treatments to facilitate optimum, rapid healing. Clearly, it seems like the best approach to me—*use what works from all forms of healing.*

I know you will find *The Complete Home Healer* a useful tool for your health and the health of your family and friends. Take care, be well, and enjoy staying healthy.

Elson M. Haas, M.D.

Elson M. Haas, M.D. is the medical director of the Preventive Medical Center of Marin, an integrated health care facility in San Rafael, California, and the author of the popular books *Staying Healthy with the Seasons* and *Staying Healthy with Nutrition*.

ACKNOWLEDGMENTS

THIS BOOK WOULD NOT HAVE BEEN POSSIBLE without the help of the many health professionals who donated their time and expertise in discussing the numerous remedies and treatments listed. In particular I would like to thank Leon Chaitow, N.D., D.O., for his invaluable contributions to the naturopathic recommendations outlined; Robert Bridge, R.S. Hom., for his guidance through the vastly complex world of homeopathic self-prescribing; Kathryn Marsden, for the latest research on dietary treatments; Helena Bridge, D.O., for her osteopathic expertise and creativity in putting massage down on paper; Shirley Price, for her aromatherapy recommendations; Dr. Julian Kenyon, for his advice on acupressure; and Bates Method teacher Anthony Attenborough. My thanks also go to Janet Balaskas, founder of the Active Birth Movement; Bob King, Director of the Chicago School of Massage Therapy; and the staff of the *Journal of Alternative and Complementary Medicine.*

I would also like to thank members of the many self-help and support groups across Britain and the United States with whom I corresponded. They provide an invaluable service by making available to the public firsthand advice, information, and a support network.

The aim of this book is to offer you an informed choice of the range of treatment available, and I am greatly indebted to consultant editor Dr. Hilary Jones for his help toward that goal. Despite a busy television schedule, he gave generously of his time, bringing a delightful blend of professionalism, practicality, and open-mindedness to the writing of the book, and demonstrating that orthodox and complementary medicine can work together.

My thanks also go to my agent, Lisa Eveleigh; and to Jane Graham-Maw and Veronica Simpson of Thorsons, and to Barbara Moulton, Terri Goff, and Naomi Lucks at HarperSanFrancisco, for their direction and editing. And last but not least, I am grateful to my husband, Ian, without whose support and encouragement the book would never have been finished.

Angela Smyth

PREFACE

THERE HAS BEEN SOMETHING OF A REVOLUTION in recent years concerning the nation's attitude to health, illness, and treatment. I have seen this develop both as a practicing GP and a television doctor and journalist, and I welcome it wholeheartedly. My surgery patients and the mail I receive from my TV viewers convey the same message: that there is intense interest now in complementary medicine, which embraces alternative therapies in conjunction with, rather than as a substitute for, orthodox medicine.

People have become better informed and more responsible for their own well-being. They recognize not only the value of orthodox medicine, but also for the first time its limitations. No longer will they obey doctor's orders without question. They realize that it is no longer satisfactory to treat symptoms merely in order to make them disappear. Instead, they expect the underlying cause of the symptoms to be accurately identified and corrected. Finally, and quite rightly, they expect some say in the treatment of their own problems. They know that their lifestyle, their temperament, their relationships, and their entire outlook on life are just as important as their medical history. And they are now more likely to welcome the dispensing of patiently thought-out advice than a hurriedly scribbled prescription for potent medication.

Complementary medicine is here to stay. Most conventionally trained physicians who retain open minds have accepted it. Even diehard surgeons whose former motto was, "If in doubt, cut it out" have changed their tune. And they have realized that a holistic approach to their patients—treating them as whole people, not just as a collection of body parts—can bear both physical and psychological rewards.

Importantly, the true scientific value of complementary medicine has been proven in carefully structured clinical trials. Many orthodox doctors like myself have subsequently widened the scope of the treatments they offer their patients, and have learned new skills such as homeopathy, chiropractic, and acupuncture. *The Complete Home Healer* encompasses a vast array of common disorders, and looks at the various alternative treatments available for them. Prevention quite logically comes first, followed by self-help in the form of various complementary therapies. Finally, almost as a last resort, comes the orthodox approach, a route that many people today will only turn to when all else has failed. The choices are yours, and *The Complete Home Healer* offers the lot.

People have seen how psychotherapy and counseling can offer considerable advantages over tranquilizers in the treatment of stress. They have seen how massage, acupuncture, and chiropractic can complement chemotherapy in the palliation of cancer, and how art therapy and light therapy can be helpful in depression and mental illness. As a result, I believe treatment has become more effective, less invasive, and safer. Patients no longer want blunderbuss therapy or a sledgehammer to crack a nut. They don't want drastic or threatening treatment. I believe that what they are really looking for these days is the kind of "gentle medicine" described in this book.

Dr. Hilary Jones

INTRODUCTION

THE LAST THIRTY YEARS have seen significant changes in the types of treatment and health advice available. Not so long ago, complementary practitioners, such as homeopaths, massage therapists, chiropractors, herbalists, and acupuncturists, were regarded disdainfully as back-street quacks. Even the links between diet, exercise, and good health were considered suspect. But today practitioners of complementary medicine are respectably established in hospitals and clinics, and many are the focus of government research grants. Nutritional recommendations have become part and parcel of mainstream medical practice, and scientific evidence leaves little room for doubting the benefits of exercise.

During this time the emphasis in health care (in both orthodox and complementary medicine) has moved toward the prevention of illness and the exploration of self-help through gentle, noninvasive methods. More and more people are seeking out information about how to protect themselves from life-threatening diseases, and increasing numbers are opting for complementary treatments to remedy chronic health problems.

The result has been an explosion of different attitudes, techniques, and information about how to prevent, treat, or deal with different ailments. A day does not go past without a new discovery being made. In writing *The Complete Home Healer,* my aim has been to bring together much of this varied and often conflicting information in an easy-to-use reference book. The result is an encyclopedia of hundreds of common health problems. Each entry has a varied range of preventive measures and complementary treatments, most of which you can carry out at home. The treatments were compiled in collaboration with practitioners of more than twenty of the most popular complementary therapies in use today. They range from simple dietary and exercise recommendations, to tried and tested homeopathic and herbal remedies, and even include the health-enhancing properties of visualization and yoga. To complete the treatment picture, you will find orthodox medical advice for each ailment, outlining what most Western medical practitioners would recommend in each case. This combination of preventive measures, complementary treatments, and orthodox advice reflects the holistic nature of today's health care and provides an opportunity for informed choice of treatment.

Presenting a holistic approach is a complex task. Well over one hundred different therapies are practiced in Britain and the United States today. The job is further complicated by rapid changes and ongoing controversies in the fields of complementary medicine. I have not attempted to include all potential treatments for every ailment: the list would be end-less. Instead, I have focused on those remedies most commonly pre-scribed and considered by health practitioners to be the most effective and applicable to home use. Should you develop a particular interest in one or more techniques, the Suggested Reading section provides an extensive listing of books on a wide range of subjects.

Due to space limitations, this book can only provide a brief description of the symptoms and causes of each ailment. It is not in any way intended to replace a medical diagnosis, and I strongly recommend that you seek out a professional assessment of your symptoms. Once you are aware of the nature of your ailment, *The Complete Home Healer* will provide you with the means to explore different approaches to prevention and treat-ment. It will guide you toward the type of complementary therapy that will be most beneficial, it will empower you with the means to take con-trol of your health, and it will offer a wealth of resources for further help, support, and information.

//////// *Gentle Treatments*

THE RANGE OF COMPLEMENTARY TREATMENTS available today is extensive. The treatments outlined in this book have been extensively researched, and are considered suitable for self-help. In cases where self-help is not appropriate, you will find advice on where to seek professional help. The following is a brief introduction to each type of treatment found in this book.

✳ ACUPRESSURE

Acupressure is a massage technique that combines fingertip massage with pressure to the acupuncture points lying along the meridians (the channels through which *qi,* the life force of the body, is thought to flow). Just as acupuncture (see below) is thought to stimulate the flow of *qi* through the meridians, so acupressure is thought to stimulate energy blockages that lead to disease and pain. However, because acupressure is done with the hands rather than with needles, it is most appropriate for self-help. Acupressure is best carried out using the thumb, exerting deep pressure so that the acupressure point feels rather achy or even slightly numb. Use a circular massage movement in the direction indicated by the illustrations.

➤ ACUPUNCTURE

Acupuncture, the placing of extremely thin disposable needles in points along the meridians (channels through which the *qi,* the life force of the body, flows), is thought to help clear energy blockages that might otherwise lead to disease. Acupuncture is not a self-help treatment—it must be performed by a licensed practitioner—but is sometimes recommended as a suitable means of professional help. In the West acupuncture is often offered as a treatment in itself, rather than as a part of traditional Chinese medicine. Some acupuncturists make dietary recommendations and prescribe herbs; others do not. Acupuncture is a diverse system of treatment that can be applied to virtually all ailments. We have indicated conditions where we feel it would be particularly helpful.

▲ ALEXANDER TECHNIQUE

The Alexander Technique is an educational therapy aimed at improving overall mental and physical well-being through changes in habitual posture. The technique aims to allow the body to have perfect balance and poise, with minimum tension and energy usage. Though difficult at first, the Alexander Technique leads to a sense of lengthening, ease of movement, reduced muscular and mental tension, and often pain relief. It can be particularly effective in helping back and neck problems and in rehabilitation following accidents.

You will need to take lessons from a professional, so the Alexander Technique is not truly a self-help method. However, you can use the exercises and information you have learned at home, without a professional.

✦ APPLIED KINESIOLOGY

Applied Kinesiology (AK) is a professional diagnostic technique that can help distinguish the location of problems and their causes. By testing different muscle groups of the body, the kinesiologist is able to identify areas of muscle weakness that indicate areas of impaired energy and function. AK practitioners believe that muscle strength and tone reflect the inner state of the organs, so AK is thought to help diagnose potential areas of disease in organs such as the heart, lungs, bowel, and kidneys. The technique is particularly useful for identifying food and substance sensitivities.

❀ AROMATHERAPY

The ultimate in gentle medicine, aromatherapy has its roots in the ancient use of aromatic herbs in Egypt, India, Greece, and the Arab world. Knowledge of how odor can be used to stimulate, relax, and heal has been passed down through the centuries and was refined in the early twentieth century in France and Germany. Since then, aromatherapy has become a widely practiced treatment, and its use in orthodox medicine is increasing. Essential oils, obtained from plants, roots, leaves, flowers, and fruit, have been shown to have powerful psychological effects. Research has shown that certain oils, when inhaled, have the power to relax or stimulate. In treatment, aromatherapy can be used to relieve conditions such as depression and fatigue. Many essential oils also have antiseptic and anti-inflammatory properties.

You can safely use aromatherapy as a self-help treatment if you follow these guidelines:

Use the purest oils available from reputable suppliers.

Essential oils are highly concentrated. When placed on the skin, they are nearly always diluted with a carrier oil (sunflower, safflower, or almond are suitable) or an emulsified oil-and-water lotion. The dilution you will need is outlined in the treatment for each ailment. When making up a dilution, add the required drops of oil to the carrier oil or lotion and shake well.

If you have sensitive skin, test a little of the diluted essential oil on a small area of your skin before you proceed with treatment.

Avoid contact with the eyes.

Keep essential oils out of the reach of children.

Always close your eyes when inhaling essential oil.

✿ BACH FLOWER REMEDIES

Flower remedies were first invented and used by Dr. Edward Bach around the turn of the century. They are now extensively used in the home and are suitable for self-help. The remedies are derived from wildflowers and one from pure stream water, which Dr. Bach believed provide subtle energy that is effective in treating emotional disharmony.

The remedies are made by picking fresh flowers, placing them on the surface of a bowl of water, and leaving them in the sun for several hours. It is thought that the action of the sun on the flowers releases their life force or energy into the water. Each of the remedies is appropriate to specific personality traits, and is administered in liquid form. The most commonly used remedy is Rescue Remedy, a combination of five flower remedies.

▶ BATES METHOD

The Bates Method is an alternative method of dealing with eyesight problems. Bates Method teachers believe that many vision defects are due to tensions and poor functioning of the muscles controlling the lens of the eyes. The method provides exercises to strengthen these muscles. Treatment should be carried out initially under the supervision of a Bates teacher, though we have included some safe and beneficial introductory exercises in the section on eyesight problems.

✳ BIOCHEMIC TISSUE SALTS

This therapy is based on the theory that the body contains twelve essential mineral salts. Imbalance or deficiency in these salts is thought to lead to disease. Biochemic tissue salts are manufactured in the same way as homeopathic remedies, in very dilute forms (see Homeopathy, below). They are available from pharmacists and health food stores and can safely be used in the home.

↕ BIOFEEDBACK

Stress and anxiety bring physical responses in the body, such as increased pulse, sweating, or muscle tension. With the help of a mechanism strapped to the body to monitor these effects, biofeedback helps you to know when your body is responding to stress, and allows you to develop strategies to reduce tension. As you become increasingly aware of what stress feels like, you learn to respond to its signs and prevent it before it occurs.

☯ CHINESE MEDICINE

Chinese medicine is a complex system of treatment that has evolved over thousands of years. It uses diet, herbalism, acupuncture, and exercise to treat a wide variety of ailments. The principle concept of traditional Chinese medicine is that disease is caused by an imbalance of the vital force or energy, also known as *qi*. The practitioner's aim is to detect imbalances in the flow of *qi* and redress them before they cause serious illness.

Practitioners of traditional Chinese medicine use diagnostic methods that are very different from those of orthodox doctors. They observe the patient as a whole, taking into consideration mind, body, and spirit, and not forgetting environmental concerns. Treatment may include dietary recommendations, exercise, acupressure, or acupuncture. Like many holistic practices, Chinese medicine is highly individual. Recommendations are made for each person's particular set of symptoms, rather than a collective treatment for each ailment. In this book we have placed herbal treatments under the general heading of Chinese medicine, and have given a separate heading for acupressure. Acupuncture is recommended where appropriate, under the heading Professional Help.

☆ CHIROPRACTIC

Chiropractors specialize in the diagnosis and treatment of mechanical disorders of joints (particularly joints of the spine). They believe in the principle that misalignments in the vertebrae can interfere with the circulation of blood, lymph, and nerve activity to vital organs, causing discomfort and sometimes disturbing bodily functions, which may result in disease. Chiropractors usually use X-rays when making a diagnosis, and treatment often involves short, direct manipulations of the spine. Some chiropractors use palpatory (feeling with the hands) diagnostic techniques and use massage, heat treatment, gentle manipulation, and exercise to "ease" misalignments back into place.

✗ DIETARY

The importance of diet in preventive medicine and treatment is becoming increasingly acknowledged. Practically every day, news hits the headlines regarding something we should or should not eat or drink. Diet is probably the area where we can make the greatest impact on general health and vitality, the prevention of disease, and the treatment of common ailments.

The dietary advice given in this book originates from different sources. First, we have incorporated the latest findings from nutritional research being carried out in universities and hospitals throughout the Western world. This work gives clinical evidence of the effects of diet on many different diseases and syndromes. Second, we have included information from naturopathic medicine, a complementary treatment founded on the principles that disease occurs when the body's inner force is suppressed through incorrect diet and lifestyle. Naturopathic treatment seeks to provide the body with the strength to heal itself through the elimination of toxins, and dietary rebalancing according to individual needs and lifestyle. Therapy may include a period of fasting, special diets, methods to encourage elimination, and supplementation with vitamins, minerals, amino acids, or other nutrients.

❖ EXERCISE

Exercise is not a therapy as such, though many who exercise regularly claim it is a drug. Over the last twenty years, the benefits of exercise in preventing disease and contributing to overall well-being have become increasingly recognized. Like diet, exercise is one of the most important factors in healthy living, for the following reasons:

It prevents weight gain and helps people lose excess weight, thought to contribute to disease.
It improves blood circulation and heart function.
It assists digestion.
It strengthens bones, increases muscle mass, and keeps joints mobile.
It reduces stress and relieves anxiety and depression.
It increases blood circulation to the brain, improving mental function and relieving fatigue.

The exercise treatments in this book range from recommendations to increase regular aerobic exercise (activity that requires increased oxygen intake and strengthens the heart, such as brisk walking, running, or swimming), to specific stretches designed to strengthen specific muscle groups. Whatever your age or strength, we suggest that you start any new exercise gently, allowing yourself to gradually build up strength and stamina. We also advise you to carry out the treatment regularly. It is better to exercise little and often than to overdo it. Always consult your doctor before beginning a new exercise routine.

🐎 HERBALISM

The value of plants in treating illness has been documented for some five thousand years. Modern herbalism stems from a variety of sources, and much has been passed down through folklore and tradition. Like many of the other gentle treatments listed in this book, herbal medicine is used to provide the body with the ideal environment for health and self-healing. Herbs are generally given fresh or dried, taken as infusions (herbs prepared like a tea), decoctions (herbs gently simmered in water), ointments (herbs made up into a cream), or compresses (prepared herbs placed in a compress and applied externally). Fresh herbs can also be incorporated into the diet. Instructions on how to prepare and administer each specific herbal remedy are given with each ailment. Follow these rules when you keep and prepare herbal remedies:

Use only herbs you can identify and that you know are safe.
Store herbs in an airtight glass jar. Do not refrigerate.
Use a glass or porcelain pot or saucepan to prepare remedies.
Do not exceed the recommended doses.
During pregnancy, is it not advisable to self-administer herbs without the supervision of a professional herbalist.

You can grow herbs in the garden from seed, or you can obtain plants from specialist suppliers. If you gather wild herbs, use caution: they may be contaminated with exhaust fumes or pesticides, or you may identify them incorrectly. The easiest access to herbal remedies is through a health food store or herbalist, some of which provide herbs by mail order.

☐ HOMEOPATHY

Homeopathy is a complete system of complementary medicine based on the principle of "like cures like." In other words, homeopathic remedies that produce a set of symptoms (mental, emotional, and physical) of an ailment in a healthy person can cure those symptoms in a sick person.

Remedies are prepared from extracts of plants, minerals, and animal and human tissues or secretions, which are diluted many times and shaken vigorously. While this dilution process greatly reduces the physical presence of the original composition of the remedy, it seems to bring out other qualities that are often more powerful than the original concentrate. Despite the fact that nobody has been able to show exactly how homeopathy works, its efficacy has been seen in clinical trials. It is extensively used in Europe, and to a growing extent in America and Australasia.

Homeopathic prescribing is highly individualized. Unlike orthodox drugs, where one remedy is prescribed for virtually all cases of a particular illness, homeopaths treat the person rather than the disease. In this book we do not have the space to provide an individualized means of prescribing for every ailment. However, we have listed remedies that professional homeopaths consider to be common to the majority of people. Consult a professional homeopath if you find that the treatments listed do not seem appropriate.

Where homeopathic treatment is appropriate, we list a selection of commonly prescribed remedies. A brief symptom picture is given with each remedy. Choose the remedy whose description is most like your symptoms. For example, when treating a child with a cold, you would look at the physical symptoms, such as a sore throat and runny nose. You would also take into consideration the mental and emotional state of the patient—whether the child is clinging and tearful, or irritable and aloof—as described in the text.

Homeopathic remedies are available as pills, granules, tinctures, and ointments. They are available in many different potencies; in this book most recommended remedies are the "6c" potency, which is the most easily obtained. Keep treatment to a minimum; once symptoms start to improve, it is not necessary to keep taking the remedy. Indeed, it is only necessary to repeat the remedy if the original symptoms recur. It is not unusual, on taking a homeopathic remedy, for symptoms initially to worsen for a few days before they get better. If this occurs, stop taking the remedy and consult a professional.

≈ HYDROTHERAPY

The relaxing, rejuvenating, and healing power of water has long been acknowledged. Hydrotherapy, or water therapy, has many applications; the treatments suggested in this book have the following effects:

Stimulation of blood circulation: Water can provide extremes of temperature, allowing the blood vessels to constrict and dilate, stimulating blood circulation. Increased blood flow provides an injured or diseased area with additional nutrients to aid healing, and helps eliminate toxins. It also increases the flow of oxygen through the body and the brain, maintaining energy and alertness.

To draw out heat: Cold compresses (cloths soaked in cold water) are sometimes used to remove heat from inflammatory conditions.

To provide support while exercising: The buoyancy of water provides support for weak limbs. Swimming in warm water is an effective means of strengthening weak muscles.

✳ HYPNOTHERAPY

Putting a patient into a trance to implant suggestions for self-cure has been used by healers throughout the ages. Although the mechanism by which hypnotherapy operates is still unclear, the method is used today by doctors, psychotherapists, and other health professionals to cure obsessive habits and relieve a number of emotional and physical disorders. It is particularly helpful in giving up smoking and dealing with substance abuse, and relieving anxiety, phobias, depression, and pain. Although methods of self-hypnosis are sometimes used, we recommend that you consult a professional.

☛ MASSAGE

Massage is based on the natural instinct to hold or rub an area that hurts, or to provide physical comfort through touch in times of stress. It is a popular and effective gentle treatment that you can easily use on yourself and others.

On a physical level, massage relaxes tense, tight, and knotted muscles. It stimulates blood and lymph flow through the body. Increased blood supply provides the tissues and organs with more oxygen, helping them to function better. Energy is increased, muscle and skin tone are improved. Increased circulation also facilitates healing. By increasing lymph flow, massage assists the elimination of waste materials, which can stagnate, contributing to stiffness and disease.

By relieving tense muscles and increasing blood flow, massage has a soothing effect on the central nervous system. This treatment is effective in preventing and treating stress and anxiety, and inducing deep relaxation. It is well known that stress compromises the immune system. Indirectly, therefore, massage can strengthen the body's resistance to disease.

The massage treatments described in this book can be carried out with a little oil (a vegetable oil, such as almond, sesame, or safflower, is suitable), lotion, or talc, unless otherwise indicated. You can use the techniques with people of any age; however, the intensity of the strokes should accommodate the physical condition of the receiver, not the giver. Take care not to "over-massage" children, the weak, and the elderly. The treatment should be felt, but should not cause pain and tension. Do not use massage when there is acute inflammation, fever, serious heart disease, a cancerous condition (unless approved by a professional), or phlebitis. Avoid massage on areas of broken skin and varicose veins.

✧ MEDITATION

Meditation is taught by trained teachers. Once you have learned the technique, you can practice it alone at home to assist in achieving a state of total relaxation. There are many varieties of meditation. Your teacher will probably recommend that you sit in a quiet room and fix your gaze on an object (a candle or crystal, for example). You will be taught to become aware of your breathing and to repeat your mantra (a word, chosen by yourself or your teacher, that is used as a mental focus). The object of meditation is to achieve a state of total physical relaxation and to empty the mind of all thought.

✤ REFLEXOLOGY

Reflexology, also known as zone therapy, is a system of diagnosis and treatment carried out by massaging the feet. Reflexologists believe that the body is divided up into ten energy zones that correspond to different areas of the feet. By massaging the relevant area of the foot, it is possible to bring a response in the corresponding tissues of the body. Although no one knows how reflexology works, it is thought to be helpful in treating a number of different ailments, from back pain to heart disorders. It is particularly useful in cases where the area of injury or disease cannot be touched or treated directly.

∼ RELAXATION TECHNIQUES

Stress is a natural response to fear. It prepares the body for "fight or flight" by tensing the muscles and constricting the blood vessels. However, most of the stress we encounter today is mental anguish and does not require us to fight or flee. The body is thus left in a state of physical tension, lead-ing to decreased energy, fatigue, and lowered immunity. Prolonged stress has been shown to be a major contributing factor to disease.

Both as a preventive measure and as a treatment, relaxation can be an important therapy, as it combats stress and anxiety and strengthens the body's resistance to disease. For some people, however, relaxation is very difficult to achieve. Often, when we think we are relaxing, our muscles remain tense and we cannot "turn off" mentally. To relax effectively, the mind should be in the present (not worrying about the past or future), barely ticking over, the body should be limp, and the breathing deep and slow. Carry out the relaxation treatments we recommend in a quiet, dimmed room where you will not be disturbed.

✿ VISUALIZATION

Many alternative and orthodox practitioners have found that visualizing a positive scene or symbol can bring mental and physical relaxation, relieve pain, help fight disease, and assist healing. To carry out visualiza-tion, you need to be in a quiet room where you will not be disturbed. Relax in a comfortable position and let your attention go to the area of your body that is injured or diseased. Focus on that area and let an image come to your mind. It may be a real-life image of the body part, or an abstract image or symbol. Allow the image to change as it will. Then start to visualize something happening to heal the body part. You may see white blood cells flowing toward it to attack disease; you may see light, energy, or warmth. Many people find that the healing image brings immediate physical or psychological relief. For those who have difficulty visualizing, autogenic training with a qualified practitioner can help. Relaxation tapes can also be beneficial.

✳ YOGA

Hatha yoga is a movement system that strives to achieve harmony of mind and body. Because the system teaches postures that encourage stretching up to one's individual capacity, yoga is appropriate to all age groups. The postures strengthen muscles and greatly increase flexibility, and improve circulation and balance. Through breathing and visualization exercises, yoga induces deep relaxation and combats stress. As a preventative therapy, yoga strengthens immunity and brings increased energy. The postures can also be used to combat specific ailments, as outlined in this book.

////////// *Medicine Cabinet*

THIS BOOK LISTS MANY REMEDIES and treatments—far too many for you to keep at home. Some remedies, however, are easy to obtain and can be used for a number of everyday ailments. Keep a supply of the following at hand for common problems and emergencies:

✗ DIETARY

vitamin C
vitamin E
multivitamin and mineral supplement
wheat germ (keep refrigerated)
live yogurt, or *Lactobacillus acidophilus* supplements

✤ AROMATHERAPY

lavender oil to relax
peppermint to rejuvenate and stimulate
tea tree oil as an antiseptic and antifungal
citronella oil to repel insects

૨૦ HERBALISM

mullein oil for earaches
meadowsweet to soothe stomach problems
ginger for nausea and vomiting
valerian for anxiety, stress, insomnia
dandelion for constipation and urinary problems
aloe vera (plant or juice) for burns

☐ HOMEOPATHY

Aconite 6c
Arnica 6c
Arnica cream
Arsenicum 6c
Belladonna 6c
Calendula cream
Calendula tincture
Chamomilla 6c
Hypericum
Ledum 6c

Nelson's Burn ointment
Nux vomica 6c
Pulsatilla 6c

❀ BACH FLOWER REMEDIES

Rescue Remedy is useful in most situations, particularly injury, shock, nervous conditions, and pain.

≈ HYDROTHERAPY

large bowl or tubs for sitz baths
cotton cloths for compresses
ice pack or bag of frozen peas (peas will be refrozen, so mark this bag and keep it purely for hydrotherapy purposes)
kitchen towels
hot water bottle or heating pad

☛ MASSAGE

light vegetable oil (safflower, sesame, almond) or lotion
a tennis ball or squash ball for those who find it hard to massage with the fingers

 **A**

ABSCESS

A collection of pus in a pocket of tissue that develops when the body traps bacteria. The pus forms from white blood cells carried to the area to fight the infection. See also **Abscess, Dental.**

TREATMENT

✕ DIETARY

Recurrent abscesses may indicate a sluggish digestive tract and inadequate elimination. To help detoxify the system and stimulate digestion:

- Reduce your intake of fatty foods, including meat, eggs, and dairy products.
- Reduce your intake of sweet foods and refined carbohydrates (white flour and sugar).
- Increase your intake of fresh fruits and vegetables.

The following supplements are recommended:

- zinc: 45 milligrams a day
- vitamin A: 50,000 iu a day for 2 weeks only

✿ AROMATHERAPY

Essential oil of tea tree is a useful antiseptic: Put 2 drops of the oil in 1 cup of water; dab on the abscess several times a day.

🐌 HERBALISM

Echinacea decoction helps rid the body of bacterial infections: Place 2 teaspoons of the root in 1 cup of water, bring to a boil, and simmer for 10 minutes; drink 3 times a day.

☐ HOMEOPATHY

Take 1 tablet every hour for 4 doses; repeat if needed:

When the abscess is very tender and causes stabbing pain: *Hepar sulphuris* 6c

In the early stage, when the abscess is throbbing, red, and inflamed: *Belladonna* 6c

☯ CHINESE MEDICINE

Abscesses are thought to be caused by excessive heat in the body. Practitioners of traditional Chinese medicine recommend these herbs to reduce heat: Chinese golden thread, dandelion, or wild chrysanthemum and violet in the form of a tea.

≈ HYDROTHERAPY

Prepare a hot compress by soaking a piece of sterile cotton in hot water. Hold it on the abscess to help expel the pus.

••• ORTHODOX

Most doctors will drain the pus from the abscess, and may recommend antibiotics to clear up further infection.

ABSCESS, DENTAL

Tender, throbbing, pus-filled gum tissue caused when bacteria invade a cavity in the root of a decaying or dead tooth. See also **Abscess.**

TREATMENT

✿ AROMATHERAPY

Essential oil of clove is a good painkiller: Add 10 drops of the oil to 2 teaspoons of a carrier oil; apply directly to the abscess.

Add 1 drop each of essential oil of tea tree and geranium to a glass of warm water; use as a gargle.

⁂ HERBALISM

Add 2 teaspoons of red sage leaves to 2 cups of water, bring to a boil, and let stand, covered, for 15 minutes. Gargle with the warm solution for 5 to 10 minutes, several times a day.

Golden seal is effective in attacking the bacteria associated with abscesses; it also stimulates the immune system and reduces inflammation: Mix ½ to ¾ teaspoon of golden seal tincture in a glass of spring water; drink 3 times a day.

☐ HOMEOPATHY

Take 1 dose every hour for 3 doses; repeat if needed:

Foul taste and offensive breath, profuse salivation, pain is worse at night: *Mercurius solubilis* 6c

Hot and throbbing, pain relieved by clenching teeth: *Belladonna* 6c

Teeth and gums excessively painful and made worse by cold drinks: *Hepar sulphuris* 6c

To promote discharge of the abscess, with sticking pains and the sensation of a hair on the tongue: *Silicea* 6c

••• ORTHODOX

If the abscess is large, your dentist will probably recommend antibiotics to prevent the spread of infection throughout the body. Once sterilized by a full course of antibiotics, the abscess is usually drained, cleaned, and the tooth filled or removed.

ACID STOMACH

A burning pain in the stomach and chest, often accompanied by belching (which seems to bring relief), and sometimes a feeling of food getting stuck; commonly known as heartburn. Causes include overeating; consuming too much rich or spicy food and alcohol; and stress (see **Stress**). Acid stomach is common in pregnant women (see Heartburn under **Pregnancy Problems**) and people who are overweight (see **Obesity**). See also **Indigestion.**

PREVENTION

Avoid rich, spicy food.

Eat small meals, but more often, and avoid heavy meals at night.

Get regular exercise to aid digestion—but not immediately after a meal.

Try to reduce stress.

TREATMENT

✗ DIETARY

Reduce your intake of food; eat smaller meals more often.

Avoid caffeine (found in coffee, tea, chocolate, cola), alcohol, sugar, carbonated drinks, spices, and fatty foods.

Counteract acidity by eating plenty of alkaline foods: fresh fruits and vegetables (but not milk).

❧ HERBALISM

Meadowsweet infusion soothes the membranes of the digestive tract: Add 1 cup of boiling water to 1 to 2 teaspoons of the dried herb, and infuse for 15 minutes; drink 3 times a day.

Take ginger in capsule form or as a decoction: Add 1½ teaspoons of the freshly grated root to 1 cup of water, and simmer for 10 minutes; drink when needed.

▢ HOMEOPATHY

Take 1 tablet every 15 minutes, for up to 4 doses; repeat if needed:

After rich foods, with gas and rancid belching: *Carbo vegetabilis* 6c

After spicy food, stimulants, alcohol: *Nux vomica* 6c

Burning pain, worse in the small hours of the morning: *Arsenicum album* 6c

☯ CHINESE MEDICINE

Acid stomach is thought to be caused by an imbalance of the spleen and liver. Practitioners of traditional Chinese medicine recommend ginseng, licorice, and orange peel. Avoid acidic and "cold" foods (bananas, grapefruit, salads, watermelon, tomatoes).

⊹ EXERCISE

Regular exercise, such as walking, running, swimming, or bicycling at least 3 times a week, can help you reduce weight, take pressure off the stomach, and relieve stress.

••• ORTHODOX

Your doctor may recommend antacids (either a mixture of magnesium hydroxide and aluminum hydroxide, or a calcium tablet), which can be bought over the counter. Take antacids 1 to 2 hours before meals, and just before going to bed. **Caution:** Do not take antacids without first consulting your doctor if you suffer from high blood pressure, kidney disease, or any type of intestinal bleeding.

ACNE

Pimples, blackheads, and whiteheads on the face, neck, or back, often due to the hormonal changes of adolescence that lead to an increase in oily sebum production and clogged pores. Acne can also occur in adults of any age, particularly premenstrual women (see **Premenstrual Syndrome**) and women who take oral contraceptives. See also **Pimples.**

TREATMENT

▬ PRACTICAL ADVICE

Avoid oil-based cosmetics.

Wash the skin well with unperfumed soap twice a day.

Do not squeeze pimples or whiteheads; this can cause scarring and may spread the infection.

✗ DIETARY

Avoid fats, sugars, refined foods, and junk foods. Eat plenty of raw fruits and vegetables, whole-grain breads and cereals, cooked dried beans, additive-free low-fat dairy products, chicken, and fish.

Increase your intake of zinc, found in poultry, fish, organ meats, and whole-grain breads and cereals. Studies have shown a daily supplement of 45 milligrams of zinc picolinate to be effective.

⟨ HERBALISM

Blue flag decoction: Put 1 teaspoon of the dried herb into 1 cup of water, and simmer for 10 minutes; drink 3 times a day to detoxify the system.

▢ HOMEOPATHY

Take 1 tablet, 3 times a day, for up to 7 days; repeat if needed:

Initially, try: *Calcarea silicata* 6c
With itchy spots: *Kali bichromicum* 6c
With red, sore, infected spots: *Sulphur* 6c
Extreme sensitivity to touch: *Hepar sulphuris* 6c

••• ORTHODOX

Gels and creams containing benzoyl peroxide are recommended to help unblock pores.

Doctors may prescribe antibiotics to reduce infection of pores.

Drugs and creams based on vitamin A reduce sebum production, but may have side effects, such as dry eyes, inflammation of the lips, and reddening of the skin.

Specially designed oral contraceptives may be offered to combat acne in women.

Doctors sometimes recommend getting out in the sunshine or using a sunlamp for short periods.

ADENOIDS, ENLARGED OR INFECTED

Larger than normal adenoids, the two swellings above the tonsils that help in resisting infection, may be natural, or they may become enlarged as a result of infection. Usually this affects children between the ages of five and seven who tend to breathe through the mouth and snore. Infection may lead to coughs, ear problems, and loss of the senses of smell and taste. The condition often disappears as children grow older.

TREATMENT

✕ DIETARY

The following guidelines help reduce congestion:

Avoid cow's milk, cream, butter, cheeses, roasted peanuts, bananas, and excessive sugar.

Avoid fatty and fried foods.

Avoid excessive salt.

Increase your intake of vitamin C to fight infection (found in citrus fruits, berries, green leafy vegetables, tomatoes, and potatoes).

Garlic helps attack infection: Incorporate raw garlic into your diet; if you do not like the taste or smell of fresh garlic, you can take garlic capsules (3 capsules, 3 times a day).

❧ HERBALISM

Infusion of cleavers reduces inflammation and tones the lymphatic system: Pour 1 cup of boiling water onto 2 teaspoons of the dried herb, and infuse for 15 minutes; drink 3 times a day.

Red sage gargle helps fight infection and soothes the throat: Pour 1 cup of boiling water onto 2 teaspoons of the leaves, infuse for 10 minutes, and allow to cool; use as a gargle 3 times a day.

☐ HOMEOPATHY

Take 1 tablet, 2 times a day, for up to 2 weeks; repeat if necessary:

Initially, try: *Agraphis nutans* 6c

Inflamed adenoids and tonsillitis, poor mental and physical development: *Baryta carbonica* 6c

Inflamed adenoids, child overweight and prone to head sweats during sleep: *Calcarea carbonica* 6c

Thick, yellow discharge from nose and throat, tearful child: *Pulsatilla* 6c

☞ MASSAGE

Massage gently down either side of the nose, using the thumb and forefinger.

••• ORTHODOX

Very large or persistently inflamed adenoids are usually removed surgically, especially if they interfere with hearing, speech, or school attendance. The adenoids are useful glands that help fight infection, so doctors generally do not recommend surgery unless the problems are persistent.

AGING

A natural process of physical and mental changes. Aging is not an ailment: Some believe the rate of aging is determined by genetic makeup; others say it is a result of cumulative damage to cells. Evidence implicates both, suggesting that there are ways to slow down the process of aging, or even reverse changes.

PREVENTIVE TREATMENT

✕ DIETARY

Studies have shown that a gradual reduction in calorie intake increases lifespan in animals. Human studies show that people who are overweight tend to live shorter lives than those who are not. Reducing calorie intake means cutting out all nutritionally empty foods (refined carbohydrates, sugar, junk food) and eating a highly nutritious diet of whole-grain cereals, low-fat protein, and plenty of fruits and vegetables.

Free radicals, found in cigarette smoke, pollution, radiation, and rancid fats, enter the body and cause some of the damaging effects of aging. You can combat them with the following:

- Increase your intake of vitamin C, found in fresh fruits and vegetables (eat these raw, if possible).
- Increase your intake of vitamin E, found in wheat germ, seeds, and seed oils.
- Increase your intake of selenium, found in whole wheat, brown rice, poultry, and low-fat dairy products.
- Increase your intake of beta-carotene, found in green leafy vegetables, and orange and yellow vegetables.

Increase your intake of the amino acids cysteine and methionine (found in beans, fish, liver, brewer's yeast, and nuts), or take a daily supplement: 250 milligrams of each between meals. **Caution:** Do not take if you are diabetic.

✤ EXERCISE

Studies have shown that exercise started early in life retards signs of aging, and helps prevent one of the Western world's biggest killers, coronary heart disease. Exercise at any age helps maintain bone and muscle strength, and preserves flexibility and balance. Exercise also aids circulation and the elimination of toxins, all of which help preserve healthy skin and hair.

Yoga exercises, done only to your own tolerance, are appropriate for people of all ages. Yoga stretches and tones the body and provides relaxation, another important ingredient for longevity.

••• ORTHODOX

Doctors recommend the dietary and exercise treatments listed above. Cosmetic surgery can repair some of the physical effects of aging.

AIDS (ACQUIRED IMMUNE DEFICIENCY SYNDROME)

A deficiency in the immune system strongly thought to be caused by infection with HIV (human immunodeficiency virus), which is spread through infected blood and semen. The most common means of transmission are sexual contact and sharing needles, and mothers who pass the virus on to the fetus. Because HIV affects certain white blood cells that are crucial for fighting disease and infection, people with AIDS fall prey to a variety of infections: from skin disorders, diarrhea, and yeast infections, to tuberculosis, neurological disorders, and cancer. Early symptoms include enlarged lymph glands or unexplained weight loss and fatigue. The syndrome is fatal; as yet there is no cure. Treatment is aimed at strengthening the immune system and dealing with the infections brought by immune deficiency.

PREVENTION

Practice safe sex:

- Limit sexual partners to those whose sexual history you know.
- Use a condom for oral, anal, or vaginal sex.
- Hugging, mutual masturbation, kissing, body massage, body kissing, and touching are safe.

Intravenous drug users should avoid sharing needles.

When traveling in third world countries, carry a supply of disposable sterile needles in case you require medical injections.

TREATMENT

Researchers are making new discoveries about AIDS every day, but there is still no cure for the syndrome. The following treatments are some of the current methods used as this book goes to press.

••• ORTHODOX

Doctors generally prescribe antiviral drugs, such as zidovudine (AZT) and acyclovir, which are thought to prolong life once symptoms have started.

◯ OTHER TREATMENTS

Many different complementary therapies are being used alongside ortho-dox treatment of HIV and AIDS. They aim to stimulate immune function and provide antivirals to resist the infection. The ones most commonly used are listed below.

✗ DIETARY

Increase your intake of beta-carotene, found in green leafy vegetables, and orange and yellow vegetables.

Vitamin C stimulates immunity and is an antiviral. Naturopaths advise taking vitamin C to bowel tolerance (that is, keep taking it until it causes diarrhea, then cut back to find the highest tolerable level).

Increase your intake of bioflavonoids, found in green leafy vegetables and in the pith and rind of citrus fruits. These enhance the action of vitamin C.

Zinc is also an immune stimulator and antiviral: Take 15 milligrams of zinc picolinate daily.

Make sure your diet is as nutritious as possible: whole grains, fresh fruits and vegetables (organic, if possible), lean meat, fish, and dairy products are recommended. Limit your intake of junk foods and refined foods, alcohol, nicotine, and recreational drugs.

≳ HERBALISM

Golden seal boosts immunity and fights microbes, such as fungal infec-tions. It is a useful remedy for diarrhea. Consult an herbalist for the appropriate dosage.

☐ HOMEOPATHY

Professional homeopathic prescribing appears to be beneficial, both to those who are HIV positive and to people with AIDS.

☻ CHINESE MEDICINE

Chinese herbs and acupuncture are extensively and effectively used to treat many of the symptoms brought by AIDS (night sweats, fatigue, neu-ropathy, diarrhea). Many people with HIV who take Chinese herbs claim that their overall health improves. Studies have also found Chinese medi-cine to be useful in relieving the side effects of orthodox drug use and radiation. The herbs commonly used are the tonic herbs (astragalus, ganoderma, and ginseng); and the blood-circulating herbs: (salvia, millet-tia, and peony).

～ RELAXATION TECHNIQUES

A diagnosis of HIV positive brings considerable mental anguish. Stress and unhappiness have been shown to weaken the immune system further.

Yoga and meditation have been shown to promote relaxation, ease stress, and relieve pain.

Massage promotes relaxation, relieves pain, and reduces muscle tension. With the right therapist, it provides intimate, caring, and pleasurable physical contact.

Joining a support group, where you can share your experience of the physical and mental effects of the syndrome with others in the same situation, is highly beneficial in helping people deal with stress and anguish. It also provides you with the latest information on research, treatment, and methods of coping.

ALCOHOLISM

An addiction to alcohol that progressively interferes with one's health and ability to function. Left untreated, alcoholism can be fatal (see **Cirrhosis**). Often alcohol becomes so much a part of daily life that we are not aware of becoming dependent on it. Anyone who abuses alcohol or drinks excessively will experience problems with physical and mental health. Personal relationships, work, and finances can also suffer.

TREATMENT

The following signs indicate that you may need help in resolving alcohol abuse:

You turn to alcohol when feeling sad or when faced with a problem.
You are sometimes unable to meet responsibilities due to heavy drinking.
Someone close to you is concerned about your drinking.
You experience unpleasant side effects when you stop drinking.
You drink in secret and feel guilty about it.

Alcohol abuse is difficult to treat alone. A number of self-help groups, such as Alcoholics Anonymous, provide treatment to sufferers and help families of alcoholics. If you prefer not to work in a group, you could seek help from a doctor or psychotherapist who specializes in alcohol abuse, a homeopath, or a hypnotherapist. Treatment should be aimed not only at helping you to stop drinking, but at bringing you to a better understanding of why you drink, and at helping you create a lifestyle where you do not need to drink. Use the following treatments to complement professional therapy.

✗ DIETARY

Nutritional deficiencies accentuate the other complications of alcohol abuse. Studies have shown that the following nutritional supplements help accelerate alcohol detoxification and prevent liver damage:

Zinc is found in lean meat, poultry, fish, and whole-grain cereals. A 15-milligram daily supplement is recommended.

Increase your intake of vitamin C, found in fresh fruits and vegetables, and vitamin E, found in wheat germ, seed oils, and nuts.

The amino acid glutamine has been shown to be helpful in decreasing the desire to drink alcohol. A between-meal daily supplement of 2 to 4 grams is recommended.

❧ HERBALISM

Alcoholics are often deficient in GLA (gamma-linolenic acid). GLA is found in evening primrose oil, which is thought to help prevent mood swings and liver damage: Take 4 capsules of evening primrose oil a day.

Infusion of skullcap, motherwort, or lavender can help you overcome withdrawal symptoms: Add 1 cup of water to 2 teaspoons of the herb, and infuse for 15 minutes; drink 3 times a day.

☐ HOMEOPATHY

Quercus mother tincture: Add 3 drops of tincture to ½ a glass of water; take 2 times a day to reduce alcohol craving.

☯ CHINESE MEDICINE

Practitioners of traditional Chinese medicine recommend herbs to clear heat from the body. Strong green tea is used to cool the liver and stomach.

✿ BACH FLOWER REMEDIES

If you turn to alcohol to overcome difficult times: Agrimony
For obsessional thoughts: Aspen
In recovery: Olive

ALLERGIC DERMATITIS

A rash or inflammation of the skin in reaction to a substance; the symptoms are the same as for eczema (see **Eczema**). The most common causes of allergic dermatitis are detergents (traces of which can be left in washed clothes, causing irritation); nickel (in watches, jewelry, and bra straps); chemicals in rubber gloves and condoms; cosmetics; plants; and some medicines. The reaction may also result from a food source see **Allergies, Food**.

TREATMENT

The best treatment is to identify the source and avoid it.

See **Eczema** for natural treatments that may be useful.

✚ PROFESSIONAL HELP

Applied kinesiology can help identify unknown allergens.

••• ORTHODOX

Allergists can perform tests to identify the suspected allergen by placing the substance on a patch of skin and observing the reaction over several days. Corticosteroid drugs or creams may be used to treat symptoms.

ALLERGIES, FOOD

Food sensitivities that produce a variety of symptoms, including cramps, nausea, vomiting, diarrhea, gas, migraine headaches, skin eruptions and irritations, hyperactivity, mood swings, fatigue, and food cravings. The most common food allergens are dairy products, eggs, strawberries, fish and shellfish, cereals, and some food additives. See also **Colitis.**

PREVENTION

Food allergies can sometimes develop when a child is weaned too early. Try to breast-feed infants for at least the first six months of life, and longer if possible. Introduce new foods slowly and carefully; make sure the baby has adapted to the new food before moving on to the next one. Start with baby rice and millet. Do not give wheat or milk during the first year.

TREATMENT
✗ DIETARY

Identify the foods or drinks to which you may be allergic. Any food that appears more than once on the following lists is a potential allergen:

- List any foods that disagree with you or produce fatigue, skin reactions, hyperactivity, irritability, and so on.
- List foods or drinks you consume every day.
- List any foods you regularly crave.
- List foods you would miss if unavailable.
- List any foods you have begun to eat recently.

You can further identify food allergens by testing your pulse. Take your resting pulse on waking, just before each meal, thirty minutes after the meal, and before going to bed. If the pulse remains constant, then the foods you are eating are probably not causing an allergy. If the pulse swings up or down more than six beats, it is likely that the food is causing an allergic reaction. Work your way through the suspected foods using this means of diagnosis.

Eliminate any food that seems suspect for at least two weeks, then reintroduce it and notice whether it produces symptoms. Replace foods that cause allergic reactions with alternative foods (for example, soy milk, goat's milk, or nondairy creamers can replace cow's milk). After six months try reintroducing the offending food: You may find you have overcome your sensitivity.

✚ PROFESSIONAL HELP

To reduce sensitivity to food allergies, naturopaths often recommend a detoxification diet. Do this in consultation with a professional.

If you are unable to identify what is causing your allergy, a kinesiologist may be able to use muscle testing to identify which foods are producing weaknesses in the body.

Professional homeopathic prescribing can boost general immunity and thus reduce sensitivity to potential allergens.

••• ORTHODOX

Doctors recommend avoiding potential allergens. Look carefully at ingredients on processed foods to make sure they do not contain substances that will trigger an attack.

ALLERGIES, HAY FEVER, AND RHINITIS

An exaggerated response of the immune system to substances such as grass or tree pollen, spores from molds, house-dust mites, or animal dander (shed dead skin and fur from pets). Symptoms include a congested, runny nose; itchy, watery eyes; headache; drowsiness; itchy throat; and sneezing. See also **Asthma; Eczema; Hives; Allergies, Food; Allergic Dermatitis**.

PREVENTION

Vacuum floors and carpets every day to eliminate indoor pollutants.

Put a net curtain over windows and wear sunglasses to reduce pollen exposure.

In hot climates air-conditioning can greatly help to prevent exposure to airborne allergens.

Ionizers help to remove pollen, dust, and other airborne allergens from the atmosphere.

TREATMENT

✗ DIETARY

Vitamin C combined with bioflavonoids acts as a natural antihistamine to control a runny nose or help unblock a congested one. Increase your intake of citrus fruits, which contain both vitamin C and bioflavonoids (bioflavonoids are found in the rind and pith).

- To make a decongestant: Slice up some grapefruit peel or orange peel, making sure to include some pith, and boil with a little water and honey for 10 minutes. Eat a piece before going to bed, and when symptoms start during the day.
- Take vitamin C with citrus bioflavonoids in supplement form: 500 milligrams, 3 times a day.

Pantothenic acid has also been shown to relieve allergy symptoms. Take a daily supplement of 200 to 500 milligrams of pantothenic acid and 50 milligrams of vitamin B-complex.

Pollen supplements are said to help prevent allergies, particularly hay fever. Take 4 to 6 tablets a day for several weeks before the hay fever season.

Licorice and beta-carotene are also helpful. If you are buying supplements over the counter, follow the instructions on the package; otherwise, consult a naturopath or nutritionist for correct dosage.

❀ AROMATHERAPY

Add 1 drop of essential oil of lavender to 1 teaspoon of a carrier oil or lotion; use to massage the skin over the sinuses on either side of the nose once a day.

Dilute 1 drop of essential oil of inula in 1 teaspoon of jojoba or sweet almond oil; rub into the skin over the sinuses once a day.

✳ ACUPRESSURE

To relieve headaches, sneezing, and itching eyes, find the highest spot of the muscle in the webbing between the thumb and index finger, and rub firmly for 1 minute; repeat on the other hand. **Caution:** Do not press this point during pregnancy.

To strengthen the immune system, find the spot on the top of the forearm between the two arm bones, two finger-widths from the wrist; firmly massage this area with a deep circular motion of the thumb.

⚜ EXERCISE

Rigorous exercise can help control allergies, which are often aggravated by stress. Try early morning jogging, brisk walking, or swimming.

••• ORTHODOX

Doctors generally prescribe antihistamines to relieve symptoms.

Sometimes inhaled medications, including steroids, can reverse and control allergy-induced asthma (see **Asthma**).

In severe cases, or where immediate re-sults are needed, a cortisone injection can provide relief for up to three months.

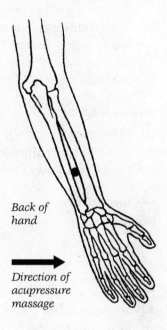

Back of hand

Direction of acupressure massage

ALOPECIA
See **Hair Loss.**

ALTITUDE SICKNESS

A condition brought on by a rapid ascent to heights above 8,000 feet; also known as mountain sickness. The reduced atmospheric pressure and oxygen at these heights lowers levels of oxygen in the blood, bringing symptoms of headache, nausea, dizziness, and impaired concentration. Severe cases result in a buildup of fluids in the lungs, leading to breath-lessness, coughing, and the production of frothy phlegm. Seizures, and sometimes coma, may follow.

PREVENTION

Make your ascent gradually, stopping for regular rests. Once you are above 8,000 feet, you should stop for a few days every 2,000 feet to acclimatize.

If you experience dizziness, nausea, shortness of breath, or if you feel faint (see **Fainting**), come down, rest, and do not climb higher until symptoms have subsided.

High altitudes can sometimes cause headaches. Taking 3,000 to 5,000 milligrams of vitamin C before the ascent can help prevent this.

TREATMENT

① **FIRST AID**

Descend to a lower altitude as quickly as possible, and seek emergency medical help. A delay may result in permanent brain damage.

••• ORTHODOX

Doctors generally administer oxygen and powerful steroids.

ALZHEIMER'S DISEASE

A progressive illness that generally occurs after the age of sixty, in which the nerve cells degenerate and the brain shrinks. Symptoms range from memory loss and forgetfulness to confusion and dementia.

PREVENTION

We do not know what causes Alzheimer's disease, but the following preventive measures have been suggested:

Avoid free radicals, found in cigarette smoke, pollution, radiation, and rancid fats, and counteract their production in the body by eating foods rich in antioxidants:

- vitamin C, found in citrus fruits, berries, green leafy vegetables, tomatoes, and potatoes
- vitamin E, found in wheat germ, seeds, and vegetable oils
- beta-carotene, found in orange and green leafy vegetables
- zinc and selenium, found in liver, lean meats, Cheddar cheese, lentils, and whole-grain bread

Avoid cooking in aluminum utensils.

Avoid antacids and deodorants that contain aluminum.

TREATMENT

People with dementia rarely ask for help themselves, and it is usually left to distraught relatives to enlist professional support. The aim of treatment is to maintain quality of life and standard of everyday function as far as possible. Drug therapy is generally kept to a minimum, but may become necessary if agitation, aggression, or antisocial behavior occurs. The following herbal treatment can complement orthodox help.

⅍ HERBALISM

Studies have shown ginkgo biloba extract to be useful in treating this condition. Ginkgo biloba increases blood supply to the brain and increases nerve impulse transmission. The recommended dose is 40 milligrams, 3 times a day, of ginkgo biloba extract containing 24 percent ginkgo heterosides.

AMNESIA
See **Memory Problems.**

ANAL FISSURE

An ulcer that develops from a tear in the lining of the anus, often as a result of straining to pass hard, dry stools. Symptoms include pain during bowel movements, and bright blood spotting on the toilet paper.

PREVENTION

Avoid becoming constipated (see Dietary suggestions). For further recommendations, see **Constipation.**

TREATMENT

▬ PRACTICAL ADVICE

Use soft toilet paper or wet wipes. Wash the anal area regularly, particularly after bowel movements, to prevent infection of the broken skin.

✗ DIETARY

Eat prunes once a day to help loosen the stools. For long-term benefit, introduce more general fiber into your diet in the form of whole-grain cereals (but not wheat bran), fruit, and raw vegetables. (See **Constipation** for more detailed advice.)

Drink at least 8 glasses of water a day.

Dab olive oil on the fissure to relieve pain and irritation.

🎿 HERBALISM

Dandelion decoction (dandelion coffee) is a gentle laxative: Mix 2 to 3 teaspoons of the root with 1 cup of water, and simmer for 10 minutes; drink 3 times a day.

For a general bowel tonic: Mix an infusion of 2 teaspoons of dandelion root, 2 teaspoons of yellow dock, and 1 teaspoon each of senna, licorice, and ginger; take before sleeping.

☐ HOMEOPATHY

Take 2 times a day for up to 7 days, and repeat if necessary:

When it feels as if the stools tear the anus: *Nitric acid* 6c

When it feels as if the anus is full of splintered glass: *Ratanhia* 6c

≋ HYDROTHERAPY

Take hot sitz baths, in combination with a high-fiber diet.

⚜ EXERCISE

Exercise is very important to maintain a healthy digestive system. Take a walk, a run, or a swim at least 3 times a week.

✳ YOGA

The following yoga position will help relieve constipation: Lie on your back. Bring the right knee up to the chest, inhale, and bring the head up and the chin toward the knee. Hold the position for 10 seconds; exhale, and lower the leg to the floor. Repeat with the left leg, and then with both together.

••• ORTHODOX

Some doctors recommend liquid paraffin to soften the stools.

For persistent fissures, your doctor may recommend anal dilation to enlarge the anal passage.

Surgery may be used to remove the ulcer.

To counteract pain, sit on a rubber or foam ring to reduce pressure on the tender area.

ANAL ITCHING

Persistent itching around the anal area, sometimes caused by fissures (see **Anal Fissure**), hemorrhoids (see **Hemorrhoids**), discharge, eczema (see **Eczema**), or a rash resulting from sweat accumulation, bad hygiene, or sitting for long periods. Itching can sometimes be caused by worms, particularly in children (see **Worms**).

TREATMENT

▬ PRACTICAL ADVICE

Once an anal irritation has started and the skin becomes broken, it is very difficult to heal. To prevent further irritation, use moist wipes instead of toilet paper. Wash the anal area gently but regularly, and always after bowel movements, and pat dry with a towel. Avoid scented soaps and talcum powder.

Allow the area to air as much as possible.

Wear cotton underwear and loose clothing. Avoid nylon stockings and tights.

Irritation is sometimes a reaction to the detergent or fabric softener you are using to wash your clothes. Try a different brand and rinse your underwear well.

Dab the anal area with olive oil to soothe the itching and make bowel movements easier.

✗ DIETARY

Constipation can sometimes lead to anal irritation. To avoid constipation, introduce more fiber into your diet in the form of whole-grain cereals, fresh fruit, and raw vegetables. Every day, eat at least 1 large serving of salad and drink at least 8 glasses of water. For more suggestions, see **Constipation.**

Anal itching is sometimes thought to be caused by a *Candida* infection of the stomach and bowel (see **Fungal Infection**). To counteract, insert live yogurt that contains *Lactobacillus acidophilus* into the rectum, using a plastic syringe applicator, once a day.

❋ AROMATHERAPY

Before going to bed, run a warm bath. Add 10 ounces of bicarbonate of soda and 5 to 8 drops of chamomile and mix well. Sit in the bath for at least 10 minutes to relieve irritation and promote healing.

☐ HOMEOPATHY

Take *Peonia* 6c, 2 times a day, for up to 7 days; repeat if needed.

••• ORTHODOX

Doctors often prescribe hydrocortisone cream for this complaint. It is effective in relieving itching and mending broken skin, but can mask the presence of infection. Use with caution—continuous use can thin the skin.

ANEMIA

A shortage of hemoglobin, the red pigment in blood cells that transports oxygen. The most common cause is lack of adequate dietary iron, although excessive loss of blood through menstruation or a stomach ulcer can contribute. Symptoms and signs of anemia include fatigue, dizziness, breathlessness, poor concentration, recurrent colds and infections, pallor, and white eyelid linings. In children, anemia can retard mental development and contribute to behavioral problems.

TREATMENT

✗ DIETARY

Increase your intake of foods rich in easily absorbed iron. Good sources include beef, pork, lamb, organ meats, poultry, fish, cooked dried beans,

IRON ABSORPTION FROM DIFFERENT FOODS

Food *(Portion size in grams)*

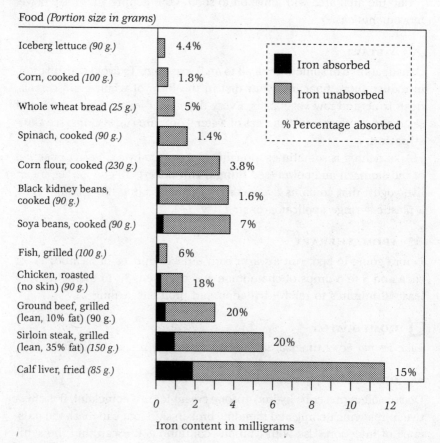

Food	Iron content in milligrams
Iceberg lettuce *(90 g.)*	4.4%
Corn, cooked *(100 g.)*	1.8%
Whole wheat bread *(25 g.)*	5%
Spinach, cooked *(90 g.)*	1.4%
Corn flour, cooked *(230 g.)*	3.8%
Black kidney beans, cooked *(90 g.)*	1.6%
Soya beans, cooked *(90 g.)*	7%
Fish, grilled *(100 g.)*	6%
Chicken, roasted (no skin) *(90 g.)*	18%
Ground beef, grilled (lean, 10% fat) *(90 g.)*	20%
Sirloin steak, grilled (lean, 35% fat) *(150 g.)*	20%
Calf liver, fried *(85 g.)*	15%

Legend: ■ Iron absorbed ▨ Iron unabsorbed % Percentage absorbed

Iron content in milligrams

dark green leafy vegetables, and dried fruits. Animal products provide more easily absorbed iron than do vegetables.

To increase iron absorption, incorporate vitamin C from citrus fruits or juices into your meals. Do not drink black tea immediately before, during, or after meals, as the tannin inhibits iron absorption.

Large doses of iron supplements may cause stomach upsets and constipation, and can be fatal in children. They can also compete with other minerals, leading to nutritional imbalances. If you have to take supplements, take a multivitamin and mineral supplement that includes copper, iron, selenium, vitamins B2, B6, and B12, folic acid, vitamin C, and vitamin E.

☯ CHINESE MEDICINE

Practitioners of traditional Chinese medicine recommend restoring the body's ability to absorb iron by stimulating the spleen with Return Spleen tablets, also known as *gui pi wan.*

✳ BIOCHEMIC TISSUE SALTS

Calc Phos 6x, 4 times a day, helps form healthy red blood cells.
Ferr Phos 6x, 4 times a day, aids absorption of dietary iron.

✚ PROFESSIONAL HELP

Acupuncture has been shown to help anemia.

••• ORTHODOX

Most doctors will look for the underlying cause of anemia and treat it. Iron injections or supplements are usually suggested if no apparent underlying cause is found.

ANEMIA, MEGALOBLASTIC

Megaloblastic anemia is caused by a deficiency of vitamin B12 or folic acid. These are two different and chemically unrelated nutrients, but deficiency of either has the same effect—interference in the production of red blood cells in the bone marrow. Sometimes the body is unable to absorb these nutrients, as in Crohn's disease and celiac disease (see **Celiac Disease; Crohn's Disease**). Symptoms include fatigue, headaches, pallor, loss of appetite, poor concentration, and a sore mouth and tongue.

TREATMENT

✗ **DIETARY**

Increase your intake of vitamin B12, found in animal products (lean meats, poultry, fish, shellfish, milk, liver, kidney, cheese, and eggs). Vegans are at increased risk of vitamin B12 deficiency, and should take yeast extract or vitamin supplements (2 to 3 micrograms a day) as a precaution.

Increase your intake of folic acid, found in green leafy vegetables, such as spinach, broccoli, and lettuce, brewer's yeast, liver, orange juice, and avocados.

Reduce your intake of alcohol, which depletes stores of vitamin B12 and folic acid.

••• **ORTHODOX**

Your doctor may suggest injections of vitamin B12 and folic acid tablets to replace the deficient nutrients.

ANEURYSM

The abnormal and permanent ballooning of a weak artery wall due to its weakened structure and the pressure of blood flow. The weakness may be a result of disease, injury, or a congenital defect. Aneurysms can exist for years without symptoms. They cannot be reversed, and therefore treatment is aimed at preventing them from becoming worse.

TREATMENT

✗ **DIETARY**

Cut down on saturated fats (red meats and dairy products).
Increase your intake of oily fish (sardines, herring, salmon).
Eat plenty of garlic.
Sprinkle brewer's yeast on your food.
Avoid salt.

▢ **HOMEOPATHY**

Take *Baryta carbonica* 6c, 1 a day for 1 month, to help tone and strengthen the arterial walls.

•❖• **EXERCISE**

Gentle regular exercise, such as walking or swimming, is good for this condition. However, avoid going out in very cold weather, and stop exercising immediately if you feel any pain.

～ RELAXATION TECHNIQUES

Attending a yoga or meditation class will help prevent this condition from worsening. Carry out the following relaxation routine at least once a day: Find a quiet place where you won't be disturbed. Lie on a firm surface, close your eyes, allow your breathing to slow, and begin to be aware of how your body feels. Consciously try to relax every part of your body in turn. Begin with your face (your eyes, your forehead, your jaw), and work down to your toes. The whole procedure should take at least 10 minutes.

Yogic breathing helps relaxation: Kneel on the floor. Place one hand on your abdomen and the other on your chest. Inhale, filling your abdomen with air and feeling it inflate. Then slowly exhale for 4 to 8 seconds, feeling it deflate. Now repeat the procedure, this time allowing your chest to inflate and deflate. Repeat this pattern for several minutes.

Relaxation tapes and biofeedback training can help teach you to relax if you find it difficult.

••• ORTHODOX

For life-threatening aneurysms, surgery to tie off the weakened area or replace it with a synthetic graft is relatively successful.

ANGINA

A tight, constricting sensation across the chest, accompanied by pain that moves up the neck and jaw and down the arms, particularly the left side. This may be accompanied by dizziness, nausea, and difficulty in breathing. Such symptoms require immediate medical attention. Angina is caused by a fall in blood supply to the heart, and occurs when the demands on the heart are increased through overexertion, excitement, stress, high blood pressure, or structural changes to the blood vessels supplying the heart. Angina is an early symptom of coronary heart disease (see **Coronary Heart Disease**).

PREVENTION

Do not smoke.

Reduce your intake of saturated fats (such as butter), and replace with polyunsaturated vegetable oils. Avoid red meat, full-fat dairy products, sweets made with fat, snacks containing fat, and fried foods. Eat moderate amounts of poultry, nonfat milk, and nonfat or low-fat cheeses and spreads.

Try to adopt a regular exercise routine. Walking and swimming are helpful.

Take measures to reduce stress (see **Stress**).

TREATMENT

■ PRACTICAL ADVICE

Stop smoking.

If you experience angina attacks at night, tilt the head of your bed up by 3 or 4 inches to reduce the pressure of blood on your heart. If an attack still occurs at night, sit on the edge of the bed with your feet on the ground, allowing the blood to flow into your legs.

✗ DIETARY

Eating the wrong foods can raise your blood pressure and promote an angina attack:

Reduce your intake of animal fats (found in meat, dairy products, and eggs).

Avoid salt.

Increase your intake of fiber, found in whole-grain cereals, and fresh fruits and vegetables.

Eat oily fish regularly (sardines, herring, salmon, trout, mackerel).

Incorporate raw garlic into your diet. If you do not like the taste or smell of fresh garlic, you can take garlic capsules (3 capsules, 3 times a day).

❊ AROMATHERAPY

Essential oil of lavender has been shown to aid relaxation: Add 4 to 5 drops of the oil to a bath or steam inhalation, or simply sprinkle 2 drops on a tissue or handkerchief and inhale it from time to time. **Caution:** If you suffer from asthma, avoid steam inhalations.

❧ HERBALISM

Infusion of hawthorn berries provides a good tonic for the heart and circulatory system: Pour 1 cup of water on 2 teaspoons of hawthorn berries, and infuse for 20 minutes; drink 3 times a day (warm or cold).

▢ HOMEOPATHY

For acute attacks, take the following:

With fear and panic: *Aconite* 6c, as often as required until symptoms are alleviated

When the chest feels as if it is squeezed by an iron band: *Cactus grandiflorus* 6c, as often as required until symptoms are alleviated

☯ CHINESE MEDICINE

Angina is believed to be a stagnation of the blood and energy in the heart. Practitioners of traditional Chinese medicine may prescribe herbal medicines such as cinnamon twigs, safflower, red sage root, or macrosten onion bulb.

✳ ACUPRESSURE

Relieve symptoms by applying deep thumb pressure to points H7, B15, and P6, as shown, for at least 1 minute.

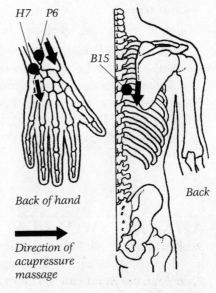

Back of hand

Back

Direction of acupressure massage

♣ REFLEXOLOGY

Heat the lung and heart areas of the foot by supporting the foot with one hand, and vigorously rubbing the areas with the other palm or fist.

To relax the central nervous system, massage the points of the toes, beginning with the little toe, until you reach the big toe. With two fingers, massage down the inside of the foot on the area of the spine and the tailbone. Repeat on the other foot.

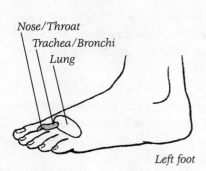

Nose/Throat
Trachea/Bronchi
Lung

Left foot

Trachea/Bronchi
Lungs
Diaphragm
Solar plexus
Waist level

Left sole

The reflex areas

✤ EXERCISE

Regular, gentle exercise has been shown to improve angina; walking is particularly good. Consult your doctor before you embark on an exercise routine.

••• ORTHODOX

Treatment varies depending on the cause of angina.

Drugs are sometimes prescribed to enlarge the blood vessels and reduce the workload of the heart muscle.

Beta-blockers are sometimes given to reduce the force of the heartbeat.

Antihypertensive drugs are sometimes given to lower high blood pressure (see **Blood Pressure, High**).

Calcium-antagonist drugs are prescribed to reduce the force of the heartbeat.

ANKLES, SWOLLEN

Swollen ankles result from an accumulation of excess tissue fluid. Flying, hot weather, standing for long periods, premenstrual syndrome (see **Premenstrual Syndrome**), kidney infection (see **Urinary Tract Infection**), varicose veins (see **Varicose Veins**), heart failure (see **Coronary Heart Disease**), thrombosis (see **Thrombosis**), pregnancy, and oral contraceptives can all contribute to this condition. It is also found in people with a protein or vitamin B deficiency. Very puffy ankles may be a sign of high blood pressure (see **Blood Pressure, High**), or preeclamptic toxemia (see **Preeclampsia**).

TREATMENT

Swollen ankles may be a sign of a serious internal disorder. Consult your doctor immediately if you suddenly notice unusual swelling. Once serious problems have been ruled out, the following treatments may help.

¿♠ HERBALISM

Parsley is a natural diuretic (it helps the body get rid of excess water); add liberally to your food. Take the following infusion 3 times a day: Pour 1 cup of boiling water on 2 teaspoons of parsley leaves, and infuse for 10 minutes. **Caution:** Do not use during pregnancy.

≈ HYDROTHERAPY

To increase circulation and reduce puffiness: Prepare two bowls of water: one with hot but not boiling water, the other with cold water (add some ice). Plunge your feet first into the hot water, then into the cold. Do this several times; finish with cold.

☞ MASSAGE

Massaging the feet, ankles, calves, and thighs can help move fluid out of the ankles.

Ask a professional or a friend to do this: Lie face down while your partner massages the back of the leg from the ankle up to the knee, using slow, firm sweeping motions up the calf. Avoid the knee area, and continue with firm, upward sweeping strokes and kneading of the thigh muscles.

You can massage your lower legs and ankles yourself according to the following routine: Sit on the floor with your knees bent. Place your thumbs on the outside of the shin bone and link your fingers around the back of the knee. Apply pressure with the thumbs, moving slowly down the outside of the leg to the ankle bone. Then move your thumbs around to the inside of the ankle and massage up the leg. Finally, place your thumbs in front of your knee and your fingers behind, and squeeze the calf muscle. Work down the back of the leg, squeezing and releasing. **Caution:** Do not massage over varicose veins.

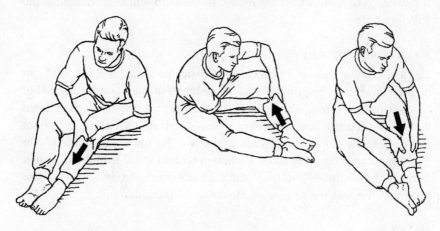

••• ORTHODOX

Doctors generally recommend the following:
    Elevate your feet whenever possible.
    Wear supportive elastic stockings.
    Take diuretic drugs (by prescription) to eliminate excess fluid.
    Follow a low-salt diet.

ANKYLOSING SPONDYLITIS

Also known as bamboo spine, this is an inflammatory disease affecting joints in the spine and pelvis, and sometimes the ribcage, which become fused, causing stiffness, rigidity, and pain, particularly after resting.

TREATMENT

✕ DIETARY

Reduce your intake of all sugars and starchy foods (pasta, potatoes). Increase your intake of legumes (peas, beans, lentils) and vegetables.

If you are regularly taking painkillers for this condition, it is advisable
to increase your intake of vitamin C, found in fresh fruits and vegetables,
particularly citrus fruits and juices; iron, found in red meat, poultry, fish,
and green vegetables; and vitamin A, found in liver, kidney, egg yolk, butter, fortified margarine, whole milk, and cream.

❋ AROMATHERAPY

Add 5 to 8 drops of essential oil of lavender, basil, or rosemary to the bath
to promote relaxation and relieve pain.

☐ HOMEOPATHY

A few drops of *Arnica* tincture placed in the bath will relieve aching and
stiffness.

≈ HYDROTHERAPY

Hot and cold compresses provide relief from pain and stiffness and can
be used as often as required: Prepare two bowls of water, one with hot but
not boiling water, one with cold. If the pain is in the back, lie face down
and have a partner fold a towel in three, roll it up, and dip it in the hot
water. Wring it out well, unroll it, and place the towel, still folded, over
the painful area for 3 minutes. Prepare a second towel in the cold water.
Remove the hot towel and place the cold one on the same area for about
1 minute. Repeat the sequence for about 20 minutes.

✛ EXERCISE

Gentle daily exercise is vital in preventing rigidity; swimming is particularly good.

✳ YOGA

Yoga helps maintain mobility by providing general stretching and breathing exercises to open up the ribcage. Do the following exercise every day:
Kneel on the floor. Place one hand on your abdomen and the other on
your chest. Inhale, filling your abdomen with air and feeling it inflate.
Then slowly exhale for 4 to 8 seconds, feeling it deflate. Now repeat the
procedure, this time allowing your chest to inflate and deflate. Repeat this
pattern for several minutes.

✚ PROFESSIONAL HELP

Chiropractic and massage help relieve pain and increase mobility. Acupuncture also helps with pain relief. Professional homeopathic prescribing has shown good results.

••• ORTHODOX

Doctors often prescribe painkillers such as aspirin or paracetamol, though long-term use can result in dietary deficiencies (bleeding of the stomach leading to loss of iron) and ulcers.

Anti-inflammatory drugs and steroids may also be recommended, along with physiotherapy to help maintain flexibility.

ANOREXIA NERVOSA

A psychological eating disorder most common in young women who have an obsessive fear of being fat. Symptoms include severe weight loss; restless energy; sometimes vigorous exercising; binge eating, which at times is followed by deliberate vomiting (see **Bulimia**); fatigue; loss of menstrual periods; depression; withdrawal; and refusal to admit to being ill. Professional treatment is vital to prevent death from malnutrition or dehydration.

The following self-treatments can be useful in conjunction with orthodox approaches aimed at helping both the sufferer and the family.

TREATMENT

▬ PRACTICAL ADVICE

Try to talk to someone outside your family and immediate circle of friends. Some support groups and women's centers have telephone hotlines that can provide immediate help and advice.

Emotional support is important in treating this illness. Try to find a counselor, therapist, friend, or relative who you can trust to talk with and express your feelings.

Becoming involved in creative activities helps express inner feelings, allowing parts of yourself that want to be recognized to come out. Activities that can help release creative energy include art activities such as painting, ceramics, or photography; playing or listening to music; dancing; gardening; and cooking.

Writing a journal of your thoughts and feelings permits you to have a private place to be honest with yourself about what is happening at an inner level.

☯ CHINESE MEDICINE

Professional treatment is necessary, and would likely be aimed at strengthening the digestive system and spleen and improving the body's capacity to absorb food, which is sometimes lost after long periods of starvation. Nutrients prescribed to increase the appetite include rice and wheat sprouts, radish seeds, or loganberries.

☛ MASSAGE

Receiving a regular massage from a therapist or learning to give massages and receive them from friends or family is a very good way to relax and unwind. It will also help you to feel more nurtured and comfortable with your body. Massage can be very healing, and can put you in touch with feelings from the past that may help you resolve psychological problems.

••• ORTHODOX

Doctors carefully assess the patient and her family, since the family can play an important role in the cause and treatment of this disorder. Specialized treatment is carried out in hospitals and clinics, where the patient is encouraged to eat and receives emotional counseling and therapeutic support.

ANXIETY

An emotional state ranging from mild unease to intense fear, often characterized by a sense of impending doom. Physical symptoms can include heart palpitations, throbbing or stabbing pains, breathing difficulties, headaches, neck and back pain, restless trembling hands, fatigue, diarrhea, upset stomach, and depression.

TREATMENT

Long-term anxiety is psychologically draining and can compromise the immune system, making you more susceptible to infection and disease. Counseling or psychotherapy can greatly assist in getting to the root of the cause of your anxiety. A simple talk with your doctor or health practitioner can also help. The following treatments help resolve short-term anxiety.

✗ DIETARY

Avoid caffeine (coffee, chocolate, cola, tea).

A deficiency in vitamin B-complex can increase symptoms of stress. Take a vitamin B-complex supplement once a day to ensure adequate intake.

❋ AROMATHERAPY

Essential oil of lavender has been shown in studies to relieve anxiety: Use a few drops in a steam inhalation or in a bath, or simply sprinkle 2 drops on a tissue or handkerchief and inhale it from time to time. Regular treatment from a professional is extremely relaxing.

For severe anxiety, add 1 drop of valerian oil to a steam inhalation or bath. **Caution:** If you suffer from asthma, avoid steam inhalations.

🦐 HERBALISM

Valerian is one of the most useful herbs taken to reduce tension and anxiety: Pour 1 cup of boiling water over 1 or 2 teaspoons of the root, and let it infuse for 15 minutes; drink when needed.

☯ CHINESE MEDICINE

Traditional practitioners of Chinese medicine see anxiety as a weakness of energy in the liver and spleen. They recommend Chinese angelica and ginseng.

❀ BACH FLOWER REMEDIES

Aspen or Rescue Remedy are useful for anxiety.

☛ MASSAGE

Stress and anxiety produce rigid and painful muscles, particularly in the neck and shoulders. A regular massage from a therapist, friend, or partner relaxes these muscles, and in turn relieves anxiety. The best way to carry out a quick neck and shoulder massage is for you to kneel with your arms and head supported on a chair or table. Your partner should firmly squeeze and stroke the muscles of shoulders and neck on either side of the spine, working upward and outward.

∼ RELAXATION TECHNIQUES

Attending a yoga or meditation class will help improve or prevent anxiety condition. Do the following relaxation routine at least once a day: Find a quiet place where you won't be disturbed. Lie on a firm surface, close your eyes, allow your breathing to slow, and begin to be aware of how your body feels. Consciously try to relax every part of your body in turn. Begin with your face (your eyes, your forehead, your jaw), and work down to your toes. The whole procedure should take at least 10 minutes.

Anxiety is often caused by hyperventilation, which can be helped by yogic breathing: Kneel on the floor. Place one hand on your abdomen and the other on your chest. Inhale, filling your abdomen with air and feeling it inflate. Then slowly exhale for 4 to 8 seconds, feeling it deflate. Now repeat the procedure, this time allowing your chest to inflate and deflate. Repeat this pattern for several minutes.

Relaxation tapes and biofeedback training can help teach you to relax if you find it difficult.

••• ORTHODOX

Your doctor may prescribe a tranquilizer, though with many (such as Valium) long-term use can lead to overreliance and serious side effects. Counseling may also be recommended.

APPENDICITIS

Acute inflammation of the appendix, a small tube branching off the large intestine. Symptoms include loss of appetite; stomach ache around the navel, shifting to sharp pain in the lower right of the belly; nausea; fever; and sometimes constipation or diarrhea. This condition requires immediate medical attention and hospital admission.

TREATMENT

••• ORTHODOX

In the early stages, after hospitalization, a fluid-only diet is recommended. This rests the inflamed bowel; it also makes it unnecessary to avoid having to wait before receiving a general anesthetic if surgery proves necessary.

Appendectomy, surgical removal of the appendix, is the only recommended treatment for advanced inflammation. If surgery is delayed, the appendix may rupture into the peritoneal or abdominal cavity, which can lead to life-threatening infection.

☐ HOMEOPATHY

After surgery, keep the wound clean by bathing with a solution of *Hypericum* and *Calendula:* Add 4 drops of each to 1 cup of warm water; or buy Hypercal.

To relieve bruising and pain, and to prevent infection of the wound: *Arnica* 6c, 2 times a day, for up to 10 days.

To relieve nausea or vomiting after the anesthetic: *Phosphorus* 6c, 3 times a day, for 3 days.

✿ BACH FLOWER REMEDIES

Take Rescue Remedy to diminish fear before surgery, and to aid recovery.

ARTERIOSCLEROSIS

A condition in which the artery walls, which are usually elastic, become hardened with age and hamper the heart's ability to pump blood through the body. This condition greatly contributes to coronary heart disease (see **Coronary Heart Disease**), and leads to high blood pressure (see **Blood Pressure, High**) and increased likelihood of strokes and heart attacks.

PREVENTION

Do not smoke.

Avoid saturated fats (see Dietary guidelines below).

Exercise regularly.

TREATMENT

▬ PRACTICAL ADVICE

Stop smoking right away. Smoking accelerates the process of arteriosclerosis by making the blood more "sticky" and likely to clot around the arteries.

✗ DIETARY

Making the following changes to your diet can prevent and reverse the illness to a significant degree:

Avoid saturated fats, found in red meats, fatty dairy products, shortening and margarine, coconut and palm oils (used in snack foods), and eggs.

Substitute fish or poultry for red meat.

Increase your intake of fiber, particularly fruits and vegetables, cooked dried beans, and oat bran.

Eat a diet rich in whole-grain cereals and fresh fruits and vegetables; avoid refined and junk foods.

Reduce your intake of salt and sugar.

Supplementation with vitamin E has been shown to help circulatory problems: Take 150 to 200 milligrams a day.

Incorporate plenty of garlic into your diet. If you do not like the taste or smell of fresh garlic, you can take garlic capsules (3 capsules, 3 times a day).

☞ MASSAGE

Regular massage promotes general relaxation, which helps lower blood pressure.

✤ EXERCISE

Regular, gentle exercise, such as daily walking or swimming, or gentle running or cycling, is helpful in treating this condition.

～ RELAXATION TECHNIQUES

Attending a yoga or meditation class will help improve or prevent this condition. Do the following relaxation routine at least once daily: Find a quiet place where you won't be disturbed. Lie on a firm surface, close your eyes, allow your breathing to slow, and begin to be aware of how your body feels. Consciously try to relax every part of your body in turn. Begin with your face (your eyes, your forehead, your jaw), and work down to your toes. The whole procedure should take at least 10 minutes.

Yogic breathing helps relaxation: Kneel on the floor. Place one hand on your abdomen and the other on your chest. Inhale, filling your abdomen with air and feeling it inflate. Then slowly exhale for 4 to 8 seconds, feeling it deflate. Now repeat the procedure, this time allowing your chest to inflate and deflate. Repeat this pattern for several minutes.

Relaxation tapes and biofeedback training can help teach you to relax if you find it difficult.

••• ORTHODOX

Doctors can generally diagnose arteriosclerosis by feeling the firmness of the arteries, by listening to blood flow with a stethoscope, or by examining the blood vessels at the back of the eye. The dietary, relaxation, and exercise treatments listed above will probably be recommended.

ARTHRITIS

Arthritis brings inflammation in one, several, or many joints of the body, leading to pain, redness, swelling, and stiffness around the joint, and sometimes symptoms in other more distant parts of the body. Different types of arthritis have specific causes, symptoms, and treatments. The following are the most common types (for treatment, see specific entries).

Osteoarthritis: Symptoms are caused by wear and tear or degeneration of the joints (see **Osteoarthritis**).

Rheumatoid arthritis: Symptoms are caused when the immune system acts against and damages joints and surrounding tissues, causing general inflammation of all structures of the body, including the joints. This is the most common type of arthritis (see **Rheumatoid Arthritis**).

Ankylosing spondylitis: Arthritis of the spine, where the joints linking the vertebrae become inflamed and the bones fuse; the hips may also be affected (see **Ankylosing Spondylitis**).

Gout: Uric acid, one of the body's waste products, accumulates in the joints, causing inflammation (see **Gout**).

ASTHMA

Recurrent attacks of breathlessness and wheezing, a dry cough, and a feeling of tightness in the chest, which often begins at night. A bad attack, which can be fatal, causes sweating, rapid heartbeat, and extreme gasping for breath. Asthma occurs when the airways in the lungs go into spasm as a result of an allergy, air irritants, lung infection, or stress. Severe attacks require professional treatment. The following self-help tips can complement professional help.

PREVENTION

Avoid cigarette smoke and wood-burning fires.

If you suddenly go out into cold weather, cover your mouth and nose with a scarf.

Remove potential allergens from the indoor environment (see **Allergies, Hay Fever and Rhinitis**).

Aspirin can sometimes trigger an attack, so avoid it if you are sensitive.

TREATMENT
✗ DIETARY

Avoid potential food allergens (milk, eggs, nuts, and seafood); and processed foods and food additives, such as monosodium glutamate (621) and sodium metabisulphite (E223), found in beer and wine and some dried fruits. Avoid the yellow coloring agent tartrazine (Yellow 5; E102).

Studies have shown that following a strict vegetarian diet reduces the incidence and severity of asthma.

Studies have shown that people taking 100 milligrams per day of vitamin B6 noticed a reduction in the frequency and severity of asthma attacks. Vitamin B6 is found in wheat germ, brewer's yeast, poultry, fish, cooked dried beans, and peas and peanuts.

❀ AROMATHERAPY

People who suffer from asthma should never take steam inhalations. Instead, put a few drops of essential oil on a handkerchief or tissue and inhale: Atlas cedarwood, eucalyptus, and peppermint help ease breathing.

🐌 HERBALISM

Elecampane infusion is recommended by herbalists: Add 1 teaspoon of the shredded root to 1 cup of cold water, let it stand for 10 hours, strain, and heat; drink hot 3 times a day.

☐ HOMEOPATHY

Professional treatment will help to reduce the frequency and severity of the attacks. The following remedies are recommended:

If very restless and anxious: *Arsenicum album* 30c, as required

Symptoms worse in late evening and night, made worse by cold weather; symptoms come on very suddenly and are accompanied by great anxiety: *Aconite* 6c, as required

Symptoms worse between 3 A.M. and 5 A.M., aggravated by damp weather: *Natrum sulphuricum* 6c, as required

☯ CHINESE MEDICINE

Treatment should be carried out by a practitioner of traditional Chinese medicine, who may offer herbs such as ephedra and bitter almond seed to calm wheezing attacks, and acupuncture to treat the lungs, kidney, or spleen.

♣ REFLEXOLOGY

Massage the area between the big toe and the second toe on both feet.

Massage the top of the foot, spreading the toes apart and loosening the toe ligaments.

✳ ACUPRESSURE

Reach with your right hand over your left shoulder to press firmly on point B13; take 5 long, deep breaths, then release. Repeat with the left hand.

Place your fists on your chest with thumbs pointing upward. Place your thumbs on the muscles that run below the collarbone, and gently feel for a sensitive spot. Press firmly and breathe deeply for 2 minutes.

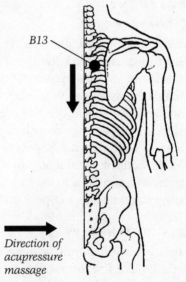

B13

Direction of acupressure massage

✳ YOGA

Do the following sequence of exercises when an attack starts. Try to relax and clear your mind of everything as you do the movements.

Sit on the floor in a comfortable position, facing the seat of a chair. Let your head, chest, and arms drop forward and rest on the seat of the chair. Inhale and let your head fall back, exhale and let your head fall forward. Repeat 5 times. Let your head fall back and forward while inhaling and exhaling, this time saying "Ahh," as you come forward exhaling.

Kneel on the floor, sitting on your heels. Move your head back and forth as above, 5 times. Then, keeping your arms straight, clasp your hands behind your back and lean forward, if possible until your head touches your knees or the floor. Hold the position for several seconds, then return to the upright position. Repeat several times.

••• ORTHODOX

Doctors generally treat asthma with drugs. Sodium cromoglycate is designed to prevent asthma, and must be taken continuously. Inhaled corticosteroid drugs, which reverse the spasm in the air tubes, are known as reverse inhalers.

ASTIGMATISM
See **Eyesight Problems.**

ATHEROSCLEROSIS

A condition in which fatty plaque deposits gradually clog up the insides of the artery walls, restricting blood flow and leading to high blood pressure and increased likelihood of stroke or heart attack. This condition is more common in men than women, and in people who smoke, are overweight, or lead a sedentary lifestyle.

PREVENTION

See Dietary recommendations, below.

Do some aerobic exercise (such as brisk walking, cycling, or swimming) at least 3 times a week. See your doctor before you begin any exercise program.

Take measures to reduce stress (see **Stress**).

TREATMENT

✗ DIETARY

Atherosclerosis is rare in countries where people eat a diet low in fat and high in fiber. The first steps in treating this disorder should therefore be dietary:

Avoid saturated fats, found in red meats, fatty dairy products, eggs, shortening, and coconut and palm oils (used in snack foods).

Substitute fish and poultry for red meat.

Use olive oil for cooking and salad dressings; replace butter with poly-unsaturated margarine.

Increase your intake of fiber, particularly fruits and vegetables, cooked dried beans, and oat bran.

Reduce your intake of salt and sugar.

Eat a diet rich in whole-grain cereals, and fresh fruits and vegetables. Avoid refined and junk foods.

Increase your intake of citrus fruits, tomatoes, potatoes, strawberries, and spinach, all rich in vitamin C, which has been shown to help prevent cholesterol buildup.

✦ EXERCISE

Exercise helps protect the body from harmful cholesterol buildup. Regular walking, running, swimming, cycling, or aerobics is the best. Check with your doctor before starting a new exercise program.

••• ORTHODOX

Doctors generally prescribe anticoagulant drugs such as aspirin to reduce clots forming in the blood. Daily small doses of aspirin have been shown to be useful in people who have already had a stroke or a heart attack.

Vasodilator drugs are designed to open up the arteries, but are not very effective and do not resolve the degeneration of the artery walls.

Surgery can widen the arteries or replace damaged areas with vein or synthetic grafts (see **Aneurysm; Coronary Heart Disease**).

ATHLETE'S FOOT
See **Fungal Infection.**

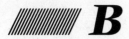 **B**

BACKACHE

Pain occurring anywhere from the base of the skull to the tailbone. The following self-assessment chart provides some indication of the many different causes and symptoms. See also **Lower Back Pain**.

1. Soft-tissue/musculo-skeletal backaches: Trouble arises from the muscles, joints, and ligaments running along the spine. May be caused by improper lifting, straining, or prolonged bad posture (driving or sitting at a desk).
2. Slipped-disc backaches: Trouble arises from a backward movement of the cartilaginous disc that cushions each vertebra of the spine from the next one. When the disc pushes against nerves in the spinal cord, it commonly produces referred pain down the back of the leg (see **Sciatica**). Common causes include lifting with a bent back or awkward twisting. See also **Slipped Disc**.
3. Inflammatory and pathological backaches: These make up the minority of backaches, but are the most serious. Bone infections, tumors, and degenerative disorders such as arthritis may all be responsible. The back pain may be the first sign of a problem arising in the back, but it may also represent the first symptom of disease somewhere else in the body.

   You should always consult your doctor about backache. However, to make an initial diagnosis, ask yourself the following questions:

   Did the pain come on suddenly? Likely to be 1.
   Was it triggered by exertion or lifting? Likely to be 1.
   Do you feel generally unwell or tired? Likely to be 3.
   Is the pain worse on coughing? Likely to be 2.
   Does the pain radiate down the leg? Likely to be 2.
   Are the pain and stiffness worse in the morning? Likely to be 1 or 2.
   Is the pain worse on bending forward? Likely to be 2.
   Is the pain worse on leaning backward? Likely to be 1.
   Is the small of the back completely straight? Likely to be 1 or 2.

TREATMENT

Severe or prolonged cases of backache require professional help. Use the following self-help treatments only after a professional has ruled out severe slipped disc or pathological causes.

≈ HYDROTHERAPY

Hot and cold treatments are very helpful for this condition, and can be repeated as often as required: Prepare two bowls of water, one with hot but not boiling water, one with cold. Lie face down and have a partner fold a towel in three, roll it up, and dip it in the hot water. Wring it out well, unroll it, and place the towel, still folded, over the painful area for 3 minutes. Prepare a second towel in the cold water. Remove the hot towel and place the cold one on the same area for about 1 minute. Repeat the sequence for about 20 minutes.

☞ MASSAGE

It is difficult to massage your own back, but treatment from a professional therapist, a friend, or a family member can provide much relief if the backache is muscular in origin. Lie face down on a firm surface, or sit leaning forward over the back of a chair. Your partner should use deep stroking movements (*effleurage*) up the muscles on either side of the spine, and small circular strokes with the tips of the fingers (*petrissage*) around areas of tension (shoulder blades and buttocks).

✳ ACUPRESSURE

Use firm pressure for at least 1 minute on the points illustrated.

⁘ EXERCISE

Exercise is helpful in some cases of backache, but it is not advised if it makes the pain worse. Swimming, gentle stretching, and yoga strengthen the back muscles without straining them, and are very helpful as a preventive measure.

The following exercises help relieve stiffness and muscular pain by "massaging" the whole of the spine:

Sit on a mat. Bend your legs and grasp your arms around your knees. Slowly rock backward and forward so that your whole spine touches the floor.

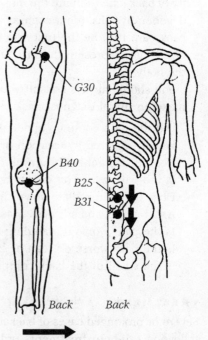

Direction of acupressure massage

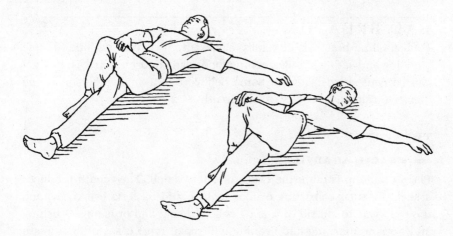

Lie on your back with your legs straight and your arms stretched out to the sides. Bend your left leg and place the foot on the outside of your right knee. Keeping your shoulders ground, lower your left knee toward the ground, and turn your head to the right. Hold the position and release. Repeat with the other leg.

～ RELAXATION TECHNIQUES

Rest on a firm mattress that supports your back.

Support the knees and hips when lying flat by placing a small cushion under the small of the back or under the knees.

Lie on your side if you have leg pain.

Place a small pillow under the neck for neck and shoulder pain.

Try to let go of the tension in your body with the following routine: Find a quiet place where you won't be disturbed. Lie on a firm surface, close your eyes, allow your breathing to slow, and begin to be aware of how your body feels. Consciously try to relax every part of your body in turn. Begin with your face (your eyes, your forehead, your jaw), and work down to your toes. The whole procedure should take at least 10 minutes.

✚ PROFESSIONAL HELP

Chiropractors specialize in diagnosing and treating back problems. Acupuncturists can often relieve severe back pain. The Alexander Technique is useful for backache resulting from poor posture; once the initial pain has gone, it will help prevent a recurrence.

••• ORTHODOX

Doctors may prescribe anti-inflammatory drugs or muscle relaxants, along with physiotherapy. They may also recommend traction, or wearing a collar or surgical corset. Surgery is a final resort.

BAD BREATH

Foul-smelling breath is generally caused by poor oral hygiene, though smoking and eating strong-smelling foods can contribute. Occasionally it can be caused by ill health. Some believe that a yeast infection of the digestive tract also results in bad breath.

TREATMENT

■ PRACTICAL ADVICE

Plaque buildup is often the cause of a foul smell. The mouth produces a sticky coating consisting of food, saliva, and bacteria every day, and the only way to get rid of it is by daily flossing and brushing. Brushing and flossing morning and evening will make most cases of bad breath disappear:

1. Using at least 5 inches of floss, wrap each end around one finger of each hand. Starting with the top right back tooth, wiggle the middle area of the floss between each tooth gently up and down several times. The aim is to remove plaque, not just bits of food caught between the teeth. Work all the way around the mouth.
2. Brush the teeth with gentle circular movements.
3. Gently brush the top of the tongue.
4. Rinse several times with cold water.
5. If desired, use a mouthwash.

✗ DIETARY

Avoid sugar, which promotes the production of plaque.

Avoid coffee, alcohol, and smoking, which all contribute to bad breath.

Chew parsley, or drink fenugreek or peppermint tea to sweeten the breath after a meal.

To combat yeast infections, eat plenty of live yogurt with *Lactobacillus acidophilus,* or take a supplement: Take ½ teaspoon *Lactobacillus acidophilus* powder, 1 teaspoon *Bifidobacteria* powder, and ½ teaspoon of *Lactobacillus bulgaricus* (available from natural foods stores), in a glass of spring water, 3 times a day.

⅔ HERBALISM

For inflamed or bleeding gums, add 2 teaspoons of red sage leaves to 2 cups of water, bring to a boil, and let stand, covered, for 15 minutes; strain and use as a mouth rinse several times a day. **Caution:** Do not use during pregnancy.

Echinacea decoction can be used as an everyday mouthwash: Add 2 teaspoons of echinacea root to 1 cup of water, simmer for 10 minutes, and allow to cool.

The Indian practice of chewing cardamom seeds after a meal has been shown to prevent tooth decay and associated bad breath.

☐ HOMEOPATHY
Take 3 times a day for 7 days:

Sour-smelling breath, particularly in the morning and after meals or drinking alcohol: *Nux vomica* 6c

Breath smells of onions: *Petroselinum* 6c

☯ CHINESE MEDICINE
Practitioners of traditional Chinese medicine recommend giant hyssop and peppermint tea to help detoxify the intestines; and radish seeds and oriental worm root to aid digestion.

••• ORTHODOX
Regular dental treatment includes professional cleaning, aimed at avoiding tooth and gum decay.

BALANITIS
Inflammation of the head of the penis and sometimes the foreskin. The area is itchy, red, and sometimes moist. In infants, balanitis can be caused by the irritation of wet diapers or damp clothing. It can also be caused by a bacterial or yeast infection; injury; and irritation from chemicals in clothing, condoms, or spermicide. The condition is most common in men with diabetes (see **Diabetes**), as sugar in the urine encourages the microbes to multiply.

TREATMENT

▬ PRACTICAL ADVICE
In infants, treat balanitis by changing diapers frequently and keeping the penis clean and dry. Disposable diapers, which retain fluid without allowing air circulation, may contribute to the problem. If you are using cotton diapers, detergent residues may be causing irritation. Perfumes or additives in the soap you use to bathe the baby, or powder you use to dry the baby, may also be a problem.

In adults, it is advisable to see a doctor for a checkup, as the symptoms of balanitis are similar to other more serious diseases.

Once a diagnosis is confirmed, the following gentle treatments may help:

- Always wear cotton underwear.
- Try changing your detergent to see if the condition is improved; always rinse underwear thoroughly.
- Avoid scented soaps and talc.
- Use hypoallergenic condoms and spermicides.
- If your doctor confirms a yeast infection as the cause of balanitis, treat it. Make sure your sexual partners are also treated, if necessary, as the infection may be passed back and forth between you (see **Fungal Infection; Thrush**).

✗ DIETARY

If balanitis is caused by a yeast infection, increase your intake of live, natural, unsweetened yogurt with *Lactobacillus acidophilus* (at least one small carton a day).

Decrease your intake of foods containing sugars and yeast (this includes fruit and alcohol).

To restore healthy bacteria to the body and help fight yeast infections: Take ½ teaspoon of *Lactobacillus acidophilus,* with 1 teaspoon *Bifidobacteria* powder, and ½ teaspoon *Lactobacillus bulgaricus* (available from natural foods stores), in a glass of spring water, 3 times a day.

❀ AROMATHERAPY

Wash the penis regularly with a solution of 4 drops of essential oil of tea tree in a basin of warm water. This is an effective antiseptic and antifungal agent.

❧ HERBALISM

Clean and dry the penis thoroughly, then apply aloe vera gel.

••• ORTHODOX

Doctors generally prescribe an antibiotic cream. For recurrent problems, circumcision may be recommended.

BALDNESS
See **Hair Loss.**

BAMBOO SPINE
See **Ankylosing Spondylitis.**

BEDSORES
Ulcers that develop on the skin as a result of spending long periods in bed or immobile. They start as tender red areas, and develop into deep sores that can become seriously infected and are difficult to heal.

PREVENTION
Turn bedridden patients regularly to distribute the pressure around the body.

Use a fleece lining or an eggcrate-foam mattress on the bed to relieve pressure.

If possible, use a water bed.

Regular massage for bedridden patients improves circulation and prevents sores from developing.

TREATMENT

▬ PRACTICAL ADVICE
Studies have shown sugar or honey to be effective in encouraging bedsores to heal: pack the sore tightly with granulated sugar or honey, and cover with an airtight dressing. Reapply each day.

✗ DIETARY
People who develop bedsores are generally in a weakened state. Good nutrition is very important to resist infection and promote healing.

Eat a whole-foods diet that includes plenty of protein, fruits, and vegetables.

Take the following supplements:

- vitamin C: 2 to 6 grams a day
- vitamin B-complex: 50 milligrams, 2 times a day
- vitamin A: 50,000 iu a day
- zinc: 25 to 50 milligrams a day

✿ AROMATHERAPY
Use a solution of 2 drops of essential oil of tea tree in 1 cup of water to clean the sore, encourage healing, and prevent infection.

☐ **HOMEOPATHY**

Take *Calendula 6c,* 3 times a day for up to 7 days; repeat if needed.

••• **ORTHODOX**

Most doctors recommend the following:

Turn immobile or bedridden patients regularly, to redistribute weight on different areas of the body.

Wash regularly to help prevent sores.

Once the sores have developed, antibiotics are given to reduce infection, and a cushioned dressing is used.

Extreme cases may require plastic surgery.

BED-WETTING

Involuntary urination in bed at night. Around 10 percent of children still wet the bed at the age of five, and some continue up to the age of sixteen or older. In most cases bed-wetting indicates that the nervous system is not yet mature enough to control the bladder. Sometimes it results from stress or anxiety. If children above the age of four have difficulty with daytime as well as nighttime bladder control, consult a professional, as this could be a sign of bladder infection or an anatomical abnormality of the kidney.

TREATMENT

■ **PRACTICAL ADVICE**

Bed-wetting in young children is perfectly normal, and most children outgrow it with time. To avoid worrying the child, change the sheets without fuss. Do not praise children if they have a dry night, or punish them when they are wet; this emphasizes the problem and can lead to stress and anxiety, which may make things worse.

Do not withhold drinks in the evening, or "lift" the child during the night to empty the bladder; neither will prevent bed-wetting.

To avoid embarrassing older children, leave out dry nightwear and sheets so that they can change themselves. This will also help them feel in control of the situation.

❀ **AROMATHERAPY**

Massage the child's stomach with 2 drops of essential oil of cypress added to 1½ to 2 teaspoons of a carrier oil or lotion.

☐ HOMEOPATHY

Take at bedtime for up to 1 week; repeat if needed:

Bed-wetting during dreams of urination: *Equisetum* 6c

Bed-wetting during first sleep; difficulty in urinating after urine has been forcibly retained: *Causticum* 6c

✿ BACH FLOWER REMEDIES

Cherry Plum has been shown to be useful in treating this condition.

✳ ACUPRESSURE

Apply deep thumb pressure to the points illustrated, 2 or 3 times a week.

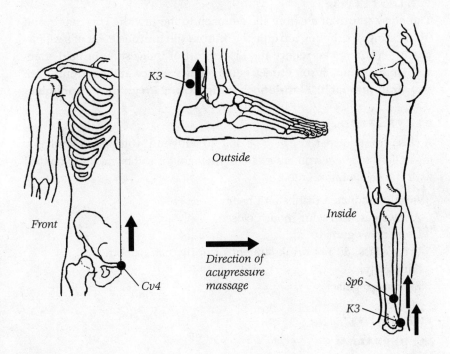

✚ PROFESSIONAL HELP

Hypnotherapy can be effective in resolving stubborn cases of bed-wetting.

••• ORTHODOX

Doctors sometimes recommend drug therapy using Tofranil (an antidepressant) or antidiuretic hormones (which suppress the urge to urinate), but this is only effective throughout the duration of the therapy.

If bed-wetting continues after the age of seven, some parents use an alarm that sets off a bell the minute the bed becomes damp, training the child to wake up and go to the toilet.

BEE STINGS
See **Insect Bites and Stings.**

BELCHING

The noisy return of air from the stomach to the mouth. This may result from eating or drinking too quickly, or from the nervous habit of swallowing air. Belching can relieve the discomfort of indigestion or acid stomach. In pregnancy it sometimes helps relieve nausea and heartburn. See also **Acid Stomach; Flatulence; Indigestion; Pregnancy Problems.**

PREVENTION

A close friend or partner may be able to tell you if you have a tendency to swallow air. Once you are aware of the habit, it will be easier to control with the following methods:

Avoid carbonated drinks and beer.
Always eat with your mouth closed.
Don't chew gum.
Use a glass; do not drink straight from the can or bottle.
Eat slowly.
Exercise regularly.

TREATMENT

HERBALISM

Fennel, peppermint, or vervain infusion aids digestion: Pour 1 cup of boiling water on 1 teaspoon of the dried herb, and infuse for 5 minutes before drinking; make when required.

Sucking a strong peppermint candy helps.

Ginger infusion helps relieve the need to belch: Pour 1 cup of boiling water on 1 teaspoon of freshly grated ginger root, and infuse for 5 minutes; drink when needed.

HOMEOPATHY

Take every 30 minutes for up to 5 doses:

If belching relieves pain or discomfort: *Carbo vegetabilis* 6c
If belching does not relieve discomfort: *China* 6c

••• ORTHODOX

Your doctor may recommend antacids to help aid digestion.

BLACK EYE

Injury to the eye area that damages the many small blood vessels beneath the skin and causes them to leak blood, which collects in the loose transparent skin around the eye. If vision is affected, seek professional attention. See also **Bruises.**

TREATMENT

▬ PRACTICAL ADVICE

Don't apply pressure to the eye or surrounding area.
Avoid aspirin, which prevents the blood from clotting.
Don't blow your nose hard, as it may rupture the blood vessels and increase the bleeding.

☐ HOMEOPATHY

Arnica 6c, every hour, for up to 4 doses; repeat the next day, if necessary. *Arnica* cream applied around the eye will help reduce bruising as long as the skin is unbroken:
If the bruising is slow to clear: *Ledum* 6c, 3 times a day, for 4 days
If the bones around the eye are very sore: *Symphytum* 6c, 3 times a day, for up to 4 days

≈ HYDROTHERAPY

Immediately place a cold compress (a cloth soaked in ice-cold water and wrung out) or an ice pack (a plastic bag filled with ice cubes or a bag of frozen peas wrapped in a dish towel) on the affected eye for 5 minutes. The cold constricts the blood vessels and decreases the bleeding that makes the eye go black. If there is swelling, repeat every 10 minutes throughout the day.

••• ORTHODOX

Doctors generally recommend the treatment listed in Practical Advice and Hydrotherapy, above. Other therapy will be recommended if vision is affected.

BLACKHEAD

A dark pore that develops when plugs of oil block the outlet of sebaceous glands surfacing through pores on the skin. On exposure to the air, the oil blackens due to oxidation and remains in the pores of the skin. Blackheads generally occur on the face, chest, shoulders, and back.

TREATMENT

■ PRACTICAL ADVICE

Avoid harsh soaps and drying creams, and alcohol-containing tonics and skin fresheners. Cleanse the face with a mild oil-in-water-emulsion cleanser, apply by hand, wipe off with tissues, and rinse the face with water.

Use an oil-in-water moisturizer.

✗ DIETARY

Avoid fatty foods and fried foods.

Increase your intake of green vegetables, particularly raw ones.

Increase your intake of vitamin B-complex, found in whole-grain breads and cereals, liver, and brewer's yeast (take 1 tablespoon added to water or fruit juice, 3 times a day).

To help to calm overactive oil glands: Make up a mixture of 2 teaspoons of brewer's yeast and 1 cup of natural, unsweetened yogurt. Use as a face mask 3 times a week for 15 minutes on freshly cleansed skin.

❀ AROMATHERAPY

For a skin freshener: Dilute 5 drops each of Atlas cedarwood and juniper berry in ½ cup of spring water; use on the skin throughout the day.

≈ HYDROTHERAPY

You can remove blackheads that are not inflamed by steaming the skin over a bowl of hot water, or applying a hot compress: Soak a clean cloth in hot water mixed with 2 teaspoons of bicarbonate of soda (this helps open up the pores); wring out the cloth and apply to the blackheads. With a clean tissue, gently squeeze out the oily plugs (never use your nails to do this). Finish by applying a small amount of antiseptic cream, or a solution of 1 cup of water and 2 drops of essential oil of tea tree.

••• ORTHODOX

Most doctors recommend the following:

Avoid makeup altogether, or change to a non-oil-based brand.

Cleanse the skin well morning and night, using a mild cleanser, and rinse well with water afterward.

Expose the skin to moderate amounts of sunlight.

Low-dose tetracycline antibiotics may be prescribed for troublesome cases.

BLADDER STONES

Hard salt collections that tend to congregate at the exit of the bladder and cause sometimes severe abdominal pain, a frequent urge to urinate, pain during urination, and occasional traces of blood in the urine. This condition is not common; it particularly affects men, especially those who have lived for any time in warm climates.

TREATMENT

୬▲ HERBALISM

Stone root is used in the prevention and treatment of bladder stones. Add 1 to 3 teaspoons of dried stone root to 1 cup of water, and simmer for 15 minutes; drink 3 times a day.

☯ CHINESE MEDICINE

Practitioners of traditional Chinese medicine recommend star fruit to promote urination and relieve the discomfort of kidney stones: Boil 3 fresh star fruit with 2 teaspoons of honey; eat the fruit and drink the juice once a day.

≈ HYDROTHERAPY

Drink plenty of fluids to help reduce urine concentrations.

If the kidneys are painful, apply a warm water bottle to the painful area.

✚ PROFESSIONAL HELP

Professional homeopathic treatment can be extremely helpful in this condition.

••• ORTHODOX

Doctors often recommend surgery to remove or break up the stones so that they can be excreted.

BLISTER

A pocket of fluid in the outer layer of skin that results from damage to the flesh, for example, burns (see **Burns**), friction, or disease (see **Chicken Pox; Eczema**).

PREVENTION: FRICTION BLISTERS

Use petroleum jelly on areas of skin likely to be rubbed by unfamiliar clothing or shoes.

Wear thick cotton socks for sports.

Use talcum powder on the feet.

TREATMENT

■ PRACTICAL ADVICE

It is best to let a blister heal on its own. However, if the blister is causing pressure or pain, or if it is likely to burst through further friction, you can puncture it with a sterilized needle (dipped in alcohol or held in a flame) and drain out the fluid, trying to leave the skin intact. During the day cover the blister with a sterile bandage. Remove the bandage at night to let the blister dry out.

❀ AROMATHERAPY

Add 2 drops of essential oil of Roman chamomile to ½ cup of water, and use as an antiseptic when the dressing is changed.

▢ HOMEOPATHY

Bathe punctured blisters in a solution of *Hypericum* and *Calendula* (Hypercal).

For red, swollen, and itchy blisters, take *Rhus toxicodendron* 6c, every 4 hours until symptoms are alleviated.

••• ORTHODOX

A blister that becomes infected and does not heal on its own may require professional draining, antiseptic cream, and antibiotics to keep the infection from spreading.

BLOOD POISONING
See **Septicemia.**

BLOOD PRESSURE, HIGH

High blood pressure occurs when there is an increase in the force of blood flow against the artery and heart walls. Smoking, obesity, too much alcohol, stress, and heart problems are contributing factors. High blood pressure, known as the silent killer, often has no obvious symptoms. Untreated, the condition can lead to stroke, heart attack, kidney failure, and sometimes damage to the eyes.

TREATMENT

✕ DIETARY

Studies show that following a vegetarian diet can significantly lower or even eliminate high blood pressure. If you decide to become a vegetarian, make sure that you replace meat with sufficient vegetable protein, such as soy products, cooked dried beans, nuts, seeds, and whole-grain cereals.

Reduce your intake of animal fat (meat, eggs, butter, cream), sugar, and salt.

Increase your intake of fiber, found in whole-grain breads and cereals, vegetables, and fruits.

Increase your intake of potassium, found in fish, orange juice, bananas, potatoes, avocados, lima beans, tomatoes, apricots, and peaches.

Increase your intake of calcium, found in low-fat milk, yogurt and cheese, sesame seeds, chickpeas, spinach, and broccoli.

Increase your intake of magnesium, found in nuts, cooked dried beans and peas, soybeans, dark green leafy vegetables, seafood, and milk.

❃ AROMATHERAPY

Lavender has been shown in studies to aid relaxation (see Relaxation/Stress Relief, below). Add a few drops to the bath, and allow yourself to relax in the soothing aroma. A professional aromatherapy treatment can be very therapeutic.

☯ CHINESE MEDICINE

Chinese herbs are effective in treating high blood pressure. Treatment should be carried out by a professional; herbs such as chrysanthemum flowers, peony root, and astragalus are likely to be prescribed.

☛ MASSAGE

Regular massage can be of great help in relieving stress. Consult a qualified massage therapist; or teach yourself and a friend or partner to do it, then exchange treatments.

✳ ACUPRESSURE

Applying deep pressure to the points illustrated 3 or 4 times a week may be helpful.

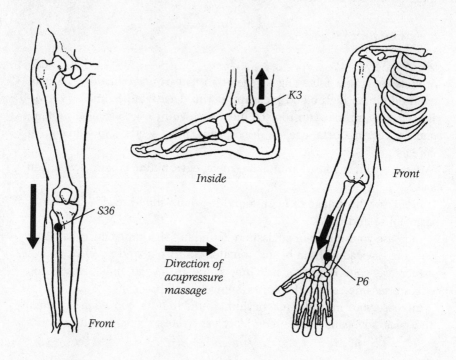

Inside

Front

S36

→

Direction of acupressure massage

P6

Front

✤ EXERCISE

Regular noncompetitive exercise is vital in treating this condition. Walking, gentle swimming, and cycling are all beneficial activities. Consult your doctor before you begin a new exercise routine.

◯ RELAXATION/STRESS RELIEF

Stress is one of the principal causes of high blood pressure. One of the first steps in treatment is learning to identify what arouses anger, anxiety, and other types of emotional stress in your professional and personal life. Consider the following questions when you think about resolving stress:

- Are you always in a hurry?
- Do you always work to deadlines?
- Do you snatch meals and eat quickly?
- Do you get less than seven hours' sleep each night?
- Do you participate in competitive sports?
- Do you often have conflict in your personal relationships?

For some people stress relief is simply a question of easing work commitments and getting more sleep. Other people need help to make necessary lifestyle changes: professional counseling, family therapy, or group therapy can be beneficial.

Do the following relaxation routine once a day: Find a quiet place where you won't be disturbed. Lie on a firm surface, close your eyes, allow your breathing to slow, and begin to be aware of how your body feels. Consciously try to relax every part of your body in turn. Begin with your face (your eyes, your forehead, your jaw), and work down to your toes. The whole procedure should take at least 10 minutes.

Relaxation tapes and biofeedback training can help teach you to relax if you find it difficult.

✳ YOGA

Attending a yoga class will help you relax and stretch, and will improve your breathing, which is vital to good circulation.

Do the following breathing exercise once a day: Kneel on the floor. Place one hand on your abdomen and the other on your chest. Inhale, filling your abdomen with air and feeling it inflate. Then slowly exhale for 4 to 8 seconds, feeling it deflate. Now repeat the procedure, this time allowing your chest to inflate and deflate. Repeat this pattern for several minutes.

✚ PROFESSIONAL HELP

Professional homeopathic treatment can treat high blood pressure successfully. The homeopath must make a personal prescription that takes account of the individual's physical and emotional situation, so self-prescribing is not recommended.

••• ORTHODOX

Doctors advise high-blood-pressure patients to stop smoking and to cut down consumption of alcohol, animal fats, and salt, and lose weight.

They may also recommend drugs, such as beta-blockers (to lower the heart rate), diuretics (to encourage the excretion of urine), or vasodilators (to enlarge the blood vessels).

BLOOD SUGAR, LOW

An abnormally low level of sugar in the blood; also known as hypoglycemia. The condition can occur in diabetics (see **Diabetes**) who take too

much insulin, skip meals, or use up their stores of sugar through unex-
pected activity. It can also occur in nondiabetics as a result of eating too
many sugary snacks, which causes blood levels to rise and fall dramatically. Symptoms include weakness, shakiness, sweating, fatigue, headaches, irritability, and confusion; in severe cases it can cause coma in
diabetics.

TREATMENT

✗ DIETARY

For emergency short-term relief of symptoms, suck a hard candy, eat a
spoonful of honey, or drink a glass of milk to boost low blood sugar.

For long-term relief, avoid sugar in any form (this includes desserts,
sweetened drinks, and breakfast cereals). Instead, eat plenty of protein
(fish, poultry, cheese, eggs, milk), fresh fruits and vegetables, beans, lentils, peas, brown rice, and whole-grain bread and pasta. Avoid alcohol, tea,
and coffee. Eat smaller meals more often—four to six small meals a day.
Do not skip meals, especially breakfast.

Chromium helps to normalize blood-sugar metabolism. It is found in
whole-grain breads and cereals, pork, kidney, molasses, lean meats, and
cheese. One of the best sources is brewer's yeast: Drink 2 scant teaspoons
mixed in water or fruit juice once a day.

••• ORTHODOX

Doctors have only recently begun to recognize the symptoms of low blood
sugar. Treatment includes recommending the dietary practices above,
and making sure that the patient is not suffering from an insulin-
secreting tumor (this is very rare).

BODY ODOR

The smell caused when stale sweat comes into contact with bacteria on
the skin. Body odor can also be caused by excessive sweating, dietary
problems, fungal infections (see **Fungal Infection**), or medication. If the
following measures do not help, consult your doctor.

TREATMENT

▬ PRACTICAL ADVICE

The most effective way to prevent body odor is to wash all over at least
once a day, and to use an underarm deodorant or antiperspirant. Deodorants work by restricting the action of bacteria on the skin; anti-

perspirants reduce the volume of perspiration that is released through the skin. (Natural practitioners do not favor antiperspirants because they interfere with the natural elimination process of sweating). Dusting the body with sodium bicarbonate provides an effective and natural deodorant.

In warm weather wear loose clothing made from natural fabrics (cotton, linen, wool). Change clothing worn next to the skin every day.

✗ DIETARY

Improper diet and deficiencies in certain vitamins and minerals can sometimes contribute to this condition:

Excess fat in the diet can sometimes cause body odor, particularly saturated fats found in meat and dairy products.

Avoid foods that contain saturated fats or list vegetable oil as one of the ingredients, but fail to mention the type of oil. Replace saturated fats with sunflower seed oil, polyunsaturated margarine, and olive oil.

Zinc deficiency is sometimes related to excessive perspiration: Take 20 to 30 milligrams of chelated zinc a day.

❀ AROMATHERAPY

Mix 6 drops of essential oil of lavender in 1 pint of distilled water, store in a bottle, and keep in the bathroom. Dab the solution onto areas of the body that perspire easily.

••• ORTHODOX

Your doctor may recommend treating excessive perspiration, also known as hyperhydrosis, by applying aluminum chloride preparations (available without prescription) to the affected areas.

BOIL

An inflamed, pus-filled lump on the skin, usually the result of a bacterial infection. Common sites are the back of the neck, armpits, groin, and buttocks. Recurrent boils could be a sign of inadequate diet or an early symptom of diabetes.

TREATMENT
✗ DIETARY

Zinc deficiency may lead to boils. To increase your intake of zinc, eat plenty of poultry, fish, liver, lima beans, pork, wheat germ, and whole-grain breads and cereals.

Naturopaths believe that boils are the body's way of cleansing itself of impurities. They also suggest that overindulgence in saturated fats (meat and dairy products) may encourage boils. They recommend a seven-day purification diet consisting of fruit juices, fresh fruits (particularly citrus) and vegetables (particularly green), along with plenty of mineral water.

Constipation can sometimes cause boils (see **Constipation**).

❋ AROMATHERAPY

Dab essential oil of tea tree on boils 4 to 6 times a day.

?❧ HERBALISM

Garlic is an effective antiseptic and helps to detoxify the body. Incorporate raw garlic into your diet as much as possible. If you do not like the taste or smell of fresh garlic, you can take garlic capsules (3 capsules, 3 times a day).

☐ HOMEOPATHY

Take every hour for up to 4 doses, and repeat if needed:

Hot, red, and throbbing: *Belladonna* 6c
Extremely sensitive, lancing pains: *Hepar sulphuris* 6c
Where the boil is slow to come to a head: *Silicea* 6c
Where other remedies have been tried without success: *Myristica* 6c

☯ CHINESE MEDICINE

Practitioners of traditional Chinese medicine recommend herbs to reduce heat in the body, which is thought to cause boils: Chinese golden thread, dandelion, or wild chrysanthemum and violet are given in the form of a tea.

❋ BIOCHEMIC TISSUE SALTS

Take *Calc Sulph* 6x, 4 times a day.

≈ HYDROTHERAPY

An Epsom salts bath stimulates circulation and encourages elimination through the skin: Dissolve 1 pound Epsom salts (available from pharmacies) in a hot bath and soak in it for 10 to 20 minutes before going to bed. Do this no more than 2 times a week. **Caution:** This treatment is not recommended for people who are weak or frail.

••• ORTHODOX

Most doctors will lance large boils and prescribe antibiotics to clear up the infection. Doctors advise against squeezing boils, which increases the risk of spreading the infection.

BREAST-FEEDING PROBLEMS

Problems associated with breast-feeding include insufficient milk production, breast engorgement, and painful nipples; see also **Breast Tenderness.** Babies benefit from receiving only breast milk for at least the first six months of life, and preferably for the first year. Learning how to breast-feed properly can make the experience much more comfortable and fulfilling for both mother and baby. La Leche League, an international support group, provides information and advice about breast-feeding. The following gentle treatments are recommended for commonly experienced problems.

PREVENTION AND TREATMENT: INSUFFICIENT MILK PRODUCTION

■ PRACTICAL ADVICE

Feed your baby regularly. The mammary glands need stimulation to produce milk.

✗ DIETARY

Make sure you are getting adequate nutrition. Eat plenty of whole-grain cereals, fruits, vegetables, and lean proteins, with plenty of fluids (especially apple and grape juice).

⅔ HERBALISM

Goat's rue infusion has been shown to increase milk production by up to 50 percent: Pour 1 cup of boiling water onto 1 teaspoon of the dried leaves, and infuse for 10 minutes; drink 2 times a day.

Nettle tea, sold in natural foods stores, is also very successful.

☐ HOMEOPATHY

Take *Annus castus* 6c, 4 times a day, for up to 3 days.

~ RELAXATION TECHNIQUES

Stress can sometimes suppress milk supply. Talking to a supportive friend or relative can help relieve anxiety; yoga, meditation, massage, or aromatherapy helps relieve tension.

PREVENTION AND TREATMENT:
BREAST ENGORGEMENT/TOO MUCH MILK

▬ PRACTICAL ADVICE

If the breasts become painfully swollen with milk, express the excess to provide relief. Store milk in sterile bottles or plastic freezer bags and use in emergencies.

⁊ HERBALISM

Nettle tea, available in natural foods stores, is useful in helping to regulate the flow.

☐ HOMEOPATHY

If engorgement is accompanied by feelings of sensitivity and tearfulness: *Pulsatilla* 6c, every 4 hours, until breasts feel more comfortable

If engorgement is accompanied by sensitivity to the cold and experiencing cold sweats: *Calcarea carbonica* 6c, every 4 hours, until breasts feel more comfortable

PREVENTION AND TREATMENT:
PAINFUL NIPPLES

▬ PRACTICAL ADVICE

See **Mastitis** for more specific details.

La Leche League advises making sure that the nipple is completely in the baby's mouth so that it does not move about, causing irritation.

Expose your nipples to the air as much as possible to let them dry naturally.

To help heal cracked nipples, allow a drop of milk to remain on the nipples after feeding.

☐ HOMEOPATHY

After feeding: Bathe nipples in a solution of 10 drops of *Arnica* tincture in 1 cup of water, dry thoroughly, and apply *Calendula* cream.

Take every 4 hours for up to 6 doses:

- Nipples inflamed and tender: *Chamomilla* 6c
- Nipples cracked and excessively sore: *Castor equi* 6c

BREAST LUMPS

The most common cause of breast lumps is fibrocystic breast disease, where fluid-filled sacs develop and the milk glands may thicken. The symptoms are tender lumps in one or both breasts, particularly one or two weeks prior to menstruation. Any lump, hard area, change in shape or hang of the breast, skin color changes, or changes in nipple size or shape should be reported to your doctor. Most lumps are benign, but some are cancerous. The following advice is for prevention and treatment of fibrocystic disease.

PREVENTION

The Dietary guidelines given below help prevent breast lumps caused by fibrocystic disease.

TREATMENT

■ PRACTICAL ADVICE

Wear a supportive bra to lessen discomfort.
Examine your breasts after every period.

✗ DIETARY

Increased intake of the following may help alleviate fibrocystic disease: vitamin A (found in liver, kidney, egg yolk, and low-fat dairy products); and beta-carotene (found in dark green vegetables and dark yellow and orange vegetables and fruits: broccoli, spinach, carrots, apricots, peaches).

Vitamin E aids absorption of vitamin A. (Vitamin E is found in vegetable oils, seeds, wheat germ, nuts, avocados, whole-grain breads and cereals, spinach, broccoli, asparagus, dried prunes). You can also take vitamin E supplements: 200 milligrams a day. **Caution:** If you are suffering from high blood pressure, check with your doctor first.

Women with low levels of selenium are at greater risk for fibrocystic breast disease. Selenium is found in whole wheat and rice, oatmeal, poultry, low-fat dairy products, lean meats, organ meat, fish, and seafood.

Evening primrose oil supplements have been shown to help reduce breast lumps: Take 500 milligrams, 2 times a day.

Breast lumps thrive in fat. Adopt a diet that is low in fat, and high in fiber (whole grains, fruits and vegetables, and beans). This will allow more estrogen to be excreted, causing less hormonal stimulation in the breasts.

If you are overweight, try to reduce your weight (see **Obesity** for suggestions).

Reduce your intake of caffeine (coffee, tea, chocolate, cola), which is thought to contribute to fibrocystic lumps.

Examining Your Breasts

Self-examination can help in the early detection of changes or lumps in the breasts that should be immediately reported to your physician. The following routine should be carried out once a month, after your period.

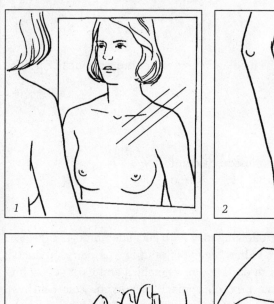
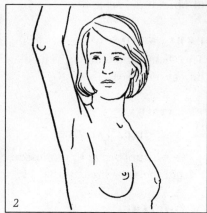
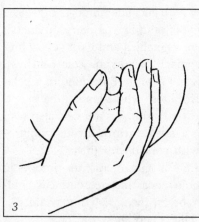
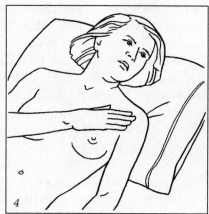

1. Examine your breasts in a mirror. Ensure that you are familiar with their general appearance (hang, shape, and size, and texture of the skin). Be alert to changes.
2. Place one arm above your head and look at the breast on that side of your body from different angles; repeat on the other side, looking for changes in appearance.
3. Examine the nipples for changes in appearance (an orange peel texture could indicate a lump). Gently squeeze the nipples to see if there is any discharge.
4. Lie on your back with the left arm by your side. With the palm and fingertips of your right hand work around the breast in a clockwise direction, feeling for lumps. Lift the left arm up above your head and feel the inner parts of the breast. Also feel along the top of the collarbone and into the armpit. Repeat on the other side.

✤ EXERCISE

Exercise stimulates blood circulation to the breasts, helping to clear toxins. Regular walking, swimming, running, racquet sports, and aerobics are all useful activities.

••• ORTHODOX

Most doctors perform routine breast examinations during physical checkups.

A mammogram may be recommended.

Cysts are usually drained of fluid; other lumps are usually surgically removed.

BREAST TENDERNESS

Tender or sore breasts, often accompanied by a feeling of heaviness or being swollen, are common in most women just before menstruation (see **Premenstrual Syndrome**), during pregnancy, or while breast-feeding (see **Breast-Feeding Problems**). If none of these causes can explain the tenderness, consult your doctor for an examination.

PREVENTION: PREMENSTRUAL BREAST TENDERNESS

✗ DIETARY

Reduce your intake of alcohol.

Reduce your intake of salt.

Eat a whole-foods diet, with plenty of fresh fruits and vegetables and low-fat protein.

Reduce your intake of coffee.

❊ AROMATHERAPY

Use 6 to 8 drops of essential oil of geranium in a hot bath.

Massage the breasts with a mixture of 15 drops of essential oil of geranium in 3½ tablespoons of a bland carrier oil or lotion.

⬩ HERBALISM

Eat plenty of chopped fresh parsley to help the body expel excess water.

☞ MASSAGE

Professional massage helps increase the circulation of the blood and lymph and prevents the buildup of toxins in the body. By improving circulation to the breasts, massage may help reduce swelling and tenderness if performed a few days before tenderness is due to begin.

✛ EXERCISE

Do regular, vigorous exercise, such as brisk walking, running, swimming, dancing, aerobics, or racquet sports.

~ RELAXATION TECHNIQUES

Reduce stress as much as possible, particularly in the week before your period. Attending a yoga or meditation class will help.

Make sure you get enough sleep and time for yourself.

TREATMENT: TENDERNESS WHILE BREAST-FEEDING

During pregnancy, prepare your breasts by massaging them with a little almond oil after a bath or shower. Avoid using soap on your nipples. Wear a cotton bra.

If you are producing more milk than the baby needs, express a little from time to time.

Make sure the nipple is completely in the baby's mouth. This will prevent the baby from tugging or pulling on the nipple, causing tenderness.

Rub a little breast milk into the nipple after feeding, to help heal any cracks. Allow the nipples to dry well. Apply *Calendula* cream if they are still sore.

••• ORTHODOX

Treatment depends on the cause of tenderness. Doctors may recommend diuretics (drugs to encourage the excretion of water from the body) for premenstrual women.

BREECH BABY

When a baby is in a breech position, the head lies beneath the mother's ribs, while the buttocks lie above the pelvis. Many babies turn themselves before birth; some remain in the breech position and are born without problems. However, if the baby is still in the breech position four weeks before the birth, it is advisable to try turn it with the techniques outlined below.

PREVENTION

Gentle exercise, such as regular walking for at least an hour a day, may help encourage the baby's head to go down.

TREATMENT

☐ **HOMEOPATHY**

Pulsatilla 200c, 1 tablet a day for 3 days, in addition to the other techniques described, may be helpful.

☛ **MASSAGE**

Before you attempt to turn the baby, consult your doctor or midwife on how the baby is lying and which way he or she is likely to turn.

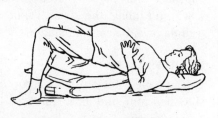

Lie on your back, placing several pillows under your hips, so that they are higher than your head. Relax and breathe deeply. Gently massage your stomach for about 10 minutes. Use gentle, circular strokes in the direction that the baby is likely to turn. Mentally, try to communicate with your baby, encouraging your baby to turn. Repeat the exercise several times throughout the day. It will probably take around two weeks for the baby to turn. At this point you will feel a change. Stop the exercises and have a checkup immediately to confirm the baby's position.

✚ **PROFESSIONAL HELP**

Chinese medicine can be helpful. Moxibustion, where a burning stick of mugwort is used to warm acupuncture points, is frequently successful in turning a baby.

••• **ORTHODOX**

Your doctor may try to turn the baby before delivery. If this is not possible, the doctor may perform an episiotomy (see **Episiotomy**) to widen the opening of the vagina, and use forceps to ease the baby's delivery.

BROKEN BONES

See **Fracture.**

BRONCHITIS

Inflammation of the airways that connect the windpipe to the lungs. Symptoms include a persistent phlegm-producing cough and breathlessness. Acute bronchitis can last from a few days to two weeks, and usually results from a virus. It can be dangerous in the elderly and in those with heart disease. Chronic bronchitis can last for months and is usually caused by smoking and environmental pollution.

TREATMENT

❀ AROMATHERAPY

Inhalations help clear chest congestion: Add a few drops of both essential oil of eucalyptus and sweet thyme to a bowl of steaming water. Sit with your face over the bowl, eyes closed. Put a towel over your head and the bowl, and inhale the steam vapor deeply. **Caution:** If you suffer from asthma, avoid steam inhalations.

🌿 HERBALISM

Elecampane infusion: Pour 1 cup of cold water onto 1 teaspoon of the shredded root, and let it stand for 10 hours; heat, and sip a cupful hot, 3 times a day.

For irritating coughs, wild cherry bark infusion: Pour 1 cup of boiling water on 1 teaspoon of the dried bark, and brew for 15 minutes; drink 3 times a day, or as needed.

▢ HOMEOPATHY

Take 3 times a day for up to 4 days:

Early symptoms accompanied by fever, tight chest, tickling cough, thirst: *Aconite* 6c

With loose white sputum, rattling cough, and irritability: *Kali bichromicum* 6c

With loss of voice, burning throat, cough, and thirst: *Phosphorus* 6c

☯ CHINESE MEDICINE

Treatment is aimed at preventing an attack by improving lung energy through herbs such as plantain seed, balloon flower root, honeysuckle flowers, skullcap root, or gardenia fruit.

••• ORTHODOX

Doctors will usually prescribe the following:

Take cough medicine to soothe the coughing.

Take inhalant drugs to open up the airways.

If you smoke, stop immediately.

Avoid places where people smoke.

Antibiotics, to eradicate secondary bacterial infections, can be life-saving in the frail and the elderly.

BRUISES

A discolored area under the skin, usually the result of an injury that damages minute blood capillaries, causing bleeding under the skin. Bruising occurs very easily in some diseases, such as hemophilia, where a blood-clotting agent is absent. See also **Black Eye.**

TREATMENT FOR BRUISES IN NONHEMOPHILIACS

✗ DIETARY

If you tend to bruise easily, increasing your intake of vitamin C, bioflavonoids, and zinc may help strengthen the integrity of the capillaries. Vitamin C and bioflavonoids are found in citrus fruits (juice, fruit, and pith), green peppers, and buckwheat. Zinc is found in meat, Cheddar cheese, lentils, haricot beans, whole-grain bread, and eggs.

🐾 HERBALISM

Bathe the bruise with a cold solution of witch hazel, available in most pharmacies.

▢ HOMEOPATHY

Arnica ointment is very effective when applied immediately to a bump or a bruise. Any household with children should have a tube handy. Do not apply to broken skin.

Arnica 6c: Take every hour after the injury for up to 6 doses, and 3 times a day the next day if pain continues.

❀ BACH FLOWER REMEDIES

Rescue Remedy cream is useful in relieving bruises. The drops help overcome shock.

≈ HYDROTHERAPY

Make an ice pack by wrapping a plastic bag full of ice cubes or a bag of frozen peas in a kitchen towel. Hold the bag on the bruise for 10 minutes to reduce swelling and pain.

••• ORTHODOX

When bruises are due to injury, treatment usually involves bathing the area in cold water or applying a cold compress. Doctors treat hemophiliacs with factor VIII, a blood protein that helps the blood to clot.

BULIMIA

An illness, most commonly afflicting women between fifteen and thirty, in which bouts of excessive eating are typically followed by self-induced vomiting, often carried out in secret. Like anorectics (see **Anorexia Nervosa**), bulimics have an obsessive fear of being fat, which is what prompts the vomiting. Some sufferers also use laxatives to expel food quickly. Bulimia may sometimes (though not always) result in significant weight loss. Frequent vomiting can lead to dehydration, weakness, and cramping. Sufferers are often depressed and sometimes suicidal.

TREATMENT

Professional treatment is essential; this illness requires psychological as well as physical support. The self-help advice given in **Anorexia Nervosa** applies equally to bulimia, and can be useful in conjunction with orthodox approaches aimed at helping both the sufferer and the family.

••• ORTHODOX

Treatment is similar to that for anorexia nervosa (see **Anorexia Nervosa**), and is best carried out in a hospital or specialized center. It involves monitoring and regulating eating habits, and counseling or psychotherapy. Some doctors may prescribe antidepressants.

BUNION

A painful, inflamed, fluid-filled area at the side of the big toe where it joins the foot. The toe joint projects outward, pushing the big toe over or under the other toes. Bunions often result from wearing narrow or pointed high-heeled shoes, although they can also be an inherited condition. The bunion forms when the projecting joint rubs against shoes, causing irritation and inflammation.

TREATMENT
≈ HYDROTHERAPY

Make an ice pack by wrapping a plastic bag full of ice cubes or a bag of frozen peas in a kitchen towel. Sit with the foot elevated. Hold the bag on the bunion for 10 minutes, and remove for 10 minutes; repeat the procedure several times, morning and night.

♣ REFLEXOLOGY

Ask a partner or friend to carry out the following massage: Have the sufferer sit on the floor, feet pointing up, soles facing you. Place one hand around the top of the foot to support it. Place the fingers of your other hand on top of the fingers supporting the foot, and your thumb underneath the big toe. Massage deeply with your thumb around the sole of the big toe, and beneath the bunion.

••• ORTHODOX

Doctors recommend wearing soft, comfortable shoes or open sandals, and may suggest a special toe pad or corrective sock to straighten the big toe. Podiatrists use a number of techniques to pad and protect the tender area. In severe cases doctors may recommend surgery to remove the inflamed tissue, or to rebuild the joint.

BURNS

Burns and scalds can be caused by heat, friction, or chemicals. Large burns (anything bigger than the palm of the hand) can lead to loss of body fluid, and require immediate medical attention.

TREATMENT

✿ AROMATHERAPY

Hold the burn under cold water, apply essential oil of lavender, and cover with a sterile dressing, if necessary. Repeat the application every 24 hours.

❧ HERBALISM

The juice of the aloe vera plant is renowned for reducing pain, preventing infection, and promoting the healing of burns. If you keep a plant in the house, remove a leaf (taking care to avoid the thorns), slit it open, and place on the skin, allowing the juice to reach the burn. Aloe vera gel is available in natural foods stores and pharmacies.

Honey is a good healing agent. For minor burns, spread a thin layer on the injured area and cover with a loose dressing. Repeat every 2 or 3 days.

☐ HOMEOPATHY

These remedies can be of great help in reducing pain and shock. Take every 30 minutes for up to 4 doses:

Immediately after the burn to relieve pain: *Cantharis* 6c

For shock, fear, and restlessness: *Aconite* 6c

A mixture of *Urtica urens* and *Calendula* is also effective.

✿ BACH FLOWER REMEDIES

Take 4 drops of Rescue Remedy immediately.

≋ HYDROTHERAPY

If the skin is not broken, immediately immerse the burn in cold water for at least 10 minutes. Add *Hypericum* and *Calendula* tinctures (10 drops of each) to the water to relieve pain. *Do not put butter or oil on the burn.* If you are taking the injured person to the hospital, wrap the burned area in a clean cloth soaked in cold water.

If the skin is broken, apply sterile, non-fluffy, dry gauze to prevent infection.

••• ORTHODOX

Doctors will dress severe burns, and prescribe painkillers and antihista-mines, along with antibiotics for infection.

 # *C*

CANCER

A general term given to the unrestrained growth of cells in an organ or tissues that interferes with the normal functioning of the body. The most common cancer sites are the lungs, breasts, intestines, skin, stomach, colon, prostate, and pancreas. Symptoms vary according to the type of cancer, though the following list shows common early signs and symptoms that warrant a checkup with your doctor:

rapid weight loss without an obvious cause
a sore that fails to heal within three weeks
a mole that itches, bleeds, or grows
severe headaches
difficulty swallowing
continual hoarseness
persistent abdominal pain
change in size or shape of testicles
change or lump in breast
discharge or bleeding from the nipple
vaginal bleeding or spotting between periods
repeatedly coughing up blood

PREVENTION

There is no single cause for cancer; however, the following guidelines have been identified as precautionary practices:

Avoid cigarette smoke.
Avoid exposing the skin to strong sunlight.
As many as 70 percent of cancers are thought to be diet-related: Eat a diet rich in fiber (fresh fruits and vegetables, especially broccoli, Brussels sprouts, and cauliflower; whole-grain cereals, dried cooked beans and peas); limit your intake of fat, meat, sugar, and alcohol; eat foods rich in beta-carotene (green leafy and orange vegetables), vitamin C (fresh fruits and vegetables), selenium (seafood, brewer's yeast, whole-grain cereals), and vitamin E (seeds, nuts, and wheat germ).
Avoid food additives.
Avoid nitrates, found in processed meats (bacon, sausage).
Avoid contaminated or moldy foods, particularly peanuts.
Avoid being overweight, as fat appears to promote cancer.
Exercise regularly and avoid excessive stress (see **Stress**).

Get regular examinations or screening for breast, cervical, intestinal, and prostate cancer. Early detection allows a greater chance of effective treatment.

TREATMENT
••• ORTHODOX

The common orthodox treatments are surgery, radiation (X-rays or internal implants), and chemotherapy (drugs that kill cancer cells). They can be very effective for some types of cancer, and less so for others. All have significant side effects, and it is advisable to seek out as much information as possible about what you can realistically expect from the treatment, regarding side effects, recurrences, and survival rates. Before you make a decision about treatment, get a second or third medical opinion. You may also find it helpful to talk to other people with cancer, or join a support group.

OTHER THERAPIES

Cancer therapy now includes a number of complementary treatments used in conjunction with orthodox medicine. The principal objective of these methods is to prepare the body and the mind to fight the disease and live in a positive way. The following approaches give some idea of the treatments you are likely to encounter.

✕ DIETARY

Dietary treatment is based on the assumption that the cancer patient is physically exhausted, and aims at restoring energy. The basic premise is to enjoy all foods and drink (including alcohol, if you like) in moderation, while increasing your intake of foods that provide the highest nutritional value.

Eat as much fresh food as possible, particularly organic produce.
Avoid processed foods.
Reduce animal fat (dairy products, meat).
Eat plenty of whole-grain cereals and fresh fruits and vegetables.

▢ HOMEOPATHY

Trials are currently being carried out in European hospitals using homeopathy to treat some types of cancer. Consult the national homeopathic organizations for further information.

☛ MASSAGE

Regular massage promotes relaxation and eases pain. It helps release pent-up emotions, and provides therapeutic physical contact, which people with cancer are often lacking. Look for an experienced massage therapist with whom you feel comfortable and who you can trust.

∼ RELAXATION TECHNIQUES

Meditation, yoga, breathing exercises, and visualization can all help relieve the discomfort, anxiety, stress, and depression associated with cancer. Achieving a relaxed state helps relieve pain and is thought to aid the healing process. See suggestions under **Stress.**

❖ REFLEXOLOGY

Reflexology can help relieve pain and promote relaxation. It is not as intimate as massage, yet can provide similar effects.

○ TALKING THERAPY

Counseling, group therapy, and psychotherapy are used to help release tension, aid relaxation, and ease anxiety. All help prepare the body to fight the disease and improve quality of life.

Research has shown that cancer patients who attend support groups have a higher incidence of survival than those who do not.

CARPAL TUNNEL SYNDROME

Pressure on the nerve where it passes from the wrist into the hand via the carpal tunnel, causing numbness, tingling, and pain in the thumb, index, and middle fingers, and pain when writing, typing, gripping, or other activities that involve repetitive use of the wrists and hands. Symptoms usually get worse at night and may affect one or both hands. This syndrome is commonly caused by repetitive movements, for example, data entry, working out with weights, or chopping vegetables. It can also appear for no obvious reason, typically in middle-aged women, or in women who are pregnant or taking oral contraceptives.

TREATMENT

▬ PRACTICAL ADVICE

Rest the hands as much as possible.

Take regular breaks from repetitive hand work. If you are working at a keyboard or machine, try to stop and do the exercises listed below every 30 minutes.

✗ DIETARY

Vitamin B6 deficiency has been linked to carpal tunnel syndrome. Studies show that taking a daily supplement of 100 milligrams of vitamin B6, along with a vitamin B-complex supplement, helps relieve symptoms after a period of 6 to 12 weeks.

Excessive protein intake, oral contraceptives, and some food additives and drugs inhibit the body's uptake of vitamin B6. Reduce your intake of protein to 50 grams daily, avoid yellow dyes in foods, and try to find an alternative means of contraception.

▢ HOMEOPATHY

Take 3 times a day for up to 2 weeks:
Symptoms relieved by heat and rubbing: *Magnesia phosphorica* 6c
Tendons feel contracted, loss of grip and sensation: *Causticum* 6c

≈ HYDROTHERAPY

Make an ice pack by wrapping a plastic bag full of ice cubes or a bag of frozen peas in a kitchen towel. Place it on the wrist for 10 minutes, then take it off for 10 minutes; repeat 4 times. Perform this procedure morning and night.

✳ ACUPRESSURE

Place your left thumb in the center of the back of the right wrist, two-and-a-half finger-widths from the crease joining the wrist to the hand. Put your fingers around the other side of the wrist. Apply firm pressure to the points shown for 1 minute; repeat on the other wrist.

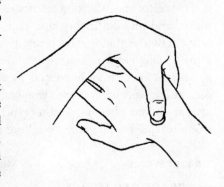

Place your left thumb on the center of the back of the right wrist, at the point where the hand joins the wrist. The fingers of the left hand should be directly behind the thumb, on the inside of the wrist. Apply firm pressure for 1 minute; repeat on the other wrist.

✛ EXERCISE

Do the following exercises at least 4 times a day to relieve numbness and tingling:
Clench your fists, then spread your fingers out; repeat 20 times.
Circle the hands, rotating from the wrist, for about 2 minutes.

Do the above exercise with your hands above your head to relieve tension in the arms and neck.

✚ PROFESSIONAL HELP

Chiropractic, massage, and acupuncture are effective treatments for this condition.

••• ORTHODOX

Doctors may give a corticosteroid injection to relieve pain.

Diuretics (drugs to expel water from the system) are sometimes used if fluid retention is the cause.

Surgery may be recommended in severe cases to sever the thick, fibrous band that presses on the nerve in the carpal tunnel.

CATARACT

The gradual loss of transparency of the lens of the eye, resulting in cloudy or distorted vision. Cataracts are most common in the elderly, though they can also occur in newborn babies as a result of infection.

TREATMENT

✗ DIETARY

Naturopaths believe that cataracts result from free radical damage to the proteins in the lens. They recommend a high intake of antioxidants to combat free radicals (cigarette smoke, air pollution, and rancid fats):

Increase your intake of vitamin C, found in fresh fruits and vegetables, particularly citrus fruits (oranges, grapefruit, lemons), Brussels sprouts, strawberries, and broccoli. Studies have shown that taking a supplement of 1 gram of vitamin C daily brings a reduction in cataract development.

Increase your intake of selenium, found in whole-grain cereals, brown rice, and oatmeal.

Increase your intake of vitamin E, found in vegetable oils, wheat germ, and nuts.

Increase your intake of beta-carotene, found in yellow, orange, and green leafy vegetables.

Avoid free radicals: cigarette smoke, air pollution, and rancid fats.

☐ HOMEOPATHY

Dilute 1 part *Cineraria maritima* mother tincture in 50 parts spring water. Bathe your eyes in this solution 2 times a day, for 3 weeks.

☯ CHINESE MEDICINE

Hachimijiogan, a combination of different herbs, has been shown to be effective in both preventing and treating cataracts, and is a common remedy used to treat this condition in China and Japan. Professional rather than self-treatment is advised.

••• ORTHODOX

Once a cataract has developed, there is no way to reverse it. Ophthalmic surgeons will surgically remove the lens and replace it with an artificial one. The results of surgery are usually good.

CELIAC DISEASE

A disease most often found in small children, where the small intestine is unable to digest and absorb food as a result of sensitivity to gluten, a protein found in wheat, rye, and other grains. Symptoms include diarrhea, failure to gain weight, bloated stomach, and fatigue. In adults it can bring symptoms of depression, mood swings, fatigue, infertility, constipation, and skin eruptions.

PREVENTION

Some doctors and complementary practitioners believe that celiac disease may be related to early weaning of infants to cereals. They recommend breast-feeding at least to the age of four months, and then limiting cereal intake to baby rice and millet. Avoid wheat products for at least the first year.

Allergy to milk and other foods may also be related to this disorder (for more information on diagnosis and treatment, see **Allergies, Food**).

TREATMENT

Avoid all foods containing gluten. This means you should exclude all grains except brown rice, millet, and corn. Use corn tortillas for sandwiches and rice cakes for crackers. Most commercially prepared foods contain gluten, so avoid prepared foods.

Eat plenty of rice, low-fat meats, fish, dairy products, vegetables, fruits, and corn.

Take a multivitamin and mineral supplement daily.

₰ HERBALISM

The protein-digesting enzyme from papaya, called papain, has been shown to digest wheat gluten and make it harmless to celiac patients. Papain supplements are available in natural foods stores.

Celiac disease can cause inflamed and irritable intestines. Slippery elm can help soothe the mucous membranes of the stomach: Take ¼ teaspoon of the ground powder dissolved in 1 cup of warm water, 4 times a day.

✚ PROFESSIONAL HELP

Applied kinesiology, a method of muscle testing, may be used to find out whether gluten is causing the problem.

••• ORTHODOX

To make sure that gluten is the culprit, doctors remove a sample of the cells of the small intestine and examine it microscopically. A life-long gluten-free diet is the recommended treatment.

CELLULITE

Puckered areas of fatty flesh, often referred to as "orange peel skin." Cellulite generally occurs around the tops of the thighs, hips, buttocks, and upper arms, and is more common in women than men. Nobody really knows what causes cellulite, yet many theories abound on how it can be treated.

TREATMENT
✗ DIETARY

Cellulite is thought by some to be caused by a buildup of toxins in the body, resulting from eating the wrong food, living in a polluted environment, and suffering from poor elimination. The following dietary recommendations may help:

Do not smoke.

Avoid caffeine (coffee, tea, chocolate, cola) and alcohol.

Drink plenty of mineral water and diluted fruit juices.

Some naturopaths advise a detoxification program that consists of eating only raw food for several weeks.

Constipation may contribute to cellulite (see **Constipation**).

❀ AROMATHERAPY

Use 4 drops each of juniper berry and rosemary, and 3 drops each of cypress and patchouli, in 2 tablespoons of a carrier oil or lotion. Massage into the cellulite twice daily in a circular motion.

🐌 HERBALISM

Fresh parsley is a rich source of vitamin C, a good detoxicant, and a diuretic (it helps the body eliminate water). Eat plenty of the herb, raw, in salads.

≈ HYDROTHERAPY

In France, a popular treatment for cellulite is to direct powerful jets of alternating hot and cold water on the body. You can do the same with a strong shower hose. Direct the water against the problem area for 5 to 10 minutes each day, finishing up with a cold spray.

☛ MASSAGE

Deep massage stimulates the circulation and the elimination of waste products and excess water thought to cause cellulite. Regular massage from a professional therapist may help eliminate cellulite.

Perform self-massage carefully, and make sure to use oil or talc. Begin with light, upward strokes, increasing the pressure gradually. Daily massage with a massage glove or brush in the shower or bath is also helpful.

⚜ EXERCISE

Cellulite seems to afflict those who lead a sedentary life. Adopt a regular exercise program that incorporates at least 30 minutes of aerobic exercise (such as walking, bicycling, or swimming), 3 times a week, to help with this problem. Always consult your doctor before beginning any exercise program.

••• ORTHODOX

Doctors recommend moderate weight reduction (see **Obesity** for suggestions), regular exercise, and a healthy diet.

Liposuction, a cosmetic surgery technique, introduces a long, thin, hollow tube into the fatty area and sucks out the excess fatty tissue. The technique holds some risks and provides only temporary relief.

CERVICAL EROSION

A reddish sore on the cervix or neck of the uterus, beside the cervical opening, which results from hormonal changes during or after pregnancy or while taking oral contraceptives; a common ailment in women of childbearing age. It can also be caused by using an IUD, or from the friction of intercourse. Symptoms include white discharge with an unpleasant odor, and sometimes a bloody discharge. A cervical smear test (Pap smear) will confirm the diagnosis.

TREATMENT

ᨠ HERBALISM

Golden seal infusion used as a douche: Add 1 cup of boiling water to 1 teaspoon of the herb, infuse for 15 minutes, strain, and allow to cool; use in a sterile douche every day for 3 or 4 weeks. (Golden seal stains, so be careful of clothing.)

≈ HYDROTHERAPY

Hot and cold sitz baths can stimulate blood circulation to the cervix and encourage healing. Using a bathtub and a tub or large bowl of water, fill one with hot water (105° F to 115° F) and one with cold tap water. Spend 30 seconds in the hot water, then 3 seconds in the cold water; repeat 3 times, finishing with the cold. Make sure to dress warmly afterward. Take sitz baths every other day.

••• ORTHODOX

Doctors generally treat severe cases with heat or freezing treatments to cauterize the area of erosion.

CHAPPED SKIN
See **Skin, Chapped.**

CHICKEN POX
A very infectious disease spread by the shingles or chicken pox virus. Symptoms include fever, rash (blisters that turn into scabs), and fatigue. The disease is common in children, and it can be serious in adults, particularly the elderly.

TREATMENT

✗ DIETARY

You may not feel like eating solid foods, but do make sure you get plenty of fluids, particularly fruit and vegetable juices that are rich in vitamin C (orange, grapefruit, lemon). When you feel ready, move on to broths, soups, and solid steamed vegetables and fresh fruit, until your appetite is back to normal.

✿ AROMATHERAPY

Essential oil of peppermint soothes the rash: Add 1 drop of the oil to 1 quart of water; apply regularly to blisters.

▢ HOMEOPATHY

If you or your child has been in contact with chicken pox or shingles: *Rhus toxicodendron* 6c, 2 times a day for 10 days, as a preventive measure.

Remedies for children during the illness, to be taken 4 times a day for up to 5 days:

- Peevish child who resents being held: *Antimonium tartaricum* 6c
- Whining child who won't be left alone: *Pulsatilla* 6c
- Feverish, restless child: *Rhus toxicodendron* 6c

☯ CHINESE MEDICINE

Practitioners of traditional Chinese medicine recommend teas made from safflower, honeysuckle flower, or cimicifuga tube.

✿ BACH FLOWER REMEDIES

To relieve the rash, try Chicory, Hornbeam, or Cherry Plum.

≈ HYDROTHERAPY

Apply cool, wet towels to soothe the rash.

Soak in a lukewarm bath to which you have added a handful of uncooked oatmeal or baking soda. This is particularly helpful to relieve discomfort before sleeping.

••• ORTHODOX

Doctors prescribe calamine lotion to relieve the discomfort of the rash; dab it on whenever needed.

Acetaminophen is sometimes given to reduce fever. (Aspirin is not recommended as it can cause Reye's syndrome.)

CHILBLAINS

Painful, itchy swellings that generally occur on the hands, feet, or ears in response to cold weather. They are generally a result of poor circulation, which can be aggravated by smoking.

TREATMENT

❃ AROMATHERAPY

Essential oil of black pepper or rosemary stimulates blood circulation. Massage the feet with 2 to 4 drops of either oil in 2 teaspoons of a carrier oil or lotion. You can also dab a few drops of the oil on the chilblain.

⅔ HERBALISM

If the skin is not cut or cracked, dust cayenne powder on the chilblains to stimulate blood circulation.

If the skin is broken, rub in *Calendula* ointment to promote healing.

☐ HOMEOPATHY

For red, swollen chilblains that burn and itch, take *Agaricus* 6c, every 30 minutes, for up to 6 doses.

☯ CHINESE MEDICINE

Bad circulation is seen as a deficiency in yang *qi*. Recommended herbs include cinnamon twigs, red sage, dried ginger, and angelica.

≈ HYDROTHERAPY

For chilblains on the feet, stimulate circulation with hot and cold treatments. Plunge the feet first into a bowl of hot water for 30 seconds, then into cold water for 30 seconds; repeat the series for 15 minutes.

☛ MASSAGE

Regular massage helps improve circulation and prevent chilblains.

★ FOLK REMEDIES

Add 1 tablespoon of honey to 1 tablespoon of glycerine, and mix with an egg white and a little flour to make a paste. Spread this over the chilblains and leave on for 24 hours.

••• ORTHODOX

Doctors advise wearing several thin layers of clothing to trap heat and protect from the cold.

Creams containing menthol and camphor can sometimes be useful.

CHLAMYDIA

One of the most common sexually transmitted diseases. In men it produces burning on urination, discharge from the penis, and swelling of the testicles, which may lead to infertility. Women may experience early symptoms of vaginal discharge, soreness, or bleeding after intercourse, and stinging or burning when urinating. Left untreated, chlamydia can lead to pelvic inflammatory disease (see **Pelvic Inflammatory Disease**) and infertility. It has also been linked to miscarriage, ectopic pregnancy, premature birth, and eye infections in newborn babies.

PREVENTION

Use a condom to help prevent transmission of the bacteria from one partner to another.

Women whose partners have symptoms should be tested—chlamydia can be symptomless in women.

Women who are planning a pregnancy should be tested for chlamydia.

TREATMENT

••• ORTHODOX

Due to the risks of infertility or miscarriage brought by this condition, doctors generally recommend antibiotics. Metronidazole, chlorhexidine pessaries, tetracycline, or erythromycin (if you are pregnant) is usually prescribed. Use the suggestions below as an adjunct to orthodox treatment, to help strengthen the immune system and restore the body to good health after medication.

✗ DIETARY

Help your body fight this infection by strengthening your immunity. Eat a whole-foods diet with plenty of low-fat protein, fruits, and vegetables.

Supplementation with vitamin E (200 iu a day) and zinc (15 milligrams a day) has been shown to increase resistance to chlamydia.

To restore healthy intestinal flora after antibiotics, eat plenty of live yogurt with *Lactobacillus acidophilus*, or take ½ teaspoon *Lactobacillus acidophilus* powder, 1 teaspoon *Bifidobacteria* powder, and ½ teaspoon *Lactobacillus bulgaricus* (available from natural foods stores) in a glass of spring water, 3 times a day.

✚ PROFESSIONAL HELP

Homeopathy and Chinese medicine are helpful.

CHOLESTEROL, HIGH

Higher than normal levels of blood cholesterol (normal blood cholesterol is considered to be between 140 to 280 milligrams per deciliter). Excess cholesterol (which usually accumulates as a result of eating foods high in saturated fat) circulates in the blood, and can deposit in fatty layers in arteries, clogging them up (see **Atherosclerosis**) and contributing to the risk of heart disease (see **Coronary Heart Disease**).

PREVENTION/TREATMENT

✗ DIETARY

Reduce your intake of animal fats (meat, dairy products, and eggs). Avoid red meat; eat moderate amounts of poultry, nonfat milk, and low-fat cheeses and spreads.

Replace saturated fats with polyunsaturated ones.

Avoid whole-milk dairy products, ice cream, confectionery made with fat, snacks containing fat, and fried foods.

Increase your intake of whole-grain bread and cereals, fruits and vegetables, cooked dried beans and peas, fruit juices, and mineral water.

Use olive oil—a monounsaturated fat—for cooking. Avoid products containing coconut or palm oil.

Oat bran and rice bran have been shown to reduce cholesterol. The recommended daily intake is ½ cup per day cooked as cereal, or incorporated into your meals.

Eat moderate amounts of nuts and avocados. These contain monounsaturated fat, which is thought to help lower cholesterol.

Try to replace the meat content of your diet with fish, particularly salmon, tuna, trout, mackerel, and sardines. Fish oil has been shown to reduce cholesterol.

?● HERBALISM

Raw garlic has been shown to reduce harmful blood fats. Use it raw in salads and make garlic bread. Eating it with parsley helps eliminate the lingering odor. If you do not like the taste or smell of fresh garlic, you can take garlic capsules (3 capsules, 3 times a day).

✦ EXERCISE

Aerobic exercise helps lower cholesterol levels. Any activity that raises the pulse and respiration rate significantly for more than 20 minutes is most effective. Jogging, swimming, skipping, and brisk walking are all good.

∼ RELAXATION TECHNIQUES

Studies have shown that simple relaxation can lower cholesterol levels. Learning to meditate, or attending a yoga class, will help you achieve deep relaxation.

Find a quiet place where you won't be disturbed. Lie on a firm surface, close your eyes, allow your breathing to slow, and begin to be aware of how your body feels. Consciously try to relax every part of your body in turn. Begin with your face (your eyes, your forehead, your jaw), and work down to your toes. The whole procedure should take at least 10 minutes.

Relaxation tapes and biofeedback training can help teach you to relax if you find it difficult.

••• ORTHODOX

Doctors recommend a low-fat, high-fiber diet. In severe cases they will prescribe drugs to lower the cholesterol content of the blood.

CHRONIC FATIGUE SYNDROME

A condition characterized by extreme exhaustion, muscle aches and weakness, headaches, digestive problems, visual disturbances, mood swings, and difficulty concentrating and speaking; also known as post-viral fatigue syndrome, or myalgic encephalomyelitis (ME). Doctors are unclear what causes the illness, though it sometimes occurs after a major viral infection.

TREATMENT

✗ DIETARY

Eat regular meals of whole-grain cereals, plenty of fruits and vegetables, and high-quality protein, at least twice a day.

Avoid caffeine and alcohol.

Reduce your intake of sugar and junk food.

Keep a supply of high-energy snacks available for times when you cannot prepare meals (soup, fruit, nuts, cereals, and juices are good).

Some chronic fatigue syndrome sufferers are unable to digest milk (see **Lactose Intolerance**). Substituting other nondairy calcium-rich foods often helps clear up digestive problems associated with this illness.

Food allergy may be a factor in chronic fatigue syndrome (see **Allergies, Food**).

Some physicians and naturopaths believe that symptoms of diarrhea, bloating, and stomach pain in chronic fatigue syndrome result from chronic yeast infection (see **Fungal Infection**).

B-complex supplements may be helpful: Take 2 50-gram supplements a day.

❧ HERBALISM

Evening primrose oil is sometimes helpful, though you must take the supplement for at least 3 months to see the effects. The recommended dose is 2 to 3 grams a day.

◻ HOMEOPATHY

Professional homeopathic treatment has shown good results with chronic fatigue syndrome.

❖ EXERCISE

Some exercise can help, but the key is not to overdo it, as this may bring a relapse. A brief walk or a short swim in a warm pool may be possible, but be aware when your body is telling you it has had enough.

～ RELAXATION TECHNIQUES

Physical and mental rest is one of the most important factors in treating chronic fatigue syndrome.

Accept that your commitments, activities, and expectations will change as a result of your illness.

Organize your activities every day to allow sufficient rest in between.

Plan for a period of bed rest in the afternoon; listen to the radio or a tape if you do not want to sleep.

Rest in a quiet place; do not answer the phone or doorbell.

If you feel tired, rest; there is no point in continuing if you feel bad.

Relaxation tapes, biofeedback, or autogenic training may help you to relax. A gentle yoga class can also be useful. Many people who suffer from chronic fatigue syndrome also find that learning to meditate improves their physical and psychological condition.

••• ORTHODOX

Your doctor may prescribe antidepressants to treat depression, sleep disturbances, and pain. People with chronic fatigue syndrome often experience increased sensitivity to many drugs, so take medication with caution.

CIRRHOSIS

A liver disease caused by cell damage and the gradual buildup of scar tissue, which prevents the liver from functioning normally to remove toxins from the blood. Heavy alcohol consumption is the most common cause.

Symptoms include jaundice (yellowish tinge of the whites of the eyes and skin), fever, loss of body hair, swelling of the stomach and ankles, breast enlargement, drowsiness, and confusion. Cirrhosis is a life-threatening disease. All treatment should be carried out in collaboration with your doctor.

TREATMENT
✗ DIETARY

Avoid alcohol.

Reduce your intake of salt.

Increase your intake of fiber, found in whole-grain breads and cereals, fresh fruits and vegetables, cooked dried beans and peas, dried fruit, and oat bran.

Reduce your intake of fats. Eat only low-fat protein, such as poultry, fish, soy, nuts, and beans. Drink only skimmed milk or soy milk.

Increase your intake of vitamin A, found in liver, and in dark yellow, orange, and dark green vegetables.

Increase your intake of zinc, found in lean meat, poultry, fish, and whole-grain cereals.

Increase your intake of magnesium, found in nuts, cooked dried beans and peas, whole-grain breads and cereals, soybeans, and dark green leafy vegetables.

Increase your intake of selenium, found in brown rice, oatmeal, poultry, and lean meat.

The amino acid cystine helps protect the liver against the damage caused by alcohol: Take 1 gram cystine, 3 times a day, with vitamin C. **Caution**: Diabetics should not take cystine.

⌘ HERBALISM

Skilled professional treatment is advised. The following remedies have been shown to protect the liver against damage caused by alcohol:

Evening primrose oil: Take 3 500-milligram capsules, 3 times a day.

LIV25 is an herbal compound that protects the liver against alcohol. It should be prescribed by a qualified herbalist.

✿ BACH FLOWER REMEDIES

Some remedies may help where alcoholism is a problem (see listing in **Alcoholism**).

✚ PROFESSIONAL HELP

Acupuncture can help stimulate the healing of the liver.

Individual homeopathic treatment has been shown to be helpful.

••• ORTHODOX

The damage to the liver in alcoholic cirrhosis is irreversible, but progression of the disease may be halted by complete abstinence from alcohol. In other types of cirrhosis, orthodox medical treatment focuses on the cause of the symptoms.

COLDS

Viral infections that lead to inflammation of the membranes lining the nose and throat, resulting in a stuffy, runny nose, sore throat, and sometimes a headache. The virus is transmitted by breathing infected droplets from someone else's sneeze or cough, or touching an infected area.

PREVENTION

The weaker your immune system, the less able you are to resist the many strains of colds viruses. Complementary treatment usually aims at strengthening the immune system in an attempt to prevent colds.

Poor nutrition is one of the most frequent causes of a malfunctioning immune system. A low-fat, high-fiber diet, comprising plenty of whole-grain cereals, green, orange, and yellow vegetables, fruits, moderate amounts of fish or poultry, and low-fat dairy products, should provide sufficient vitamins and minerals to nourish the immune system. During and immediately after a cold, when immunity is low, add a multivitamin and mineral supplement, and a vitamin C supplement (500 milligrams, 2 times a day).

TREATMENT

✗ DIETARY

When you have a cold, drink plenty of mineral water and juice to replace lost fluids.

Eat extra citrus fruit (oranges, lemons, grapefruit), or take vitamin C supplements (500 milligrams, 3 times a day) to fight infection.

❀ AROMATHERAPY

Essential oil of tea tree and lemon are useful in combating infection: Use 1 drop of each in steam inhalations (add oil to a basin of steaming water, cover the head and basin with a towel, and inhale deeply).

If the chest is congested, steam inhalation with 1 to 2 drops of essential oil of eucalyptus or peppermint is beneficial. **Caution:** If you suffer from asthma, avoid steam inhalations; instead, put a few drops of the oil on a handkerchief or tissue and inhale.

ᶓᶔ HERBALISM

Ginger promotes perspiration and soothes the throat. Pour 1 cup of boiling water onto 1 teaspoon of the peeled and shredded fresh root, and infuse for 5 minutes; add honey if you like, and drink whenever needed.

▢ HOMEOPATHY

Take every 2 hours, for up to 4 doses:

Feeling tired, shivery, with aching limbs: *Gelsemium* 6c

Feeling irritable, nose runs during the day, but congested at night: *Nux vomica* 6c

Thick, greenish mucus, stabbing pains in ears and throat, irritable, chilly: *Hepar sulphuris* 6c

Frequent sneezing with burning nasal discharge, streaming eyes, better in open air: *Allium cepa* 6c

Hot and cold, offensive sweats, metallic taste: *Mercurius solubilis* 6c

••• ORTHODOX

Generally, doctors do not treat colds, which usually clear up without medication within a week or two, although some prescribe mild pain-killers, antihistamines, or decongestants. Antibiotics are useless against viruses and should only be prescribed if secondary bacterial infection has occurred.

COLD SORES

A blister or clump of blisters around the mouth, which erupt into a sore. They are caused by the herpes simplex virus (see **Herpes, Genital**), which lies dormant in the body and is activated by sudden exposure to hot or cold weather, exposure to direct sunlight, or viral infections. Low immunity and stress may trigger an eruption.

TREATMENT

▬ PRACTICAL ADVICE

Keep the sore clean and dry to prevent bacterial infection.

Your toothbrush may carry the virus. Once the blister has formed, change your toothbrush. Change it again once the attack has cleared up.

Use a potent sunblock lip salve to protect from the harmful effects of sunlight.

DIETARY

Studies have shown that the amino acid L-lysine may help reduce the frequency and severity of cold sores. L-lysine is found in kidney beans, split peas, corn, and wheat.

The herpes simplex virus thrives off arginine, found in nuts, chocolate, and seeds, so avoid these foods.

A diet that incorporates whole-grain cereals, low-fat dairy products, and meat, fish, and plenty of fruits and vegetables is essential to resist infection.

AROMATHERAPY

Apply geranium oil or eucalyptus oil externally to cold sores every hour to reduce pain and accelerate healing.

HOMEOPATHY

Take 1 tablet, 3 times a day, as soon as the blisters start to develop; continue dosage for up to 4 days:

Deep cracks in dry, burning lips, with several blisters, or when provoked by sea air: *Natrum muriaticum* 6c

When not provoked by sea air: *Rhus toxicodendron* 6c

••• ORTHODOX

Doctors frequently prescribe idoxuridine and acyclovir, two commonly used antiviral medications that can be applied to the affected areas as soon as symptoms begin. They will not cure the outbreak on the lips, but will reduce the duration and severity of the attack. Acyclovir may also be prescribed to be taken orally as a preventive treatment.

COLIC

A general term describing the ailment of a baby who cries or screams excessively, often drawing up his or her legs and passing gas. Colic is generally worse in the evening, and is not eased by the usual means of comforting—holding, feeding, or diaper changing. Colic usually appears in the third or fourth week of life, and clears up by the twelfth. It is thought to be due to intestinal spasm. If the baby is sick between bouts of colic, or has diarrhea, constipation, or a fever, consult your doctor.

TREATMENT

✗ DIETARY

If the baby is being breast-fed, it is possible that something the mother is eating is causing the colic. Cow's milk may be a culprit, so try cutting out dairy products. Make sure you get enough calcium by eating plenty of green leafy vegetables, chickpeas, canned fish, and cooked dried peas and beans. Other foods that may provoke colic in breast-fed babies include caffeine (coffee, tea, cola, chocolate), wheat, citrus fruit, strawberries, and spices.

Make sure your baby eats slowly by taking regular pauses while breastfeeding.

If colic continues after the baby is weaned, avoid bananas, yogurt, lettuce, and gassy foods, such as turnips, green peppers, and beans.

Some children have difficulty digesting cow's milk; try mixing formula with soy milk or goat's milk. See **Allergies, Food,** for other suggestions.

☐ HOMEOPATHY

Take, when required, by breast-feeding mother, or crush and put into formula:

Fractious and inconsolable, quieted by being carried around: *Chamomilla* 6c

Better in the open air and soothed by gentle rocking: *Pulsatilla* 6c

Colic improved by arching back: *Dioscorea* 6c

Gurgling sound as fluid goes down, clenches thumbs and toes: *Cuprum metallicum* 6c

☞ MASSAGE

Lay the child on his or her back. Using almond oil as a lubricant, gently massage the abdomen in a clockwise direction with two or three fingers. Gently massaging the back can also help.

∼ RELAXATION TECHNIQUES

Anxiety and tension in the mother can sometimes be the cause of a colicky baby. This is a stressful period, so it is important that you get support and help from family or friends. If possible, take time off from the baby to do something that helps relieve tension: a yoga class or regular exercise may help.

••• ORTHODOX

Doctors no longer prescribe medication for small babies with colic. They advise against overfeeding, and recommend rhythmic, soothing activities.

Colicky babies are sometimes calmed by "white noise"—continuous vibratory noises, such as the drone of a vacuum cleaner, a washing machine or dryer, or a fan.

Some doctors suggest swaddling—wrapping the baby up in a baby blanket so that movement of limbs is restricted, and carrying the baby around the house.

A warm water bottle, wrapped in a towel and placed on the baby's stomach, may also help.

COLITIS

Inflammation of the large intestine, causing diarrhea, abdominal pain, and sometimes mucus and blood in the stools. The cause of colitis is unknown, though its prevalence in industrialized nations suggests it may result from lack of fiber in the Western diet.

TREATMENT

✕ DIETARY

Food allergies may sometimes cause colitis. The most common food allergens are milk products, cereals (wheat, oats, barley, rye), and caffeine (coffee, tea, cola, chocolate). See **Allergies, Food,** for details on determining food allergies.

Adopt a high-fiber diet, provided by whole grains (or brown rice, if you are allergic to other grains), and plenty of fruits, vegetables, and lean protein.

❧ HERBALISM

Garlic supports the growth of natural bacterial flora in the intestines, while killing infection. Use copiously in cooking, and chop and spread it raw on bread. You can take garlic capsules (3 capsules, 3 times a day) if you do not like the taste or smell of fresh garlic.

Slippery elm helps soothe the irritated mucous membranes of the intestine: Add ¼ teaspoon to a glass of warm water; drink 4 times a day.

☐ HOMEOPATHY

Take every 30 minutes, for up to 4 doses:

Where there is a lot of blood and mucus in the feces and the feeling that the bowel is not completely emptied: *Mercurius corrosivus* 6c

Profuse diarrhea accompanied by burning and colicky stomach, restlessness, anxiety, and chilliness: *Arsenicum album* 6c

Greenish, painless diarrhea with gurgling and stomach cramps, worse early morning: *Podophyllum* 6c

✳ ACUPRESSURE

Using the thumb, apply deep pressure to the points illustrated for at least 1 minute, 3 or 4 times a week.

⁙ EXERCISE

The following exercises strengthen the muscles of the abdomen and help reduce distension. Try to do the exercises at least twice a day. Start gently, and gradually build up strength:

Lie on your back on the floor. Keeping your legs straight, slowly lift them 12 inches off the ground; then slowly lower and relax; repeat 5 to 10 times.

Lie on your back on the floor. Keeping your legs straight, lift them until they are vertical, then open the legs apart and bring them together; repeat 5 to 10 times.

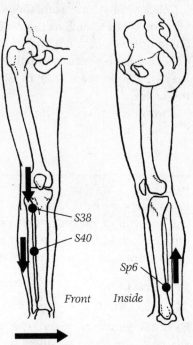

Front   Inside

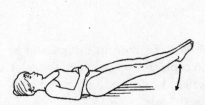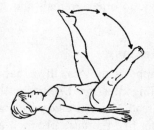

Direction of acupressure massage

Sit-ups also strengthen abdominal muscles. Don't anchor your feet, and sit only halfway up. An even better method is to do "curl-downs": Sit on the floor, bend your knees, and round your back down halfway to the ground, hold for a count or two, then curl back up again.

••• ORTHODOX

This disease can be confused with many others, so doctors make a diagnosis by examining the rectum and colon through a viewing tube (sigmoidoscopy). Treatment is with steroid drugs, and in severe cases, surgical removal of part of the intestine.

CONJUNCTIVITIS

An inflammation of the delicate lining covering the outer eye and eyelid, generally due to bacteria or a virus that gets rubbed into the eye; also known as pinkeye. Sometimes the condition can be triggered by allergies or environmental irritants, such as smoke or chlorine from a swimming pool. Symptoms include sticky yellow discharge from the eye, especially on waking, and red, itchy eyes.

TREATMENT

■ PRACTICAL ADVICE

Conjunctivitis is very infectious, so make sure that you do not share towels, bedding, or clothes. Wash your hands frequently.

To soothe red, itching eyes, lie down and place a cool, moist tea bag on each closed eye for about 10 minutes.

࣌ HERBALISM

Wash the eye with eyebright tea: Add 1 teaspoon of the herb to 1 cup of boiling water, allow to cool, and strain. With an eye cup, use the solution to rinse the eye.

☐ HOMEOPATHY

Take hourly, for up to 4 doses; repeat if needed:

- Gritty sensation in the eye, which is worse in a warm atmosphere and very bloodshot: *Argentum nitricum* 6c
- Burning sensation, swollen puffy lids, better for cool bathing: *Apis* 6c
- Itching eyes with thick yellow discharge: *Pulsatilla* 6c

Bathe the eyes several times a day in a solution of 10 drops of *Euphrasia* mother tincture and 1 teaspoon of salt to 1 cup of warm water.

☯ CHINESE MEDICINE

Chrysanthemum tea is very beneficial.

For children aged four and over: Take 1 sachet in water, 3 times a day.

For babies: Take 1 teaspoon of crystals in water, 3 times a day.

••• ORTHODOX

Wash the eyes gently with warm water.

If infection is the cause, doctors will prescribe antibiotic eye drops or ointment.

Allergic conjunctivitis is helped by antihistamine or allergy-arresting sodium cromoglycate drops (Opticrom).

CONSTIPATION

Irregular, infrequent, or difficult bowel movement, generally caused by not eating enough fiber, or by lack of sufficient fluid or exercise. Stress (see **Stress**) and irregular bowel habits can also play a role. Consult your doctor if you have a sudden and unusual change in bowel habits that lasts more than a few days and has no obvious explanation.

TREATMENT

■ PRACTICAL ADVICE

Never resist the urge to move your bowels. Make a regular habit of trying once a day, to get the body into the rhythm of regular elimination.

Avoid using over-the-counter laxatives. They weaken the muscles of the digestive tract and ultimately make the condition worse.

✗ DIETARY

Introduce more fiber into your diet (whole-grain bread, pasta, brown rice); sprinkle bran (not wheat bran) on desserts and breakfast cereal; eat oatmeal and unpeeled fresh fruits and vegetables.

Drink at least 6 glasses of water every day. A warm glass of water on waking sometimes helps stimulate bowel movement.

Constipation in children is often related to excess milk. Try reducing milk intake, replacing it with water, fresh fruits and juices, lots of green and root vegetables, and whole-grain foods.

✿ BACH FLOWER REMEDIES

Walnut, Holly, and Larch are all useful.

☛ MASSAGE

Do the following massage to help loosen the bowels: Oil your hands lightly and lie down on a comfortable surface. Place one hand over the other and, with the fingers flat, begin pressing about 1 inch into the abdomen at (1), as shown. Make small, slow circles. Move up a little, and repeat. Continue up the left side, across above the navel, and down the right side. Make large, slow, sweeping movements along the path just covered, going in the

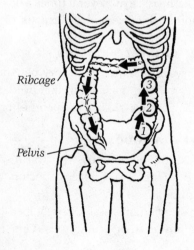

Ribcage

Pelvis

reverse order. Repeat the whole procedure several times, then try to move your bowels.

✳ ACUPRESSURE

With your right thumb and index finger, press firmly on the webbing between your left finger and thumb, as shown, for 1 minute. Switch sides and repeat.

Lie on your back and place the fingertips of both hands directly between your navel and your pubic bone. Press in 1 inch; maintain the pressure for 30 seconds, while breathing, then release.

Press firmly on the point Liver 2 on the top of the foot, as shown.

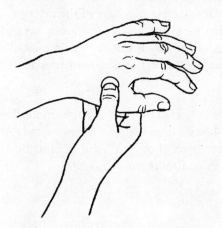

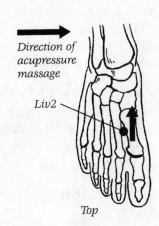

Direction of acupressure massage

Liv2

Top

✥ EXERCISE

Constipation is more common in those who are sedentary. Regular exercise, such as walking, jogging, bicycling, or swimming, helps improve bowel function.

✳ YOGA

Every morning, start the day with 2 glasses of lukewarm water, then do the Half Shoulder Stand: Lie on your back with your legs straight, and raise your legs as you inhale. Exhale, bringing your hips off the ground. Bend your knees if you want to, and place your hands under your hips to support yourself. While in this position, take 10 breaths quickly, in and

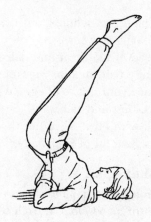

out, letting your abdomen move in and out rhythmically with the breathing. Bend your knees, and slowly lower your feet and hips to the ground.

••• ORTHODOX

Doctors recommend establishing a regular routine for moving your bowels. For some, a regular routine may be once a day, for others it may be once a week. Glycerin suppositories may be prescribed to help soften the bowel movements.

CORONARY HEART DISEASE

Malfunctioning of the heart due to narrowing or blockage of the arteries supplying the heart muscle. Heart disease brings chest pain during overexertion, stress, or anxiety (see **Angina**). It may result in a heart attack, where shortage of oxygen causes damage to part of the heart muscle.

PREVENTION/TREATMENT

Although coronary heart disease does not generally show symptoms until after middle age, its foundations are laid early in life. The following measures, implemented early in life, have been shown to help prevent this condition. They can also be useful in controlling the disease.

■ PRACTICAL ADVICE

Do not smoke.

✗ DIETARY

If you are overweight, try to lose weight, or at least avoid putting on more weight. Research shows that excess weight puts significant pressure on the heart and increases blood cholesterol levels. For suggestions, see **Obesity.**

Eat plenty of whole-grain cereals, fruits and vegetables, and cooked dried beans and peas.

Instead of red meat and dairy products, eat more poultry, fish (especially oily fish, such as mackerel and salmon), and vegetable proteins.

Reduce your intake of eggs; whole-milk dairy products; cakes, pastries and cookies; and salt.

Cook with olive oil rather than butter or lard.

Eat a handful of nuts daily.

🍃 HERBALISM

Research from Thailand shows that hot red peppers help prevent the formation of blood clots. Introduce chili or capsicum into your diet.

Onions and garlic also help reduce blood clotting. Use these herbs liberally in your meals. If you do not like the taste or smell of fresh garlic, you can take garlic capsules (3 capsules, 3 times a day).

Fresh ginger added to the diet helps reduce the stickiness of blood platelets and thus reduces clotting.

⚕ EXERCISE

Aerobic exercise (brisk walking, jogging, or an exercise class) for 20 to 30 minutes, 3 times a week, should be a minimum for everyone. It strengthens the heart, opens the arteries, and burns off excess cholesterol.

∼ RELAXATION TECHNIQUES

Stress relief is important in prevention and treatment:

Yoga and meditation help reduce stress and induce relaxation.

Massage and aromatherapy are effective methods of relaxing mentally and physically.

Biofeedback is a useful tool if you are unable to relax.

••• ORTHODOX

Drugs are prescribed to improve blood flow and reduce the work of the heart.

Surgery may be recommended to bypass a diseased artery.

Angioplasty passes a type of balloon through the narrowed part of the artery to stretch it and enlarge the volume, allowing for easier blood flow.

COUGH

A reflex that occurs to clear the chest airways of mucus, phlegm, or irritant. Coughing is often a symptom of a common cold (see **Colds**). It may also be a sign of whooping cough, asthma, or croup (see **Asthma; Croup; Whooping Cough**). Coughs that persist for more than a month may be bronchitis (see **Bronchitis**). Consult your doctor about any unusual cough, with or without phlegm, that persists for longer than 7 to 10 days.

TREATMENT

❀ AROMATHERAPY

Massage essential oil of eucalyptus and sandalwood or frankincense onto the chest and back.

If there is a lot of mucus: Massage essential oil of myrrh onto chest and back, and put a few drops on the pillow at night.

If there are breathing difficulties: Place a few drops of essential oil of frankincense on a tissue or handkerchief and inhale regularly.

☐ **HOMEOPATHY**

For early symptoms, 1 dose an hour for up to 5 doses; for persistent symptoms, 2 times a day for 4 days:

Cough with hoarseness, much rattling in the chest, difficulty breathing: *Antimonium tartaricum* 6c

Painful dry bouts of coughing, which are worse with slightest movement, patient thirsty: *Bryonia* 6c

Tickling in throat, paroxysmal bouts of coughing as soon as one lies down: *Drosera* 6c

Hollow, crowing cough like a saw going through wood: *Spongia* 6c

Machine-gun cough culminating in vomiting of mucus: *Corallium rubrum* 6c

Barking cough with fever after getting chilled: *Aconite* 6c

Tickling cough set off by the least draft of cold air: *Rumex crispus* 6c

✳ **ACUPRESSURE**

During a fit of coughing the muscles in the upper back can go into spasm. To relieve coughing, apply pressure to the point between the shoulder blade and the spine at the level of the heart, as shown.

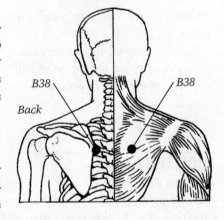

B38   B38

Back

••• **ORTHODOX**

Antihistamine cough remedies may be prescribed if the patient has trouble sleeping, since one of their side effects is drowsiness. Cough suppressants are not recommended because they prevent the body from expelling mucus or phlegm.

CRAMP

A painful muscle spasm that results from excessive contraction of the muscle fibers. Cramps usually occur during or after exercise due to a buildup of lactic acid in the muscles. They can also result from repetitive action (writer's cramp), or being in an awkward position. Night cramps may be caused by poor circulation. See also **Cramp, Calf; Cramps, Menstrual.**

PREVENTION

Do at least 15 minutes of warm-up stretches before exercising.

Start exercising slowly and gradually build up exertion.

TREATMENT

▬ PRACTICAL ADVICE

Moving and stretching the affected part relieves spasm.

✗ DIETARY

If you are susceptible to cramping, increase your intake of calcium. Good sources are milk, cheese, and yogurt, dark green leafy vegetables, broccoli, canned fish, and sesame products (tahini, halvah).

Increase your intake of vitamin D, essential for the absorption of calcium. The vitamin builds up in the skin on exposure to sunshine, and is found in vitamin-fortified milk, liver, egg yolk, and fish.

Vitamin E supplements (300 iu a day) have been shown to help night cramps.

☐ HOMEOPATHY

Cuprum metallicum 6c, sucked slowly when cramp occurs, helps relieve spasm and the ache that follows.

≈ HYDROTHERAPY

A hot shower increases circulation and brings relief.

☛ MASSAGE

Massage quickly relieves cramp by stimulating circulation in the veins and flushing out lactic acid. It also prevents the muscles from becoming stiff later. Gently knead the affected muscles, or ask a friend or partner to do it.

••• ORTHODOX

Doctors generally recommend massage; they may prescribe a calcium-containing drug or quinine for frequent night cramps. Consult your doctor if a cramp lasts for longer than an hour.

CRAMP, CALF

Spasmodic calf cramps may occur for a number of different reasons: wearing uncomfortable or high-heeled shoes, sudden strenuous exercise, or dietary deficiencies. More constant calf pain with redness and puffiness may be a sign of deep vein thrombosis (see **Thrombosis**), which needs immediate medical attention. See also **Cramp.**

TREATMENT

✗ DIETARY

Increasing your intake of calcium may help you avoid calf cramps. Good sources of calcium include milk, cheese, and yogurt; dark green leafy vegetables; broccoli; canned fish; cooked dried beans and peas; almond butter; and sesame products (tahini, halvah).

Vitamin D is essential for the absorption of calcium. It builds up in the skin on exposure to the sun, and is found in vitamin D–fortified milk, liver, egg yolk, cod liver oil, and fish.

Vitamin E supplements have been found to help night calf cramps. Increase your vitamin E intake by eating wheat germ, sunflower seeds, soybeans, olive oil, eggs, and parsley. Alternatively, you may choose to take a daily 300-iu vitamin E supplement.

☐ HOMEOPATHY

Cuprum metallicum 6c, sucked slowly when the cramp occurs, helps relieve the spasm and ache that follow.

☞ MASSAGE

Massage stimulates circulation in the veins of the legs: Sit on a flat surface and bend your knees. With the heels of both hands, massage the muscles of the back of the calves, starting in the middle and working outward. Then, with your thumbs, make small, circular movements to soften the muscles all over the backs of the calves. You can also do this in the bath, with soap lather on your hands.

✳ ACUPRESSURE

Acupressure can be useful in relieving the symptoms of cramps. Apply deep pressure to the points illustrated.

⠕ EXERCISE

Regular walking, bicycling, or swimming helps prevent cramps.

To stretch the calf muscles during a cramp, stand facing the wall, with your feet together, about 2 to 4 feet from the wall. Place your forearms flat on the wall and lean forward, keeping your heels down. You should feel a stretch in the back of the calves. Move the feet back to intensify the stretch.

✳ YOGA

The Sun Salutation exercise is useful for general stretching, particularly the legs (see **Stiffness** for instructions).

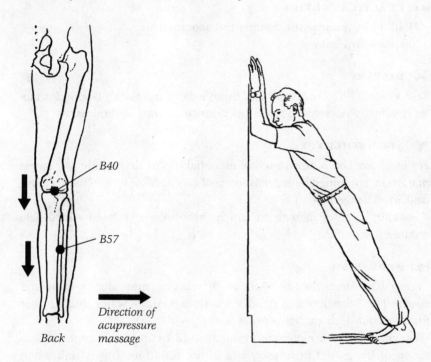

B40

B57

Direction of
acupressure
massage

Back

••• ORTHODOX

Doctors generally recommend massage; they may prescribe a calcium-containing drug or quinine for frequent night cramps.

CRAMPS, MENSTRUAL

Stomach cramps and discomfort associated with menstruation; also called period pain or dysmenorrhea. Menstrual cramps are categorized by doctors into two types: (1) Primary dysmenorrhea, which tends to occur in young women when they begin their periods, results from the contractions of the uterus; (2) secondary dysmenorrhea, more common later in life, brings stomach cramps a week or two before the period starts, along with other premenstrual symptoms (see **Premenstrual Syndrome**). Secondary dysmenorrhea may result from pelvic infections (see **Pelvic Inflammatory Disease**), endometriosis (see **Endometriosis**), fibroids (see **Fibroids**), polyps (see **Polyp**), or other gynecological abnormalities.

TREATMENT

■ PRACTICAL ADVICE

Hold a hot water bottle against the abdomen.
Take a warm bath.

✗ DIETARY

Take vitamin B6 (50 milligrams, 2 times a day), and a daily B-complex tablet (gradually decrease dose as occurrence of cramps diminishes).

❀ AROMATHERAPY

For massage: Use 3 drops each of essential oils of chamomile and sweet marjoram, combined with 2 teaspoons of carrier oil or lotion (use as lubricant in massage below).

Soaking in a warm bath to which these oils have been added also reduces discomfort.

❧ HERBALISM

Cramp bark decoction is effective in relaxing muscular tension and spasm: Put 2 teaspoons of the dried bark in 1 cup of water, and simmer for 15 minutes; drink hot 3 times a day.

Ginger infusion is a common remedy: Add 1 cup of hot water to 1 teaspoon of the grated fresh root, and infuse for 10 minutes; drink when needed.

☐ HOMEOPATHY

Take every 2 to 4 hours, as needed:

Cramping pain, better from hard pressure and bending double: *Colocynth* 6c

Waves of labor-like pains with a terrible temper: *Chamomilla* 6c

Heavy bearing-down pains with tiredness and irritability: *Sepia* 6c

Bright blood with dark clots, and pain stretching from sacrum to pubes: *Sabina* 6c

✳ BIOCHEMIC TISSUE SALTS

Dissolve 2 tablets *Mag Phos* 6x in 1 cup of warm water; sip frequently.

☞ MASSAGE

Massage of the lower abdomen, the sacrum, the lower back, and the legs relieves menstrual cramps: First, massage the uterus to help relieve spasm and encourage blood flow. Lie on the floor or a bed with your knees bent. Place your right palm on the lower right side of your abdomen (just above the pubic hair) and place your left hand on top of it. Press in with the fingers of both hands, and make small circular movements. Gradually, move your hands up the right of the abdomen to the waist, across under the ribs and back down, and across the lower abdomen above the pubic hair. Then have a partner massage your legs and back, using large, stroking, upward movements.

✳ ACUPRESSURE

Lie face down on a firm surface and ask a friend or family member to press with the flat of the thumb on either side of the spinal column, from the tailbone to the waist. Do not exert pressure directly on the spine, but on the muscles on either side.

Massage the other points illustrated, using deep pressure, for at least 1 minute.

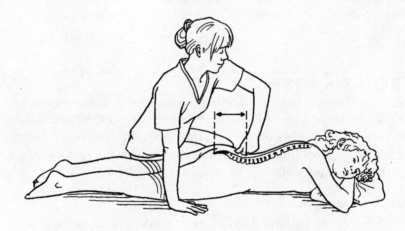

✳ YOGA

Menstrual cramps can be exacerbated by stress and unexpressed emotions. Regular yoga practice helps reduce stress and, in turn, pain. The following yoga exercise is suggested for cramps: Sit on the floor with your back straight, your knees bent, and the soles of your feet together so your knees fall outward. Clasp your feet in your hands, and gently bounce your knees up and down. Slowly lean forward, bending from the hips as far as you can comfortably go. Hold the position for several minutes and relax.

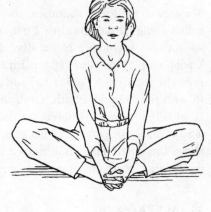

✚ PROFESSIONAL HELP

Chinese medicine: acupuncture and moxibustion are very helpful in treating this problem.

Menstrual cramps can often be relieved by chiropractic treatment of the pelvis, spine, and abdomen.

Homeopathy can help when cramps are a recurrent problem.

••• ORTHODOX

For primary dysmenorrhea, doctors advise aspirin to relax the muscles of the uterus, and drugs that inhibit uterine contractions. Oral contraceptives are sometimes recommended. Low-dose Danazol is also effective, although not without side effects, such as unwanted hair growth. Treatment of secondary dysmenorrhea depends on the underlying cause.

CROHN'S DISEASE

Recurrent attacks of inflammation of the gastrointestinal system, causing pain, fever, diarrhea, and weight loss. In between attacks the inflamed tissue heals, leaving scars, which can obstruct the intestine and reduce nutrient absorption. Inflammation may also occur in the eyes and joints, and the skin may be affected by eczema (see **Eczema**).

TREATMENT

Treatment should be carried out in consultation with a professional.

✗ DIETARY

Many find that Crohn's disease, like colitis, can be relieved by eliminating foods that produce an allergic reaction. The most common ones are dairy products and grains (wheat, oats, barley, rye, and corn). Try eliminating these foods for at least 2 weeks to see if symptoms improve. (See **Allergies, Food,** for further suggestions.)

Crohn's disease is often accompanied by deficiency in the following nutrients: vitamin A (found in liver, kidney, egg yolk, butter, whole-milk cheese, and cod liver oil); beta-carotene (found in dark green, orange, and yellow fruits and vegetables); and vitamin D (obtained through exposure of the skin to sunlight, and eating fortified milk, egg yolk, cod liver oil, and fish).

Take a vitamin B-complex supplement once daily.

✾ AROMATHERAPY

Essential oil of lavender has been shown to induce relaxation and relieve stress. Use it in steam inhalations, a diffuser, a bath, or sprinkled on a handkerchief. **Caution:** If you suffer from asthma, avoid steam inhalations.

Put a few drops of Roman or German chamomile in warm water, dip a towel in to make a compress, and place on the abdomen.

❍ STRESS RELIEF

Crohn's disease is made worse by stress.

Learning yoga or meditation can help you to counteract stress.

Hypnotherapy, autogenic training, and biofeedback can also help.

Regular massage and exercise are also beneficial.

••• ORTHODOX

Your doctor may prescribe the following drugs:

Sulphasalazine, a combination of anti-inflammatory agents, may be given to relieve the inflammation. It sometimes causes nausea, headaches, and abdominal pain.

Corticosteroid drugs are also used to reduce inflammation. Side effects may be swelling, high blood pressure, diabetes, or peptic ulcer.

CROSS-EYE

See **Strabismus.**

CROUP

Inflammation and narrowing of the air passages in children as a result of infection or obstruction. The symptoms are a barking cough, hoarseness, and stridor (a wheezing, grunting noise when the child inhales). See also **Cough.**

TREATMENT

■ PRACTICAL ADVICE

Provide as much humidity in the child's room as possible, by means of a humidifier or by placing bowls of water near radiators.

During a severe attack of coughing, take the child to a steamy bathroom: the humidity will help relieve the attack. Stay with the child and try to keep him or her calm.

ᨠ HERBALISM

Elecampane infusion is helpful in expelling phlegm and soothing the larynx and lungs: Pour 1 cup of cold water onto 1 teaspoon of the shredded root, and let it stand overnight; heat, and drink hot 3 times a day.

☐ HOMEOPATHY

Night coughing, if the child is breathless and panicked: Give 1 dose of *Aconite* 6c, and another 30 minutes later if the child is still awake.

For a very dry, barking cough that sounds like sawing wood: *Spongia* 6c, 1 dose, and another 30 minutes later.

••• ORTHODOX

Most cases of croup are mild and pass quickly. If the infection persists, your doctor will probably prescribe antibiotics. If the child is unable to breathe, or is turning blue, obtain medical help immediately.

CUTS AND SCRATCHES

Mild cuts and scratches heal quickly on their own, provided they are kept clean and the patient is healthy. Deep, penetrating cuts, particularly those contaminated by soil, may contain tetanus spores, so full immunization against tetanus is vital. The following treatments will soothe pain, ensure cleanliness, and speed healing of small wounds.

TREATMENT

■ PRACTICAL ADVICE

Wash the broken skin with warm soap and water and remove all debris.

To stop the bleeding, put a clean, absorbent cloth over the cut and apply pressure.

Elevate the wound if possible.

Once the bleeding has stopped, apply a bandage.

✿ AROMATHERAPY

Essential oil of tea tree is a powerful antiseptic, while geranium helps to heal. Add a few drops of each to the water when washing a wound.

☐ HOMEOPATHY

Calendula ointment prevents the formation of sepsis and helps to soothe scrapes and wounds.

Take *Ledum* 6c hourly for 6 doses if concerned about the risk of tetanus infection.

✿ BACH FLOWER REMEDIES

Rescue Remedy helps relieve the shock of an injury.

★ FOLK REMEDIES

Sugar accelerates healing and helps prevent scarring: Pack a cleaned cut or wound with granulated white sugar and cover with gauze. Rinse and repeat 4 times a day.

CYSTITIS

A condition commonly found in women that causes inflammation of the inner lining of the bladder, usually due to a bacterial infection. Antibiotics, oral contraceptives, stress, diet, and bruising during intercourse can also cause inflammation of the bladder. Symptoms of cystitis include a frequent or constant urge to pass urine with little success. Urination is accompanied by burning or stinging pain. Sometimes the urine has blood in it. There may also be fever, chilliness, and stomach pain.

TREATMENT: TO RELIEVE DISCOMFORT

✗ DIETARY

Drink at least 8 glasses of water a day to flush the infection out of the bladder.

Drink sugar-free cranberry juice 2 times a day, or eat the fresh-cooked fruit. Cranberries acidify the urine, and prevent the growth of bacteria.

Avoid tea, coffee, and alcohol.

Take vitamin C, 1 gram a day, until symptoms are relieved.

✿ HERBALISM

Yarrow infusion: pour 1 cup of boiling water onto 1 teaspoon of the dried herb, and leave to infuse for 15 minutes; drink warm at least 3 times a day.

☐ HOMEOPATHY

For recurrent cystitis, professional treatment will reduce the frequency and the severity of the episodes. For occasional cystitis, take every 30 minutes for up to 5 doses; repeat if necessary:

Urine feels like scalding water; violently painful: *Cantharis* 6c
Burning pain at the end of urination and afterward: *Sarsaparilla* 6c
Stinging pains better from cold bathing: *Apis* 6c
Violently painful with blood in the urine: *Mercurius corrosivus* 6c
Cystitis after sex, pain eased by urinating: *Staphysagria* 6c

≋ HYDROTHERAPY
❄ AROMATHERAPY

Take a warm bath, and add a few drops of essential oil of lavender, juniper, or sandalwood to the water for further relief.

Massage the abdomen and lower back with 5 drops of one of the above oils, diluted in 4 or 5 teaspoons carrier oil or lotion.

Rest with a warm water bottle over the abdomen.

PREVENTING RECURRENT ATTACKS

▬ PRACTICAL ADVICE

Do not try to hold your urine; use the toilet as soon as you feel the urge.

After passing water or bowel movements, always wipe from front to back, not the other way round, to avoid contamination.

Shower before intercourse (both partners).

Make sure you are sufficiently lubricated before intercourse; use KY jelly if necessary.

Empty the bladder as soon as possible after intercourse.

Avoid douches, vaginal deodorants, and powders.

••• ORTHODOX

Doctors generally prescribe antibiotics to alleviate the infection. They provide quick relief, but often promote a yeast infection (see **Thrush**) because they kill off healthy bacteria as well as harmful ones. If you take antibiotics, make sure you eat plenty of live, unsweetened yogurt that contains *Lactobacillus acidophilus,* to restore healthy bacteria to the digestive system. Alternatively, take ½ teaspoon of *Lactobacillus acidophilus,* with ½ teaspoon of *Bifidobacteria* powder, and ½ teaspoon of *Lactobacillus bulgaricus* (available from natural foods stores), in a glass of spring water, 3 times a day.

 **D**

DANDRUFF

A dry, flaky scalp, or itchy, waxy scales that stick to the hair and cause severe irritation. Dry dandruff usually indicates insufficient brushing (which usually removes the flakes), poor circulation of the scalp, or the use of alkaline products that irritate the scalp. Waxy dandruff may result from overactivity of the sebaceous, oil-producing glands, or from dietary deficiencies. It may also be a symptom of a fungal infection. Severe dandruff could be due to psoriasis (see **Psoriasis**).

TREATMENT

■ PRACTICAL ADVICE

Brush your hair well every day with a natural-bristle brush.
Avoid harsh dyes and scented hair products.

✗ DIETARY

Dandruff may result from food allergies (see **Allergies, Food**).

Increase your intake of vitamin A, found in liver, kidney, egg yolk, butter, whole milk and cream, and cod liver oil.

Take a vitamin B-complex supplement: 50 milligrams, 2 times a day.

Cut down on sugar.

Some naturopaths believe that excess consumption of citrus fruits and juices (orange, lemon, grapefruit) contributes to dandruff. Limit your intake of these fruits; instead, eat plenty of bananas, avocados, and raw and cooked vegetables.

Increase your intake of zinc, found in lean meat, poultry, fish, and organ meats.

Massage vitamin E oil directly into the scalp at night for 2 to 3 weeks.

Take a supplement of evening primrose oil: 500 milligrams, 6 times a day.

❧ AROMATHERAPY

For greasy dandruff, apply the following mixture to the scalp and leave on overnight: 4 drops of essential oil of cedarwood mixed with 2 drops of juniper or lemon, in 2 teaspoons of a carrier oil. Shampoo thoroughly in the morning and rinse. Repeat this procedure 3 times a week until symptoms are relieved.

૭& HERBALISM

Infuse 1 ounce each of fresh or dried rosemary and sage in 2 cups of water for 24 hours; use as a hair rinse daily.

☛ MASSAGE

Massage your scalp to improve circulation: With the tips of your fingers, rub firmly in circular movements all over the scalp, as if washing the hair. Try to move the loose skin of the scalp back and forth. Pick up clumps of hair and tug a little.

••• ORTHODOX

Your doctor will probably recommend a medicated shampoo, containing zinc pyrithione or selenium sulphide, for flaky dandruff. Shampoos containing coal tar or selenium sulphide are better for waxy dandruff. Allow the shampoo to soak into the scalp for at least 5 minutes before rinsing.

DEAFNESS

Hearing loss, complete or partial, can result from a number of different causes: ear blockage, disease, injury, degeneration of the hearing mechanism brought by loud noise or old age. In children, deafness may be caused by ear infections (see **Earache and Ear Infections**).

PREVENTION

One of the most common causes of hearing loss is exposure to loud noise. Always protect your ears with ear plugs when exposed to noisy machinery, loud music, or gunfire (soft foam ear plugs that mold themselves to the ear provide the best protection).

TREATMENT

▬ PRACTICAL ADVICE

If you are having hearing problems, have your doctor check for a buildup of excess ear wax: this causes temporary deafness but is easily treated (see **Tinnitus** for details).

◉ CHINESE MEDICINE

Acupuncture is often used in China to treat deafness, particularly when it occurs following an infection. Herbs that may be prescribed to clear the infection include peppermint, thorowax root, plantain seed, and chrysanthemum flowers. A kidney tonic may be prescribed for elderly patients.

••• ORTHODOX

Deafness caused by infection is treated by an operation to drain the middle ear.

Wax is successfully removed by flushing the ear canal with water.

Hearing aids are recommended for those with permanent deafness.

DEEP VEIN THROMBOSIS
See **Thrombosis, Deep Vein.**

DENTURE PROBLEMS
Problems can range from having a very sore mouth to experiencing difficulty talking, or even keeping the dentures in place. The following tips will help you to get used to the dentures, and ensure healthy gums.

■ PRACTICAL ADVICE

Break your dentures in gradually. Don't try to wear them all the time; rest your gums frequently.

Eat soft foods until your mouth is used to the dentures.

To get used to talking with dentures, practice reading out loud in private. It may take a little time to learn, but practice makes perfect.

Even with dentures, you still need to clean your mouth regularly. Use a very soft brush over the gums, followed by a mouthwash (see below).

You may want to use a dental adhesive (available over the counter in pharmacies) to hold the dentures in place while you are getting used to them.

❀ AROMATHERAPY

Essential oil of lavender helps soothe sore gums, while oil of tea tree is a good antiseptic: Add 2 drops of each to a glass of warm water; use as a mouth rinse, morning and night.

❧ HERBALISM

Red sage mouthwash is effective in soothing inflamed or bleeding gums: Pour 1 cup of boiling water onto 2 teaspoons of the leaves, and allow to infuse for 15 minutes; use as a mouth rinse, as required.

••• ORTHODOX

Consult your dentist if you are suffering long-term discomfort. Ill-fitting dentures, gum ulcers, and infection are common problems that can be remedied.

DEPRESSION

An emotional disorder characterized by pervasive feelings of sadness that affects people in different ways. Common symptoms include intense misery, negativity, and self-doubt; tearfulness, guilt, and bouts of crying; lethargy; difficulty sleeping; loss of appetite; loss of sex drive; constipation; headaches; and in extreme cases, suicidal thoughts.

TREATMENT

■ PRACTICAL ADVICE

Get help. Depression is a physiological and psychological illness that you cannot treat by yourself. One of the first steps is to seek out a trusted friend, relative, or health professional with whom you can share your feelings and get advice on how to cope. Many HMOs have counselors on staff, or your doctor will be able to recommend counseling services. Self-help groups may also be able to offer support or recommend professional help.

Try to avoid spending long periods alone, even though you may not feel like socializing. Seek out new activities and people with whom you can share your feelings.

✗ DIETARY

Depression can sometimes result from nutritional allergies (see **Allergies, Food**) or deficiencies.

Avoid junk food and sugar, and increase your intake of whole-grain cereals, fruits, vegetables, lean meats, low-fat dairy products, and fish. Take a multivitamin and mineral supplement daily.

The amino acid tryptophan has been found to relieve depression. Natural sources include turkey, chicken, fish, cooked dried beans and peas, brewer's yeast, peanut butter, nuts, and soybeans. Make sure you eat plenty of these foods, and eat them with a carbohydrate (potatoes, pasta, rice), which facilitates the brain's uptake of tryptophan. **Note:** Synthetic drugs containing tryptophan have been withdrawn from the market. Natural food sources such as those given above are, however, completely safe.

The amino acid D,L-phenylalanine (DLPA) has been shown to relieve depression. Take 100 to 500 milligrams a day. **Caution:** Do not take DLPA if you have high blood pressure.

AROMATHERAPY

Essential oil of clary sage is both a powerful relaxant and mentally uplifting. It eases mental fatigue and depression and helps bring good sleep.

Put 2 to 3 drops into a bowl of steaming water and inhale. If you are asthmatic or cannot inhale steam, inhale 4 to 6 drops from a tissue or handkerchief.

Add 5 to 6 drops to a bath.

Place 1 to 2 drops on the edge of your pillow.

BACH FLOWER REMEDIES

Use together or separately, as needed: Rescue Remedy, Sweet Chestnut, Mustard. (All the remedies may be of use, depending on the particular case, but these three are specifically for depression.)

EXERCISE

Exercise diverts the mind and alleviates mental stress. It also increases blood flow to the brain. Studies have shown that jogging for 30 minutes, 3 times a week, is as effective as psychotherapy in treating depression. Establish a routine of regular exercise, such as walking, jogging, swimming, or playing a sport. Start gradually, building up to a more energetic pace as you go on. If you can find someone to exercise with, it will encourage you and provide more pleasure. Always consult your doctor before beginning any exercise program.

••• ORTHODOX

Your doctor may suggest counseling or psychotherapy. In some cases drugs may also be prescribed, such as tricyclic antidepressants. These can be very effective, but they are not without side effects. Discuss the potential effects and the expected duration of antidepressant medication with your doctor.

DERMATITIS

See **Allergic Dermatitis; Eczema.**

DIABETES

A condition where the body produces very little or no insulin, the hormone needed to transform carbohydrates into energy, causing sugar to accumulate in the blood; also known as sugar diabetes or diabetes mellitus. Symptoms include the constant need to urinate, thirst, recurrent infections, fatigue, and weight loss. There are two types of diabetes: insulin dependent diabetes (IDD) usually begins in childhood and requires regular intake of insulin; noninsulin dependent diabetes (NDD) typically begins later in life. Consult your doctor before you begin any type of treatment.

TREATMENT

✗ DIETARY

Professional dietary treatment from a registered dietitian or a naturopath is recommended, and can be effective in treating diabetes. In mild cases of noninsulin dependent diabetes, the following dietary recommendations may help:

Make sure that 50 percent to 60 percent of your diet is high-fiber, whole-grain complex carbohydrates (whole-grain bread, rice, pasta, oatmeal, bran, and other unrefined cereals).

Replace red meats with fish and chicken. Eat soybean products as often as possible.

Eat plenty of beans, peas, and root vegetables.

Replace whole-milk products with nonfat milk products.

Cut out all foods containing sugar.

Avoid all sweet fruits and juices.

Eat plenty of vegetables (raw when possible), especially cucumbers, garlic, soybeans and tofu, avocados, Jerusalem artichokes, and Brussels sprouts.

Cut out alcohol and caffeine (coffee, tea, cola, chocolate).

Take 2 tablespoons of brewer's yeast daily. This contains chromium, which helps to normalize blood sugar metabolism.

Research studies show olive oil to be helpful. Incorporate it into your diet as much as possible.

❧ HERBALISM

Onion and garlic have been shown to lower blood sugar levels significantly. Eat as much cooked and raw garlic as possible. If you do not like the taste or smell of fresh garlic, you can take garlic capsules (3 capsules, 3 times a day).

Fenugreek seed is known to have antidiabetic effects; incorporate it liberally into your diet.

☯ CHINESE MEDICINE

Diabetes has been documented in Chinese literature in ancient medical texts. Practitioners of traditional Chinese medicine generally recommend lilyturf root, grassy privet, lotus seed, and Chinese yam. Insulin dependent diabetics may find help with professional treatment.

⚜ EXERCISE

Regular exercise is very important in treating diabetes. It reduces the need for insulin injections, prevents the accumulation of cholesterol, and limits weight gain. Aerobic exercise (swimming, brisk walking, jogging, or bicycling), 30 minutes a day, 3 times a week, is a good routine.

••• ORTHODOX

Regular injections of insulin are essential for insulin dependent diabetics. Your doctor will also make dietary recommendations.

DIAPER RASH

Redness and soreness of the skin around the diaper area. It often results when the baby's delicate skin is irritated by prolonged contact with damp urine and stools.

TREATMENT

▬ PRACTICAL ADVICE

Change the diaper as soon as it is dirty. Clean the skin gently and thoroughly, and allow the diaper area to air. Try to let the baby go without a diaper for a period of time each day. Cloth diapers may be gentler to the skin than disposable ones.

Use the minimum amount of detergent possible for washing diapers, and rinse well to avoid irritants.

✗ DIETARY

Acidic urine and strong-smelling stools are often signs of digestive disturbances that bring diaper rash.

Limit your intake of rich and spicy foods. If you are breast-feeding, avoid spicy foods, red meat, and alcohol.

If the baby is not breast-fed, give easily digestible foods and allow at least 2 hours between feedings.

If the weather is hot and the baby perspires more than normal, increase the baby's intake of water.

✿ AROMATHERAPY

To help disinfect diapers: Add 8 drops of essential oil of tea tree to the final rinse when washing diapers.

To alleviate the rash: Add 2 drops each of essential oil of sandalwood, peppermint, and lavender to 4 teaspoons of carrier lotion; apply to the diaper area.

❧ HERBALISM

Apply *Calendula* cream to the rash.

Make a strong infusion of chickweed: Add 1 cup of boiling water to 3 teaspoons of the dried herb, and infuse for 10 minutes. Add to the bathwater to relieve pain and itching; use to clean the baby during each diaper change.

☐ HOMEOPATHY

Give bottle-fed babies 1 dose, 4 times a day, for up to 5 days; breast-feeding mothers can take the remedy themselves:

Red, dry, and hot rash: *Sulphur* 6c

Accompanied by green-yellow diarrhea in angry and irritable babies: *Chamomilla* 6c

••• ORTHODOX

Most pediatricians recommend barrier creams and emollients, along with soothing antifungal agents.

In severe cases doctors may prescribe corticosteroid drugs or creams to suppress inflammation.

DIARRHEA

Urgent and watery bowel movements commonly caused by a food intolerance, a virus, or bacteria; it may also result from a change of diet or anxiety. Consult your doctor if diarrhea is accompanied by vomiting and lasts for more than 24 hours.

PREVENTION

When traveling in hot countries where refrigeration is lacking, avoid eating meat, dairy products (including ice cream), and raw fish. Peel all fruit and eat only cooked vegetables. Drink only bottled drinks or boiled water, and avoid ice cubes in drinks. Eat plenty of live yogurt before the trip to provide your digestive system with healthy bacteria (see Dietary, below).

TREATMENT

✗ DIETARY

Diarrhea is one of the most common symptoms of food allergy (see **Allergies, Food**).

During an attack, do not eat solids. To replace lost salt and water and to avoid dehydration (this is particularly important in infants and the elderly), add 1 teaspoon of salt and about 1 tablespoon of sugar to 1 quart of boiled water and 1 pint of orange or lemon juice. Drink 1 pint of the mixture every hour until symptoms subside.

Grated apple that has been left in the air to go brown is an effective folk remedy to settle the stomach.

Eat live yogurt that contains *Lactobacillus acidophilus,* both as a preventive measure and as an effective treatment for diarrhea. Alternatively, take ½ teaspoon of *Lactobacillus acidophilus* powder, with 1 teaspoon of *Bifidobacteria* powder, and ½ teaspoon of *Lactobacillus bulgaricus* (available from natural foods stores) in a glass of spring water, 3 times a day.

❧ HERBALISM

Golden seal infusion: Pour 1 cup of boiling water onto 2 teaspoons of the dried root, and infuse for 15 minutes; drink 3 times a day.

☐ HOMEOPATHY

Take every 30 minutes for up to 4 doses; repeat if necessary:

Profuse diarrhea accompanied by burning and colicky stomach, restlessness, anxiety, and chilliness: *Arsenicum album* 6c
Vomiting and diarrhea with profuse cold sweats: *Veratrum album* 6c
After rich foods, stomach feels like a stone, thirstless: *Pulsatilla* 6c
After stimulants (coffee, alcohol, spices) alternating with fruitless urging: *Nux vomica* 6c

☯ CHINESE MEDICINE

Practitioners of Chinese medicine generally recommend dandelion, golden thread, or skullcap root for acute diarrhea.

✳ ACUPRESSURE

Pressure on the points shown may be helpful in treating diarrhea.

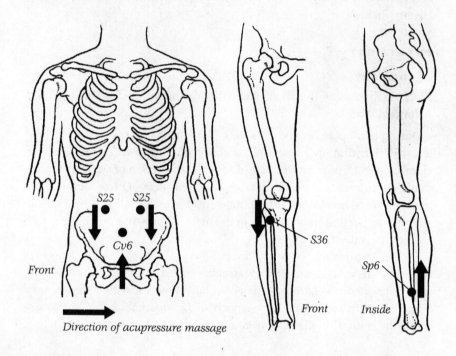

S25   S25

Cv6

Front

Direction of acupressure massage

S36

Front   *Inside*

Sp6

••• ORTHODOX

Diarrhea is nature's way of getting rid of bacteria or an infection, so anti-diarrhea drugs are no longer recommended, as they may prolong the problem. Consult your doctor if diarrhea recurs or persists for longer than a week, or is accompanied by blood in the stools. Always consult your doctor about diarrhea in infants, children, and the elderly.

DISC, SLIPPED OR PROLAPSED
See **Slipped Disc.**

DIVERTICULITIS
The inflammation of small finger-like bulges (see **Diverticulosis**) of the lining of the intestines, which causes pain in the lower left side of the abdomen, constipation, and sometimes fever.

PREVENTION

Constipation is often the underlying cause of diarrhea. See **Constipation** for prevention.

TREATMENT

✗ DIETARY

Initially, low-bulk foods may be required while the bowel is very inflamed and sensitive. However, it is important to incorporate more fiber into the diet gradually to help soften the stools and prevent constipation, which makes the condition worse. Gradually increase your intake of cooked vegetables, brown rice, and pasta, and later raw fruits and vegetables and other whole-grain cereals.

Drink at least 6 glasses of water a day.

Avoid foods with seeds that may lodge in the diverticula.

⅔ HERBALISM

Garlic helps combat infection. Incorporate fresh garlic liberally into your diet. If you do not like the taste or smell of fresh garlic, you can take garlic capsules (3 capsules, 3 times a day).

Decoction of slippery elm helps soothe the inflamed diverticula: Add 1 teaspoon of the powder to ½ cup of water, bring to a boil, and simmer for 15 minutes; drink 3 times a day.

☞ MASSAGE

Lubricate your hands with a light vegetable oil. Gently massage your lower abdomen with circular strokes in a clockwise direction for several minutes before rising in the morning. Follow this by drinking a glass of warm water or herbal tea.

••• ORTHODOX

Your doctor may prescribe antibiotics to remedy the infection, and anti-spasmodic drugs to reduce pain.

DIVERTICULOSIS

A condition in which small pouches, known as diverticula, develop in the bowel tube in areas where there is muscle weakness. Spasm occurs in the intestine around the diverticula, leading to bloating, pain in the lower abdomen, constipation or diarrhea, or both alternately. The pouches may get clogged up with debris and become infected, leading to diverticulitis (see **Diverticulitis**). This is one of the most common causes of stomach pain in anyone over the age of sixty.

TREATMENT

■ PRACTICAL ADVICE

Diverticulosis is often caused by irregular bowel movements and constipation. Try to establish a regular routine for moving your bowels, and don't delay or ignore the urge to go to the toilet when you need to (for suggestions, see **Constipation**).

✗ DIETARY

Avoid refined foods (white flour, rice, and other processed cereals).

Gradually increase your intake of fiber, found in whole-grain cereals, fruits and vegetables, and cooked dried beans and peas.

Drink at least 6 glasses of water daily.

Avoid eating seeds that may lodge in the diverticula.

ᛒ HERBALISM

Raw garlic helps combat infection. Eat 1 clove of garlic 3 times a day, chopped in food or made into garlic bread. If you do not like the taste or smell of fresh garlic, you can take garlic capsules (3 capsules, 3 times a day).

Decoction of slippery elm helps soothe the sensitive or inflamed mucous membrane of the digestive tract: Add 1 teaspoon of the powder to ½ cup of water, bring to a boil, and simmer for 15 minutes; drink 3 times a day.

☞ MASSAGE

Lubricate your hands with a light vegetable oil. Gently massage your lower abdomen with circular strokes in a clockwise direction for several minutes before rising in the morning. Follow this by drinking a glass of warm water or herbal tea.

••• ORTHODOX

Your doctor may want to perform a simple barium X-ray or sigmoidoscopy (the passing of a specialized telescope into the sigmoid colon) to make a diagnosis.

Most doctors prescribe antispasmodic drugs to ease stomach pain, and antibiotics for severe pain and fever caused by infection.

DIZZINESS

A sense of being unbalanced and spinning. It may be a mild, brief symptom, or a more prolonged attack of vertigo, which usually brings nausea, sweating, or fainting. Dizziness is commonly caused by:

a fall in blood pressure on rising too quickly from a lying or sitting position
fatigue (see **Fatigue**)
stress (see **Stress**)
anemia (see **Anemia**)
low blood sugar (see **Blood Sugar, Low**)
Ménière's disease (see **Ménière's Disease**)
brain hemorrhage or tumor
phobias (see **Phobia**)
side effects of drugs

TREATMENT

Report severe, prolonged, or recurrent dizziness to your doctor. The treatments listed below will help brief dizzy spells.

■ **PRACTICAL ADVICE**

Sit down, put your head between your knees, and breathe deeply.

✗ **DIETARY**

If you live in a hot climate, take vitamin B-complex supplements and extra salt to help prevent recurrent attacks.

◻ **HOMEOPATHY**

Take 2 doses 10 minutes apart; repeat if necessary:
Worse on rising from a seat, better for keeping absolutely still: *Bryonia* 6c
Made worse by loud noise: *Theridion* 6c
Feeling trembly and dizzy, head feels heavy: *Gelsemium* 6c
Room seems to turn in a circle, sees stars before the eyes: *Cyclamen* 6c

◉ **CHINESE MEDICINE**

Treatment will depend on the cause; mulberry fruit, Chinese angelica, wolfberry, and dasdrodia tube are common herbal remedies.

✳ **ACUPRESSURE**

Pinch hard between your eyebrows with the index finger and thumb.

✚ **PROFESSIONAL HELP**

Sometimes spinal misalignments can result in dizziness. It may be worth seeing a chiropractor to check whether this is the cause. If so, treatment involving massage and adjustments to the spine may help.

••• **ORTHODOX**

Treatment is aimed at resolving the cause of dizziness. If the condition is caused by a disorder of the inner ear, your doctor may prescribe anti-emetic or antihistamine drugs.

DYSENTERY

A severe intestinal infection caused by bacteria or parasitic amoebae. Symptoms include diarrhea that can quickly lead to dehydration, fever, and abdominal pain.

TREATMENT

▬ **PRACTICAL ADVICE**

Always wash your hands after going to the toilet, and before touching another person or preparing food.

✗ **DIETARY**

Replacement of salts and fluid lost through diarrhea is essential to prevent dehydration (see **Diarrhea**). Add 1 teaspoon of salt and about 1 tablespoon of sugar to 1 quart of boiled water and 1 pint of orange or lemon juice. Drink 1 pint of the mixture every hour until symptoms subside.

When symptoms have subsided, introduce small quantities of wholegrain solids and vegetables.

Make sure you get enough potassium, found in potatoes, avocados, bananas, apricots, orange juice, and cooked dried beans and peas.

Take 1 25-milligram vitamin B-complex supplement a day.

☐ **HOMEOPATHY**

Take 1 dose every 10 minutes for up to 6 doses; repeat if necessary:
Burning in the rectum and anus with involuntary evacuations: *Aloe* 6c
Exhausting diarrhea with cold sweats and vomiting: *Veratrum album* 6c
Feverish and anxious with burning pain in stomach, better from warm covers: *Arsenicum album* 6c

Greenish, painless diarrhea with gurgling and stomach cramps, worse early morning: *Podophyllum* 6c

⟨⟩ HERBALISM

Decoction of slippery elm or marshmallow soothes an inflamed digestive system: Add 1 teaspoon of chopped marshmallow root or slippery elm powder to 1 cup of water, and boil for 15 minutes; drink 3 times a day.

⟨⟩ CHINESE MEDICINE

Dysentery is considered to be caused by heat and damp poison in the intestine. Practitioners of Chinese medicine generally recommend treatment with anemone, white peony root, and golden thread.

••• ORTHODOX

Doctors will generally prescribe antibiotics if bacteria is the cause.

Amebic dysentery is eradicated by a course of the amoebicide metronidazole or a derivative.

DYSMENORRHEA
See **Cramps, Menstrual.**

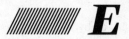 **E**

EARACHE AND EAR INFECTIONS

Pain in the ear that can be caused by a number of mechanical and pressure-related problems, by a bacterial or viral infection resulting from a cold or sore throat, or by a buildup of ear wax. Earaches often start at night, and can be accompanied by fever. They can lead to severe infection and permanent ear damage and should always be investigated by a doctor. See also **Tinnitus.**

PREVENTION

Research has shown that children who are breast-fed experience fewer ear infections than children who are not.

TREATMENT

✕ DIETARY

Recurrent earaches can sometimes be resolved by eliminating dairy products from the diet. Use goat's milk or soy milk products in place of cow's milk.

🌿 HERBALISM

St. John's wort infusion helps reduce pain, inflammation, and fever: Pour 1 cup of boiling water onto 2 teaspoons of the dried herb, and infuse for 15 minutes; sip as required.

☐ HOMEOPATHY

Take every 15 minutes for up to 4 doses; repeat if necessary:

In the early stages of infection with sudden onset, feverish restlessness, and painful sensitivity to noise: *Aconite* 6c

Throbbing and stitching pains, external ear is red and hot, children become wild-eyed and delirious: *Belladonna* 6c

Inconsolable and furious from the pain, cannot be soothed, pain worse from cold air and drafts: *Chamomilla* 6c

✿ BACH FLOWER REMEDIES

If a child is panicked and frightened, try Rescue Remedy.

≈ HYDROTHERAPY

For immediate pain relief, hold a warm hot water bottle wrapped in a towel to the ear.

✳ ACUPRESSURE

For uninfected earaches caused by sensitivity to cold, or by a change in air or water pressure:

Press firmly with 3 fingers on the area directly in front of the ears for 3 minutes.

Place your middle fingers in the hollows behind the ear lobes; hold lightly for 2 minutes while breathing deeply.

Apply firm pressure to the point between the inside of the ankle bone and the Achilles tendon. Hold for 1 minute on each side.

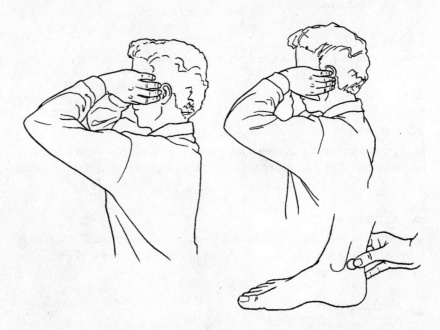

••• ORTHODOX

Inflammation or infection in the ear canal itself can be very painful, and your doctor will probably recommend cleaning and antibiotics. Eardrum tension or the presence of infected fluid behind the eardrum is generally relieved by painkillers and antibiotics.

EATING PROBLEMS IN CHILDREN

Problems with eating, including children who eat too much, too little, and the "wrong" foods, are usually experienced by the parents rather than by the children. Parents often tend to worry about the amount of food their children eat; they have fixed ideas about how much children should and should not eat, and about what is a "normal" weight and a "normal" growth rate. Eating problems usually begin at the age of about six months, when weaning from milk to solids takes place.

■ **PRACTICAL ADVICE**

Encourage children to experiment with new foods, but don't force them to eat certain things. Some toddlers tend to play slowly with their food, while others are happy to be spoonfed by the parents.

Never allow children to see that you are concerned over what and how much they eat. Once they see a crack in your defenses, they are likely to play on it for the sake of gaining attention. Any parent worried about true nutritional deficiency, food allergy, or failure to grow properly should consult a health professional.

Children generally know what kinds of foods are good for them, though they do not know what is bad for them. If children repeatedly refuse a food, it probably does not agree with them. Parents should exercise some restraint, however, with a child who constantly demands sweet and sugary foods and junk foods.

☐ **HOMEOPATHY**

Feeding problems respond well to individualized prescribing.

ECZEMA

Inflammation of the skin (often in creases: elbows, knees, and armpits) accompanied by itchiness, redness, and sometimes the formation of blisters, scales, or scabs. Eczema may result from a number of underlying factors: dietary problems, emotional stress, chemical irritants, or allergies (see **Allergic Dermatitis**).

PREVENTION

Avoid harsh detergents and soaps.

Eczema can sometimes be caused by metal in jewelry or bra straps.

Wear plastic or cotton gloves for all household and garden work if eczema affects your hands.

TREATMENT

✗ **DIETARY**

Increase your intake of vitamin A, found in liver, kidney, egg yolk, butter, whole milk and cream, and cod liver oil.

Take 1 25-milligram vitamin B-complex supplement a day.

Increase your intake of niacin, found in lean meat, fish, cooked dried beans and peas, and peanut butter.

Remove potential food allergens (dairy products, wheat, corn, soybeans, and all food and drink preservatives, colorants, and additives). Replace cow's milk with goat's milk or soy milk. See also **Allergies, Food**.

To relieve inflammation, vitamin C and bioflavonoids act as a natural antihistamine. Take them in supplement form; or eat the fruit, pulp, and rind of organic citrus fruits (shred the peel and simmer gently in a little water and sugar until soft).

¿♣ HERBALISM

Evening primrose oil has been shown to be successful in relieving the itching related to eczema: Take 4 to 6 500-milligram capsules, 2 times a day (children should take 2 to 4 500-milligram capsules, 2 times a day). This treatment may take 3 to 6 months to show any effects.

☐ HOMEOPATHY

Eczema requires professional treatment, although the following remedies may be helpful to alleviate symptoms temporarily. Take once a day for up to 7 days:

With burning, red, hot, and itching skin: *Sulphur* 6c

Skin cracked, with thick, yellow, oozing discharge: *Graphites* 6c

Deep cracks in skin with a watery discharge: *Petroleum* 6c

☯ CHINESE MEDICINE

Medical trials carried out at Great Ormond Street Hospital, London, have shown Chinese herbs to be very beneficial in treating eczema. Chinese doctors recommend individual prescribing, as eczema can result from a number of different causes. Some of the herbs used are oriental wormwood, Chinese gentian, peony root, and rumania.

✻ ACUPRESSURE

Massage the illustrated points several times a week, using deep pressure.

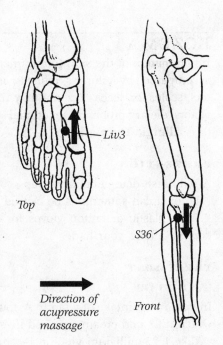

Top

Liv3

S36

Front

Direction of acupressure massage

∼ RELAXATION TECHNIQUES

Eczema can sometimes be made worse by stress.

Exercise daily (walking, swimming, jogging).

Set aside time each day for relaxation (see **Stress**).

Take a daily bath to which you have added 2 drops of essential oil of lavender.

••• ORTHODOX

Doctors commonly recommend short-term therapy with steroid creams. However, the condition often returns, and constant use of these creams can lead to thinning of the skin.

EDEMA
See **Ankles, Swollen.**

EJACULATION PROBLEMS

Conditions in which ejaculation either occurs too soon (premature ejaculation), does not occur at all (inhibited ejaculation), or the ejaculate is forced backward into the bladder (retrograde ejaculation).

PREVENTION AND TREATMENT: PREMATURE EJACULATION

Premature ejaculation is a common problem, particularly in young men in new relationships. It is often due to incomplete control of the ejaculatory impulse, anxiety, or being unaware of techniques that can delay orgasm and the need to prolong sex to fulfill a partner. Frequent premature ejaculation can lead to dissatisfaction for both partners, resulting in loss of sex drive.

▬ PRACTICAL ADVICE

The squeeze technique: This is a form of biofeedback that allows the development of control over what is normally an automatic function. Either partner gently squeezes the head of the penis between the thumb and finger when the man is about to ejaculate, until the urge to climax has passed. This can be done several times. Ejaculatory control will gradually become automatic.

Another method is for both partners to stop thrusting a moment before ejaculation. Again, if partners practice this technique routinely, the man will gradually achieve automatic control.

～ RELAXATION TECHNIQUES

Stress and anxiety can sometimes make ejaculatory control even more difficult. Try to relax during lovemaking and focus more on giving each other pleasure than on penetration.

✚ PROFESSIONAL HELP

Homeopathic remedies have been found to be helpful. An effective prescription necessitates an understanding of the individual's emotional and physical situation, so professional treatment is recommended.

PREVENTION AND TREATMENT: INHIBITED EJACULATION

Inhibited ejaculation is a rare condition in which erection is normal but ejaculation does not occur. It may result from taking medication, or it may be a symptom of an underlying disorder, such as diabetes, so discuss the problem with your doctor.

PREVENTION AND TREATMENT: RETROGRADE EJACULATION

In retrograde ejaculation the valve at the base of the bladder fails to close during ejaculation. It can result from a neurological disease or from surgery on the bladder, prostate, or pelvis. Avoid going to the toilet just before intercourse—having a full bladder can sometimes help resolve the problem.

EMPHYSEMA

Chronic difficulty breathing due to air sacs deep in the lungs that become damaged (usually due to smoking or air pollution) and enlarge and burst, reducing the area that absorbs oxygen. Symptoms include difficulty breathing, and consequently limited exertion and expansion of the chest, and chest infections.

TREATMENT

Consult your doctor before beginning any type of treatment.

❀ AROMATHERAPY

Massage the chest with 4 teaspoons of light vegetable oil mixed with 2 drops each of the following essential oils: Atlas cedarwood, peppermint, or eucalyptus.

☐ HOMEOPATHY

Take 2 times a day for 7 days; repeat if necessary:

Great rattling and suffocative wheezing but unable to produce phlegm: *Antimonium tartaricum* 6c

Worse on cloudy days, in warm rooms, and in the early morning: *Ammonium carbonicum* 6c

Worse in cold air and drafts and in the late evening: *Hepar sulphuris* 6c

◯ HYDROTHERAPY/AROMATHERAPY

Steam inhalations help the body to expel phlegm when the chest is congested. Fill a basin with boiling water, and add 3 drops of essential oil of eucalyptus. Keeping the eyes closed, put your head over the basin with a towel over you to trap the steam. Inhale deeply for 2 to 5 minutes. **Caution:** If you suffer from asthma, avoid steam inhalations; instead, put a few drops of the oil on a handkerchief or tissue and inhale.

❖ REFLEXOLOGY

The lung area is on the upper surface of both feet, just below the toes, stretching from the second to the fourth toe. Gently massaging this area facilitates breathing.

❖ EXERCISE

Studies have shown that daily bicycling (stationary or outdoors) can greatly relieve the symptoms of emphysema. Walking and swimming are also very good. Exercise should be gentle to begin with, building up exertion gradually. Try to breathe deeply while exercising. Ideally, people with emphysema should exercise in this way for 5 minutes, 3 times a day. Always consult your doctor before you begin any new exercise program.

✳ YOGA

Attending a yoga class will help teach you to breathe better. The following movements aid expansion of the chest. Do them as often as is comfortable:

Arm rotation: Place your fingertips on your shoulders. Inhale, and bring your elbows together in front of you. Lift them as high as possible, then bring them back to your sides in a circle while exhaling. See figure on next page.

Sit on a stool, or stand. Stretch out your arms in a breaststroke action, bringing the arms back behind you. Clasp your hands, stretch your arms down below your buttocks, and pull back your shoulders. Inhale, and lift your arms up, hands still clasped behind you, as far as possible. Exhale, lower the arms, and release your hands.

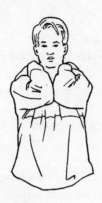 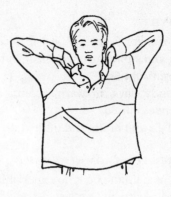

••• ORTHODOX

Regular courses of antibiotics are recommended for repeated chest infections.

Bronchodilator drugs may be given to open up the remaining healthy airways linking the windpipe to the lungs.

Corticosteroid drugs are sometimes given to reduce inflammation of the lungs and dispel phlegm.

Oxygen therapy is usually necessary in the later stages of the disease.

ENDOMETRIOSIS

A sometimes painful condition caused when fragments of the lining of the uterus, shed during menstruation, lodge elsewhere in the pelvic cavity, in the reproductive areas, and sometimes in the urinary tract. They respond to the menstrual cycle and bleed, causing growths of varying sizes to build up. Symptoms include heavy periods, often with abdominal or back pain (generally most severe toward the end of the period), painful intercourse, and sometimes constipation or diarrhea. Endometriosis can be a cause of infertility.

TREATMENT

■ PRACTICAL ADVICE

Tampons can sometimes inhibit menstrual flow; sanitary napkins may be more comfortable.

If sexual intercourse is painful, use a lubricant, such as KY jelly. KY jelly is not recommended if you are trying to get pregnant, but egg white is a good lubricant, and is said to help sperm motility.

✗ DIETARY

Cramps are caused by the production of prostaglandins, which activate the uterine muscles. Oily fish, such as sardines, salmon, or mackerel, contain natural antiprostaglandins, which help reduce cramps. You can also take fish oil supplements or cod liver oil.

The British Endometriosis Society recommends the following dietary supplements:

- Take vitamin B6, 100 milligrams a day, with 25 to 50 milligrams of vitamin B-complex a day.
- Calcium and magnesium improve muscle tone and reduce the pain of cramps. Take a multivitamin and mineral supplement containing them daily.
- Vitamin E naturally balances estrogen and has an important part to play in the management of hormone levels. It helps keep scar tissue soft and flexible, reducing the pain caused by adhesions. Take 400 to 600 iu a day. (Consult your doctor first if you suffer from high blood pressure.)

✳ BIOCHEMIC TISSUE SALTS

Take 4 tablets dissolved on the tongue 2 times a day, for 2 weeks:

For premenstrual syndrome and depression: *Kali Phos*

For heavy periods: *Kali Phos* and *Silica*

For painful periods: *Mag Phos*

✳ ACUPRESSURE

To relieve cramps: Press firmly on the point that is located on the inside leg, 2 inches above the ankle bone.

◉ VISUALIZATION

Do this visualization at least 2 times a day: Find a quiet place where you won't be disturbed. Sit or lie quietly and start breathing down into your stomach. Relax each part of your body in turn. When you are relaxed, visualize yourself in pleasant surroundings. Then visualize the weak, confused endometriosis cells, lost in the wrong place, and the strong, purposeful army of white blood cells flooding in to attack the endometriosis. Imagine the scar tissue disintegrating and the internal organs pink and healthy.

✚ PROFESSIONAL HELP

Endometriosis responds well to individual homeopathic prescribing. You may also call the Endometriosis Association directly for information at: (800) 992-3636.

••• ORTHODOX

Regular examinations rarely discover endometriosis. Diagnosis can only be made through surgery and a laparoscopy (visual examination of the area through a scope inserted into the abdomen). Oral contraceptives or other drugs, such as Danazol, Lupron, and Synarel, inhibit ovulation and thereby prevent the changes that occur in the second half of the menstrual cycle and lead to bleeding.

EPILEPSY

Excessive electrical discharge from nerve cells in the brain leads to partial seizures, where consciousness is maintained, or general seizures, where consciousness is lost.

TREATMENT

Do not try to treat seizures on your own. Consult your doctor before you begin any treatment.

■ PRACTICAL ADVICE

Allergy to chemicals, pesticides, or certain foods (peanuts and tea, for example) has been found to trigger some epileptic attacks. See **Allergies, Food,** for further information on the identification and treatment of food allergies, or consult a naturopath, applied kinesiologist, or clinical ecologist.

✗ DIETARY

Some studies show that vitamin D and vitamin B6 deficiency can prompt epileptic attacks. Vitamin D is obtained through exposure to sunlight and eating fish or drinking fortified milk. You should only take supplements of these vitamins under the supervision of your doctor.

Magnesium, zinc, and calcium have all been found to have anticonvulsant properties. In studies, a magnesium supplement of 450 milligrams a day successfully controlled attacks. You can maintain an adequate intake of zinc and calcium by taking a daily multivitamin and mineral supplement.

Low blood sugar may also be a causative factor. See **Blood Sugar, Low.**

The amino acid taurine has been shown to help control seizures: The recommended dosage is 50 milligrams to 1 gram a day.

✤ **EXERCISE**

Exercise is beneficial, providing the condition is stable. Walking, swimming, and gentle aerobics are good activities. Consult your doctor before beginning any exercise program.

••• **ORTHODOX**

Doctors usually prescribe anticonvulsants and sedatives to maintain the minimum level of drug in the bloodstream sufficient to control the seizures.

Some cases of epilepsy can be treated by the surgical removal of part of the brain.

EPISIOTOMY

A cut made in the skin and muscles between the vagina and the anus, to enlarge the vaginal opening during childbirth. Until relatively recently, episiotomies were performed routinely in order to avoid natural tearing and, it was thought, to prevent damage to the baby's head. Current research shows that the procedure is only necessary in rare cases of fetal distress. Studies show that natural tears generally heal more quickly than surgical incisions, which cut through deeper layers of tissue and can take a long time to heal.

PREVENTION

During pregnancy, practice pelvic floor exercises: While lying, sitting, or standing, tighten and release the muscles that control urine flow 10 times. Do this as many times as possible every day.

In the last 6 weeks of pregnancy, massage the perineum (the area between the vagina and the anus) and the outer vaginal area with olive oil.

Upright births: Crouching, kneeling, squatting, standing, or being on all fours when giving birth helps prevent or minimize tearing and the need for an episiotomy. Lying or sitting puts more strain on the perineum.

Do not rush or push forcefully in the second stage of birth. Giving yourself time allows the perineum to expand, preventing tears.

Avoid the use of disinfectant to wash the vagina, as this washes away natural lubrication and dries up the skin.

Apply a hot towel or diaper to the perineum. This brings blood to the area and relaxes the tissues.

When you feel the baby's head, ease the tissues of the perineum, or massage them with a little oil. Use your own hands to help the baby out.

TREATMENT

Stitching is generally required after a tear, and always after an episiotomy. The following remedies help speed healing and reduce discomfort.

✿ AROMATHERAPY

To aid healing and avoid infection: Take a daily bath to which you have added 2 drops of essential oil of both cypress and lavender.

☐ HOMEOPATHY

Apply *Calendula* cream locally, as often as needed.

After surgical incision where there is great sensitivity: Take *Staphysagria* 6c, 3 times a day, for up to 7 days.

❖ EXERCISE

The following stretches will help bring blood to the perineum, to promote healing:

Lie face down on the floor. Tighten and relax the pelvic floor muscles (the muscles that control urination) 10 times. Repeat as often as possible.

In the same position, lift one leg and tighten the pelvic floor muscles, then do the same with the other leg. Repeat on each side 10 times.

••• ORTHODOX

Doctors recommend keeping the area as clean as possible after an episiotomy, to prevent infection.

Avoid constipation and straining.

EYESIGHT PROBLEMS

Problems with eyesight include nearsightedness, farsightedness, presbyopia (old-age sight), and astigmatism.

TREATMENT

Orthodox medicine nearly always corrects defective sight with glasses or contact lenses, though some new surgical techniques with lasers are now being used to correct the lens itself. The Bates Method is a complementary technique that uses exercises to change the way the eyes focus. This is generally done through individual sessions with a Bates teacher.

▶ BATES METHOD

Below are some techniques a teacher would use to help common eye problems:

Daily relaxation: Palming. Sit in a chair, with your elbows on a table or desk. Cover the eyes with the palms of your hands for at least 10 minutes a day. It may be helpful to listen to the radio while doing this, to allow you to forget about your eyes and relax.

Get into the habit of using your glasses only when you really need them. Leave them off as often as possible, but do not strain your eyes. However, always put the glasses on when driving or using machinery or tools.

Make a point of looking at things that interest you and give you pleasure (flowers, children, water, and so on). The aim of this exercise is to amplify your appreciation of sight.

Become aware of your whole range of vision. Sports, particularly racquet games, help with this.

Head swing: Hold your forefinger in front of your eyes, about 6 to 10 inches from your face, and move it from the left to the right shoulder following it with your eyes; your neck should be loose and the head should follow the finger around. Focus on the finger, but be aware of the moving background behind.

Do the head swing exercise, but now focus entirely on what is behind the finger. This generally brings double vision.

Follow an imaginary finger, letting your eyes rest as far in your line of vision as they want to.

Do these exercises as often as possible, for 10- to 30-second intervals.

○ IF YOU HAVE DIFFICULTY READING

Try reading the different print sizes in a newspaper. First start with the large headlines, then move on to the smaller bold print, and finally the ordinary text.

Use a postcard or ruler to separate the lines.

Read a paragraph, then visualize its contents (the place, the people, the events), then read the next paragraph.

Scan a paragraph looking for words you recognize. Then scan it again looking for words with tails (p, q, y). Piecing the paragraph together in a jigsaw fashion may make reading easier.

○ FOR TIRED EYES

Make sure you are getting adequate sleep.

Lighting that is too bright or too dim can cause eyestrain. Fluorescent lighting is often harsh on the eyes. Replace any flickering lights.

If you are working at a computer, take a 5-minute break every hour. Try to glance up and across the room, or look out of the window at regular intervals to change your range of focus.

☐ HOMEOPATHY

Take *Ruta graveolens* 6c, every 15 minutes, for 3 doses; repeat if needed.

☛ MASSAGE

Look down, close the eyes, and gently massage the tops of the eyeballs through the eyelids. Make tiny circles on any tender areas.

◯ TO SOOTH ACHING EYES

Make a pot of tea with two tea bags. Leave until it is cold, then place a tea bag on each eyelid, lie back, and relax. A piece of freshly cut cucumber over the eyes has a similar soothing and refreshing effect.

✳ ACUPRESSURE

Place your thumbs on the upper part of the eye socket near the bridge of the nose. Press upward and breathe deeply for 1 minute.

Place your index fingers in the center of your cheeks, below the lower ridges of your eyes. Place your middle fingers directly underneath, below the cheekbone. Apply light pressure, close the eyes, and breathe deeply for 1 minute.

••• ORTHODOX

Have a checkup with an optometrist or ophthalmologist to exclude serious eye conditions, such as cataracts or glaucoma (see **Cataract; Glaucoma**). The assessment will also identify the need for glasses or contact lenses.

FACIAL PAIN

May be caused by injury, infection (see **Sinusitis**), tooth or jaw problems, or a nerve disorder (trigeminal neuralgia is the most common type, producing a sharp, knife-like pain). Sometimes facial pain may come from a disease or injury to another area of the body, or may have no apparent cause.

TREATMENT

Many factors may lead to facial pain. The following self-help techniques provide some immediate relief, but you should always consult a professional to rule out serious disorders.

☛ MASSAGE

Thorough, slow neck, scalp, and face massage, while lying down, is very beneficial.

Place your fingertips together in a line on the middle of your forehead, resting your thumbs on your temples. Draw your fingertips outward across the forehead. Repeat several times, then gradually move your fingers higher up your forehead and into the scalp. Continue this procedure across the scalp, always starting from the middle and working outward.

Massage the whole of the scalp, as if washing your hair, for about 1 minute.

Work across the scalp, gently tugging at your hair from the roots.

Placing your middle and fourth fingers on your temples, and your thumb under your jaw, gently massage the temples in a circular motion.

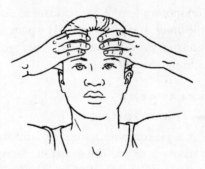

Move your fingers to just above your ears and repeat the above procedure. Continue massaging down in front of the ears and on top of the jawbone.

Using the same two fingers, massage the area just below your cheekbones. Work your way along the edge of the cheekbones to the ears, using very small circular movements, then massage down the upper edge of the jawbone into the chin.

Massage around the chin and the mouth.

Finally, hook the fingers of both hands over the corresponding shoulder, and sink the fingers into the large muscle running along the shoulder blades. Press down deeply for about 1 minute. Stroke the muscles of the neck from the top and side of the neck down and out to the shoulder joint.

~ RELAXATION TECHNIQUES

Facial pain is often a result of tension—gritting the teeth, or smiling through difficult situations—and muscle spasm. Yoga, meditation, and biofeedback are methods that help to reduce tension.

✚ PROFESSIONAL HELP

Facial pain resulting from stress, tension, or a history of head or spinal injury can often be greatly helped by chiropractic. Acupuncture can also be very effective.

••• ORTHODOX

Treatment depends on the cause of the pain. Sinusitis is treated with antibiotics; teeth problems with dental treatment and painkillers; trigeminal neuralgia with the anticonvulsant carbamazepine.

FAINTING

Temporary loss of consciousness due to lack of sufficient blood reaching the brain. It is often caused by pain, shock, fear, hunger, or lack of oxygen. Consult your doctor if you have recurrent fainting; this can be a sign of a more serious illness.

TREATMENT

▬ PRACTICAL ADVICE

For a person who is feeling faint, with symptoms of dizziness, nausea, weakness, or profuse sweating: Sit on a chair and drop the head between the knees. Loosen clothing and keep cool. Give water to drink and open the windows to allow more oxygen.

Do not make a person who has fainted sit up. Lying down allows the blood to return to the brain. Providing the patient is breathing normally, raise the feet slightly and allow to remain lying down for 15 minutes after regaining consciousness. Call emergency medical help immediately; if the person is not breathing, give CPR.

❀ **BACH FLOWER REMEDIES**

Give 4 drops of Rescue Remedy once the person begins to stop feeling faint.

✳ **ACUPRESSURE**

The following points stimulate the body to rebalance and rejuvenate. You can stimulate these points yourself if you are feeling faint, or use them to revive someone who has fainted:

Press firmly between the base of the nose and the upper lip, applying pressure for 1 minute.

Rub your fists against the lower back for 1 minute.

Rub the groove between the big toe and the second toe for 30 seconds.

••• **ORTHODOX**

Repeated attacks of fainting require medical investigation. Treatment will be aimed at resolving the cause.

FALLEN ARCHES
See **Flat Feet.**

FARSIGHTEDNESS
See **Eyesight Problems.**

FATIGUE

Tiredness that is not relieved by a few good nights' sleep may be due to anemia (see **Anemia**); ME (see **Chronic Fatigue Syndrome**); mononucleosis (see **Mononucleosis, Infectious**); depression (see **Depression**); grief; anxiety (see **Anxiety**); dietary deficiencies; toxicities derived from polluted food, smoking, drinking, or medication; or lack of fresh air and exercise. It can also be one of the very early signs of pregnancy, or a symptom of an underlying illness. For persistent fatigue that is not relieved by some of the recommendations below, consult your doctor.

TREATMENT

▬ **PRACTICAL ADVICE**

Be sure to get at least 8 hours of sleep a night. (If you are unable to sleep, see **Insomnia**.) Get into the routine of going to bed early and getting up early.

Set yourself goals each day, but make them attainable ones. Knowing you are in control of your activities will help you achieve them without getting overtired.

Involve yourself in active projects in the evening, such as reading, sewing, knitting, playing a game, drawing, and so on, rather than watching television.

✗ DIETARY

Low blood sugar is a common cause of fatigue that manifests midmorning or afternoon. See **Blood Sugar, Low,** for treatment.

Iron deficiency is also a common cause of fatigue. See the dietary section under **Anemia** for a list of easily absorbed iron-rich foods.

Make sure you start the day with a nutritious breakfast.

Eat a whole-foods diet that incorporates plenty of fresh fruits and vegetables, lean protein, and low-fat produce. Eat a number of small meals spread throughout the day, rather than one or two huge meals a day.

Make sure you get enough complex carbohydrates (whole-grain bread, potatoes, pasta, rice). Avoid nutritionally empty carbohydrates, found in sugar (soft drinks, chocolate, cakes, and so on).

Avoid alcohol.

❋ AROMATHERAPY

Essential oil of peppermint is stimulating and strengthening: Place 2 drops of peppermint oil in a bath with 4 to 6 drops of essential oil of rosemary; or place 2 drops of peppermint oil on a handkerchief or tissue and inhale.

☐ HOMEOPATHY

At night, take *Arnica* 6c every 10 minutes for 3 doses, to help you relax from the day's exertion and improve the quality of your sleep.

❀ BACH FLOWER REMEDIES

Take Olive several times a day for 4 to 7 days.

✛ EXERCISE

For nonspecific fatigue that is not related to a viral infection, moderate exercise will help you sleep better and boost energy. Any aerobic exercise that works up a sweat is beneficial.

∼ RELAXATION TECHNIQUES

Fatigue is often caused by an ongoing concern or stress. If you know what is worrying you, try to discuss it with someone you trust and respect.

If you cannot resolve the problem immediately, set aside some time each day when you will not think about it, or decide to give yourself a break from it and address the problem in a week or a month. Professional psychotherapy or counseling can help you look at issues that cause ongoing anxiety or stress.

Learning meditation or biofeedback will help you become aware of stresses in your life and how to deal with them.

Getting a massage is an excellent way to relax, and is very restorative.

✳ YOGA

Yoga is an incredibly energizing activity. It enhances your breathing, allowing more oxygen into the system; it improves blood circulation by stretching the muscles; and it relaxes the mind. Attending a class regularly will help relieve fatigue. Perform the following routine first thing in the morning:

Stand with your feet apart and your arms outstretched to the side. Swing both arms as far as you can to your right, turning your head and shoulders in the same direction, then back to the left. Repeat this movement 5 times.

Let your arms, head, and trunk drop down to the floor in front of you. Remain in this position for a moment, allowing the weight of your body to stretch you even further down. Inhale, and gradually lift your trunk and head, coming up with a rounded back, and reach up as high as you can with your arms. Remain in the stretch for a few seconds, exhale, and repeat.

••• ORTHODOX

Fatigue is one of the most common ailments reported to doctors. A routine checkup will probably be required to rule out serious illness. Treatment is generally aimed at relieving the cause of the problem.

FEEDING PROBLEMS IN CHILDREN
See **Eating Problems in Children.**

FEET, ACHING
Fallen arches (see **Flat Feet**) or varicose veins (see **Varicose Veins**) can cause aching feet, as can walking or standing for long periods. Ill-fitting shoes, corns, calluses, and bunions (see **Bunion**) can all contribute.

PREVENTION

Being overweight puts more strain on the feet; try to maintain your recommended weight.

Avoid wearing high-heeled or ill-fitting shoes for long periods. Alternate with well-fitting, flat-heeled shoes, and periods of going barefoot.

TREATMENT

▬ PRACTICAL ADVICE

Go barefoot when you are at home.

Put your feet up whenever possible.

Try not to stand for long periods without taking regular breaks.

Wear support tights for varicose veins (see **Varicose Veins**).

Use shock-absorbing insoles in shoes, especially if you are pregnant or suffering from arthritis of the knees, hips, or spine.

❁ AROMATHERAPY

Add 6 drops of essential oil of both eucalyptus and rosemary, or 4 drops of these oils and 2 drops of peppermint essential oil, to a bowl of hot water. Soak your feet in it for 5 to 10 minutes. Then alternate running hot and cold water (30 seconds of each) over your feet to improve circulation. Finish up with cold water.

☛ MASSAGE

Sit on the floor. Bend your knee so that your left foot is flat on the floor. Place the fingers of both hands under the foot and your thumbs on top, below the ankle. Use your thumbs to press down and out from the ankle bones to the toes; try to run your hands between the bones of the feet rather than on them.

Still using the thumbs, use small circular motions to massage the area just above the toes.

Take hold of the big toe with thumb and fingers, circle the toe several times and gently pull it away from you. Repeat with the other toes.

Turn your foot over to one side and massage the ball of the foot underneath, using the thumbs.

Use a foot roller to massage the bottoms of the feet.

✚ PROFESSIONAL HELP

Foot pain can be helped by professional reflexology or chiropractic.

••• ORTHODOX

Treatment will depend on the cause of the pain. Podiatrists specialize in dealing with foot problems.

FEVER

A body temperature over 98.6° F measured by mouth (many people normally run temperatures a degree above or below), often accompanied by shivering, thirst, and hot skin. Fever is generally a sign that the body is fighting infection, though it can also result from overexposure to heat or cold, or, in children, from a shock or emotional disturbance. If fever lasts longer than three days, consult your doctor. Consult your doctor immediately if your child has any of the following symptoms:

a temperature of over 104° F
becomes vague and confused
starts to twitch

TREATMENT

Practitioners of complementary medicine consider fevers to be a sign of healing rather than a symptom of disease. In children, fever often restores balance, making them feel much better afterward.

✗ DIETARY

Eat the minimum, drink plenty of fluids. Lemon and honey mixed with warm water prevents dehydration and provides energy.

Fever leaves the body exhausted; once the temperature has gone down, build strength with plenty of vegetables, given as soups, fresh fruits and juices, and later whole-grain cereals and lean protein.

?? HERBALISM

Catmint infusion reduces body temperature: Pour 1 cup of boiling water onto 1 teaspoon of the dried herb, and infuse for 15 minutes; drink 3 times a day.

☐ HOMEOPATHY

Take every 15 minutes for 4 doses; repeat if needed:

Sudden fever after getting chilled, worse around midnight, frightened: *Aconite* 6c

Hot, flushed skin and bright, staring eyes, delirious, hot head with cold limbs: *Belladonna* 6c

Cold to the touch but complains of burning pains, wants small amounts to drink at frequent intervals, restless and anxious: *Arsenicum album* 6c

❀ BACH FLOWER REMEDIES

Rescue Remedy is helpful, particularly if the fever results from a shock, or the child is frightened. Place 2 drops under the tongue.

≈ HYDROTHERAPY

Apply cold, wet compresses, or sponge down the skin with tepid or cool water to reduce heat.

••• ORTHODOX

Doctors generally recommend acetaminophen or aspirin for adults and children over 12 years.

FIBRILLATION

One of the most common types of irregular heartbeat, seen in 5 percent to 10 percent of all people over the age of sixty-five. Symptoms may be totally absent (often this condition is discovered at routine physical examination), though occasionally palpitations (see **Palpitations**), shortness of breath, and faintness occur. These symptoms may also indicate thyroid disorders (see **Hyperthyroidism** and **Goiter**), which need to be ruled out. Diagnosis is generally made by taking an electrocardiogram (ECG).

TREATMENT

▬ PRACTICAL ADVICE

The following techniques can help reduce palpitations:
  Hold your breath.
  Slowly drink a glass of water.
  Bathe your face in cold water.
  Pinch your nostrils and blow through your nose.

✗ DIETARY

Reduce intake of caffeine (coffee, tea, chocolate, cola), sugar, spices.
  Stop smoking.
  Avoid alcohol.
  Take 50 to 100 milligrams of magnesium a day, as part of a multimineral supplement.

☛ MASSAGE

Regular massage from a friend, partner, or therapist is helpful in promoting relaxation and taking pressure off the heart.

⊹ EXERCISE

Gentle walking or swimming for 30 minutes several times a week is good for this condition.

~ RELAXATION TECHNIQUES

Learning to meditate, attending a yoga class, or practicing biofeedback will all help you to relax, and will prevent this condition from worsening.

Perform the following routine at least once a day: Find a quiet place where you won't be disturbed. Lie on a firm surface, close your eyes, allow your breathing to slow, and begin to be aware of how your body feels. Consciously try to relax every part of your body in turn. Begin with your face (your eyes, your forehead, your jaw), and work down to your toes. The whole procedure should take at least 10 minutes.

If anxiety prevents you from relaxing, try to find a friend or professional you can talk to and resolve the problems. Counseling or psychotherapy may help.

✚ PROFESSIONAL HELP

Acupuncture can help restore the heart's rhythm to normal.

••• ORTHODOX

Doctors will usually prescribe drugs to regulate the heartbeat.
Sometimes electric shock treatment is given to regulate the heart.
An artificial pacemaker may be inserted surgically.

FIBROCYSTIC BREAST DISEASE
See **Breast Lumps.**

FIBROIDS

Noncancerous growths in the womb that often produce no symptoms. As they grow, fibroids may cause heavy and long menstrual periods, painful intercourse, and bladder or bowel pressure. Sometimes fibroids can cause infertility.

TREATMENT

▬ PRACTICAL ADVICE

The growth of fibroids appears to be related to hormonal imbalance, particularly the overproduction of estrogen. Coming off oral contraceptives or hormone replacement therapy (both of which provide synthetic estrogen) may help prevent further growth.

✕ DIETARY

Reduce your intake of animal fat and increase your intake of fiber. This helps reduce the production of estrogen and restore hormonal balance.

Increase your intake of vitamin C and bioflavonoids (found in the skin, pith, and outer layer of fruits and vegetables, such as citrus fruits, and in leafy vegetables and red onions).

Increase your intake of vitamin E (found in wheat germ, vegetable oils, seeds, and nuts).

Increase your intake of vitamin A (found in liver, kidney, egg yolk, butter, fortified margarine, and milk).

✿ VISUALIZATION

The following visualization is suggested for reducing the size of fibroids, or eliminating them altogether. If you find you are unable to do visualization alone, a practitioner of autogenic training or a counselor, psychologist, or psychotherapist can teach you: Lie or sit in a relaxed position and a quiet atmosphere. Let your attention go to the area of the fibroids. Focus your attention on them and experience how they feel. Try to create an image of the fibroids (it can be what you think they really look like, or an abstract); keep focusing on that image, allowing it to change and evolve. Then try to form an image of something that could be done to make the fibroids reduce in size. Finally, visualize what the womb looks like without the fibroids.

✚ PROFESSIONAL HELP

Fibroids respond well to professional homeopathic treatment.
Acupuncture can also be effective.

••• ORTHODOX

Small fibroids tend to cause no problems, and often disappear after menopause. Fibroids that cause problems may be removed surgically, an operation that may or may not involve a hysterectomy (removal of the uterus).

FIBROSITIS

Pain and stiffness in the muscles and ligaments around joints, most commonly in the neck and shoulder area. This can be caused by overuse or injury. Most commonly, it is a result of bad posture and tension in the body. See also **Frozen Shoulder; Neck Pain and Stiffness.**

TREATMENT

❋ AROMATHERAPY

Add 4 drops of essential oil of lavender to your bath to relieve pain and reduce inflammation. Add lavender to your massage oil for further effect.

☐ HOMEOPATHY

Take every 30 minutes for 4 doses; repeat if necessary:

Stiffness and pain after unaccustomed physical exertion: *Arnica* 6c

Stiffness after rest, improved by continued motion: *Rhus toxicodendron* 6c

Stiffness and discomfort that worsen with continued motion: *Bryonia* 6c

≈ HYDROTHERAPY

Make an ice pack by wrapping a plastic bag full of ice cubes or a bag of frozen peas in a kitchen towel. Apply to the painful area for 10 minutes. Follow this with 10 minutes of heat provided by a hot water bottle wrapped in a towel. Repeat. Carry out this treatment twice a day.

☛ MASSAGE

Turn your head slightly to one side. Take hold of the large muscle (the sternocleidomastoid) that runs from the base of the skull to the collar bone, hold it with fingers and thumb, and squeeze firmly up and down the muscle. Turn your head the other way and repeat on the other side.

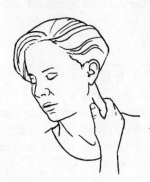

✳ ACUPRESSURE

Lie face down on a comfortable surface. Your partner should place the pads of the thumbs on either side of your spine, and apply gentle pressure (by leaning a little weight over the thumbs), starting at the top vertebra and working down each one.

✦ MEDITATION

Learning to meditate will help relieve tension, and make you aware of situations or positions that cause you to tense the muscles.

✳ YOGA

Gently lift your shoulders up as high as you can. Hold the position for 5 seconds, then release. Repeat 5 times, morning and evening.

Circle your shoulders forward 5 times and backward 5 times. Repeat morning and evening.

Stand facing a wall, with your feet about 2 to 3 feet away from the wall. Place the palms of your hands on the wall just above your head. Keeping your arms and legs straight, and without moving your feet or hands, let your head and chest fall forward between your arms. Hold the position for as long as is comfortable. You should feel a stretch in the arms and shoulders. Do this exercise whenever you experience shoulder pain or stiffness.

✚ PROFESSIONAL HELP

Massage or chiropractic will all help.

The Alexander Technique is helpful in correcting postural problems, which often lead to fibrositis.

Acupuncture can be effective in reducing pain.

••• ORTHODOX

Your doctor may recommend painkillers or physiotherapy.

FLAT FEET

The absence of arches in the feet, which means the sole rests flat on the ground. The arch simply may never have developed, or it may be as a result of weight gain, lack of exercise, weak muscles in the feet, or wearing badly fitting shoes. Flat feet may cause aches and pains in the feet, calves, and legs.

TREATMENT

☛ MASSAGE

Massage for flat feet is best carried out by an experienced massage therapist, physiotherapist, chiropractor, or reflexologist. Treatment should concentrate on the Achilles tendon, calves, and upper legs, as well as the feet.

⁘ EXERCISE

Stand on a hard floor, rise up onto the toes, and jump into the air. Repeat 20 times, morning and night.

Rock heel to toe for 3 minutes.

While sitting, scrunch the toes up inside your shoes, allowing the foot to arch. Repeat 10 times, 10 times a day.

Practice picking up things with your toes: for example, a squash ball or a marble.

✚ PROFESSIONAL HELP
Chiropractic is helpful for adults.

••• ORTHODOX
Surgery is sometimes used to correct the bones of the feet in children. In adults, podiatrists often recommend arch supports for the shoes.

FLATULENCE
The buildup of excessive air in the intestine due to nervous swallowing, or gulping food and drink; also called gas, or wind. Some foods, when they ferment, also produce an accumulation of gas in the intestine. Symptoms include stomach pain and a swollen belly.

TREATMENT
✗ DIETARY

For those who are lactose intolerant (see **Lactose Intolerance**), milk can cause excessive gas. Replacing cow's milk with goat's milk or soy milk may help.

Reduce your intake of fiber, particularly beans and peas.

Reduce your intake of fermented foods: cheese, soy sauce, alcohol.

Charcoal tablets provide immediate relief by absorbing gas.

Reduce your intake of carbonated drinks.

Try the Hay Diet, which avoids mixing protein and carbohydrate at the same meal. It is described in several books, including *Food Combining for Health* (see Suggested Reading).

Eat fruit before meals, not as a dessert or with other food.

༄ HERBALISM
Infusion of sweet flag: Pour 1 cup of boiling water on 2 teaspoons of the dried herb, and infuse for 10 minutes; drink ½ cup before meals.

Ginger infusion: Pour 1 cup of boiling water onto 1 teaspoon of the grated fresh root, and infuse for 5 minutes; drink as needed.

☐ HOMEOPATHY
Take every 30 minutes for up to 4 doses:

Stomach feels constantly full of gas: *Argentum nitricum* 6c

Burning discomfort, with some fluid reflux in the throat: *Arsenicum album* 6c

Painful stuck gas, made worse by onions and garlic: *Lycopodium* 6c

☯ CHINESE MEDICINE

Flatulence is thought to be caused by stagnation of stomach energy. Practitioners of traditional Chinese medicine recommend magnolia bark, orange peel, or lemon peel.

❖ REFLEXOLOGY

Apply pressure to the stomach point, located on the soles of both feet, above the midline, below the ball of the foot.

Apply pressure to the large intestine point, located on the soles of both feet in the area over the lower tarsal bones.

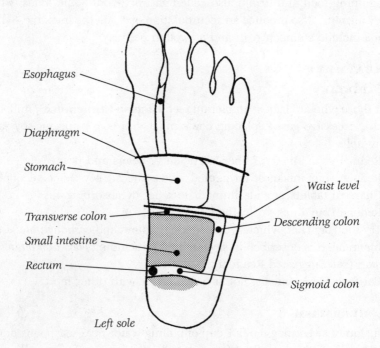

Esophagus

Diaphragm

Stomach

Transverse colon

Small intestine

Rectum

Waist level

Descending colon

Sigmoid colon

Left sole

⁘ EXERCISE

Regular exercise stimulates the digestion and promotes the reabsorption and expulsion of gas. Do not exercise within 2 hours after eating.

✳ YOGA

The Shoulder Stand can help relieve the pain and discomfort of flatulence: Fold a firm blanket two or three times. Lie on your back, with your shoulders on the blanket and your head and neck on the floor. Inhaling, raise your legs, bending your knees if necessary. Exhale, and lift your hips off the floor. Support your hips with your hands, resting your weight on your elbows. Exhale, and lift your legs as high as you are able to do comfortably. Hold the position while breathing normally for several minutes, then gradually reverse the process, bringing your legs down.

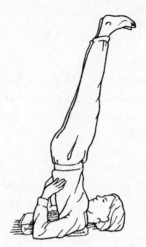

••• ORTHODOX

Usually, dietary adjustment is all that is necessary. Doctors advise reducing fiber intake, and sometimes recommend charcoal tablets.

FLU

A condition caused by an influenza virus that produces multiple symptoms, including fever, headache, joint pains, stomach upset, and a stuffy or runny nose.

TREATMENT

✗ DIETARY

Eat and drink plenty of vitamin C–rich foods: fresh fruits and vegetables, especially citrus fruits, black currants, Brussels sprouts, and strawberries.

Increase your intake of zinc, found in lean meat, fish, and whole-grain breads and cereals.

❀ AROMATHERAPY

If others around you have the flu: Gargle daily with 1 drop each of essential oils of tea tree and lemon in a glass of warm water. Stir well before each mouthful.

To treat the flu: Gargle with 2 drops each of essential oil of tea tree and geranium in a glass of warm water. Stir well before each mouthful.

If your nose is blocked or the chest is congested: Add a few drops of essential oil of eucalyptus or peppermint to a steam inhalation. **Caution:**

If you suffer from asthma, avoid steam inhalations; instead, put a few drops of the oil on a handkerchief or tissue and inhale.

﹩ HERBALISM

Boneset infusion is one of the best remedies for flu, relieving aches and fever and clearing congestion: Pour 1 cup of boiling water on 2 teaspoons of the dried herb, and infuse for 15 minutes; drink, as hot as possible, several times a day.

▢ HOMEOPATHY

Take every hour for 3 doses; repeat if needed:

Tired and aching, apathetic, irritable, with a heavy headache and aching, heavy limbs and chills up and down the spine: *Gelsemium* 6c

With intense aching in the bones: *Eupatorium perfoliatum* 6c

Chilly and very sensitive to drafts, restless and wants to stretch: *Rhus toxicodendron* 6c

Heavy and aching, foul breath and diarrhea, confused and bewildered: *Baptisia* 6c

••• ORTHODOX

Aspirin may be recommended to relieve aches and pains, but should never be given to children under twelve, except under close medical supervision (acetaminophen should be given instead). For those who become chronically ill with the flu (the elderly, the disabled and the immune-compromised), complications may arise that require antibiotics.

FLUID RETENTION

Retention of water in the tissues that may be caused by heart problems (see **Coronary Heart Disease**), kidney infection (see **Urinary Tract Infection**), premenstrual syndrome (see **Premenstrual Syndrome**), varicose veins (see **Varicose Veins**), or drugs. Sometimes there is no apparent cause. Symptoms include increased weight, and swollen areas of the body, particularly the ankles and lower back.

TREATMENT

It is important to try to find the cause of fluid retention so that treatment can be appropriate. In cases where the underlying cause is not remediable, the following measures may help the body to excrete excess water and make you more comfortable.

■ **PRACTICAL ADVICE**

Water retention in pregnancy is common and should not be a cause for concern. Lying down with your feet raised several times a day helps. Gentle exercise, such as swimming or walking, is also helpful. Reduce your intake of refined carbohydrates and get as much rest as possible.

Avoid tight clothing and shoes.

Put your feet up whenever possible.

✗ **DIETARY**

Reduce salt intake: Salt causes the body to retain water.

Eat plenty of potassium-rich foods—fresh fruits and vegetables, salads, and juices.

❄ **AROMATHERAPY**

Add 6 drops of essential oil of lavender to a warm bath.

Dilute 10 drops of essential oil of lavender in 5 teaspoons of a carrier oil or lotion. Massage the abdomen using firm, clockwise circles; massage the backs of the calves and thighs in an upward direction, and then move on to the lower back.

❧ **HERBALISM**

Parsley is an effective diuretic (it helps the body to excrete water). Eat plenty of the raw herb, or make a parsley infusion: Pour 1 cup of boiling water onto 2 teaspoons of the chopped herb, and infuse for 10 minutes in a closed container; drink 3 times a day. **Caution:** Do not use during pregnancy.

Eat dandelion leaves in salads.

Drink dandelion decoction (dandelion "coffee"): Mix 2 to 3 teaspoons of the root with 1 cup of water, and simmer for 10 minutes; drink 3 times a day.

☛ **MASSAGE**

Massage helps increase blood and lymph flow, and prevents the stagnation or pooling of blood in the legs and ankles. Always massage toward the heart.

✳ **ACUPRESSURE**

Lie on your back on the floor. Place all your fingers between the top of the pubic bone and the navel. Press 1 or 2 inches into the abdomen while taking deep breaths. Hold for 1 minute.

Lie on the floor, bend the knees, and bring the right foot onto the left thigh. With the right thumb, press on the inside leg where the tibia indents, just below the knee. With the left thumb, press on the point 3 inches above the ankle bone. Hold for a minute, then do the same on the left leg.

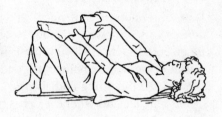

✤ EXERCISE

Muscular activity helps pump blood in the veins back to the heart, which encourages elimination of waste and prevents the blood pooling in the limbs. Walking, running, cycling, swimming, dancing, and aerobics are all good.

••• ORTHODOX

Diuretic drugs, in oral or injectable form, are effective in eradicating all but the most resistant forms of fluid retention. However, you should use them with caution, especially if you are taking other medication.

FOOD POISONING

Acute stomach pain, vomiting, and diarrhea that usually occur within 48 hours of consuming food or drinks contaminated by bacteria, a virus, or a chemical toxin. Salmonella, listeria organisms, and streptococcus are some common contaminants.

PREVENTION

You can help to prevent food poisoning when traveling by making sure that your stomach has a rich supply of healthy bacteria to fight infections: Take ½ teaspoon of high-potency *Lactobacillus acidophilus* powder, 1 teaspoon of *Bifidobacteria* powder, and ½ teaspoon of *Lactobacillus bulgaricus* (available from natural foods stores) in a glass of spring water, 3 times a day. Supplement this with plenty of live yogurt that contains *Lactobacillus acidophilus*. During your trip, continue to take the *acidophilus* mixture in a glass of water before meals. If you get symptoms of food poisoning, increase the dosage to 1 teaspoon in water every hour, until symptoms subside.

When traveling in third world countries, drink only boiled or sterilized water. Avoid eating food that is not freshly cooked, or that is inadequately heated. Avoid meat, raw vegetables, unpeeled fruit, fruit juices (unless bottled), and ice in drinks (it is usually made with tap water).

Contaminants are often stored and activated in prepared food that is inadequately reheated. Avoid prepared, chilled, and frozen foods.

Buy organic meat and free-range eggs, and be sure to cook them thoroughly.

Wash fruit and vegetables thoroughly.

Avoid eating raw fish or raw meat.

TREATMENT

Vomiting and diarrhea, though unpleasant, are the body's natural way of eliminating the poison from the body as quickly as possible. Do not attempt to suppress them unless advised by a professional. The following remedies help calm the stomach, restore strength after the attack, and prevent recurrences.

■ PRACTICAL ADVICE

Be sure to wash your hands thoroughly after going to the toilet, and before touching food, to prevent passing on the infection to others.

✗ DIETARY

Do not eat solids during the attack. To replace lost salt and water (this is particularly important in children and the elderly), add 1 teaspoon of salt and 2 scant teaspoons of sugar or honey to 1 quart of boiled water and 1 pint of orange juice or lemon juice. Drink 1 pint of the mixture every hour until symptoms subside.

Once the diarrhea and vomiting have subsided, eat plain whole-grain foods, and vegetables. Bananas help settle the stomach. Live yogurt and *acidophilus* powder (see above) help restore the protective bacteria in the stomach.

Take the *acidophilus* mixture given above in a glass of water 3 times a day for several weeks after the attack.

⅔ HERBALISM

Meadowsweet infusion soothes the irritated mucous membranes of the digestive system: Pour 1 cup of boiling water on 2 teaspoons of the dried herb, and infuse for 15 minutes; drink 3 times a day.

☐ HOMEOPATHY

Take 1 dose every 10 minutes for up to 6 doses; repeat if necessary:

Profuse diarrhea accompanied by burning and colicky stomach, restlessness, anxiety, and chilliness: *Arsenicum album* 6c

Vomiting and diarrhea with profuse cold sweats: *Veratrum album* 6c

After stimulants (coffee, alcohol, spices), alternating with fruitless urging: *Nux vomica* 6c

Burning in the rectum and anus, with involuntary evacuations: *Aloe* 6c

Greenish, painless diarrhea, with gurgling and stomach cramps, worse early morning: *Podophyllum* 6c

••• ORTHODOX

In persistent and extreme cases, drugs are recommended to alleviate exhaustion from diarrhea and vomiting.

FOOT ODOR

Smelly feet, often a result of athlete's foot. If your feet are itchy, particularly between the toes, or if the skin is crumbling or broken, see **Fungal Infection.** Heavy perspiration is the other major cause of foot odor. People who spend a lot of time on their feet are more susceptible.

TREATMENT

■ PRACTICAL ADVICE

Wash your feet often—several times a day, if possible. Use warm water and soap and clean well between the toes. Dry thoroughly. Dust feet with sodium bicarbonate.

Wear cotton socks, and change them several times a day, if necessary.

Do not wear the same shoes every day. Give them a chance to dry out and air. Dust the insides with sodium bicarbonate.

Wear leather shoes, never rubber, plastic, or canvas. Wear open sandals when possible.

✗ DIETARY

Increasing your intake of zinc and magnesium can sometimes help alleviate foot odor. These minerals are found in whole-grain breads and cereals, poultry, fish, and organ meats, nuts, cooked dried beans and peas, and dark green leafy vegetables.

❊ AROMATHERAPY

To reduce perspiration and act as a natural deodorant: Dilute 10 drops of essential oil of cypress (or 8 drops of cypress and 2 drops of peppermint) in 5 teaspoons of a carrier oil or lotion. Massage into the feet morning and night.

••• ORTHODOX

Daily application of aluminum chloride lotion drastically reduces sweating and may be effective in reducing foot odor. (Sweating can be prevented altogether by surgically cutting the autonomic nerves to the feet, but this operation is rarely carried out today.)

FRACTURE

A break in a bone, generally caused by a fall. The bone usually breaks horizontally, but it can also fracture lengthwise, diagonally, or in a spiral. Women with osteoporosis (see **Osteoporosis**) are particularly susceptible to fractures.

TREATMENT

A person with a suspected fracture should be taken to the hospital immediately. If the person cannot walk, call an ambulance. While awaiting medical care, prepare an ice pack. Make an ice pack by wrapping a plastic bag full of ice cubes or a bag of frozen peas in a kitchen towel. Place it on the fracture to reduce swelling. Do not try to move the broken bone or push it back in place.

✗ DIETARY

To help build new bone cells:

Increase your intake of calcium: add nonfat milk to sauces, milkshakes, casseroles, and soups; eat plenty of legumes (peas, beans, lentils), leafy green vegetables, and yogurt.

Increase your intake of phosphorus, found in red meat, organ meats, poultry, fish, and eggs.

Increase your intake of magnesium, found in nuts, cooked dried beans and peas, whole-grain breads and cereals, dark green leafy vegetables, and seafood.

Increase your intake of vitamin A, found in eggs, liver, butter, milk, and cod liver oil.

☐ HOMEOPATHY

For shock following a fracture: Take *Arnica* 6c, every 10 minutes, up to 3 doses.

For bruising around fracture: Take *Arnica* 6c, 3 times a day, for 3 days; repeat if needed.

To aid bone repair: Take *Symphytum* 6c, 2 times a day, for 2 weeks.

✿ **BACH FLOWER REMEDIES**

Rescue Remedy is useful in treating the shock caused by a fracture.

✚ **PROFESSIONAL HELP**

Chiropractic, physiotherapy, and massage can help restore muscle and ligament activity after a fracture.

••• **ORTHODOX**

After initial pain relief or anesthetic, X-rays are taken. Then the broken bones are put back in position and immobilized by means of a bandage, splint, sling, or cast. Healing may take between two weeks and six months, depending on the age of the patient and the bone broken.

FROSTBITE

Damage to the tissues caused by very low temperatures. Symptoms include pins and needles, followed by numbness. The skin first becomes white and hard, and later red and swollen. Blisters may form and, in severe cases, black areas may appear.

TREATMENT

━ **PRACTICAL ADVICE**

Frostbite is often accompanied by hypothermia (see **Hypothermia**); both require medical attention. While waiting for help, carry out the following first aid techniques:

Shelter from the cold and cover the head and body with extra clothing; drink warm drinks, not alcohol.

Do not rub the frostbitten area.

Do not burst blisters.

Do not attempt to walk on a frostbitten foot or move the affected area.

Remove restrictive jewelry.

Gradually warm the frostbitten area by covering it with clothing; place hands under the armpits, and feet under the armpits of a companion; do not expose to direct heat.

If warm water is available, immerse the affected area for several minutes, then cover with a sterile dressing. Keep the area warm afterward to prevent refreezing.

••• **ORTHODOX**

Emergency hospital treatment is required in severe cases.

FROZEN SHOULDER

Restricted movement and pain in the shoulder joint that may be caused by torn muscle fibers and inflammation. The surrounding "capsule" or covering of the joint itself becomes irritated. An obvious symptom of frozen shoulder is pain that occurs when lifting the arm sideways, making tasks such as brushing one's hair or dressing difficult.

TREATMENT

≈ HYDROTHERAPY

Make an ice pack by wrapping a plastic bag full of ice cubes or a bag of frozen peas in a kitchen towel. Prepare a hot water bottle, and wrap a towel around it. Hold the ice pack over the area of pain for 3 minutes, followed by the hot water bottle for 3 minutes. Repeat the procedure 3 times, and carry out several times a day.

Gentle swimming in warm water is a good way to loosen the shoulder and allow for more movement. Some hospitals have swimming pools in their physiotherapy units.

☞ MASSAGE

If your right shoulder is affected, support the left elbow with your right hand, and pass the left hand over the affected shoulder. Starting close to the neck, squeeze the large muscle that passes over the shoulder blade. Try to lift the muscle as you squeeze, working all the way down to the shoulder. Repeat several times. If the left shoulder is affected, reverse the process.

With your elbow still supported, use your fingertips to stroke firmly down from the side of the top of the neck all the way along the shoulder to the shoulder joint. Repeat the procedure several times.

✳ ACUPRESSURE

Make a fist and gently pound on the tops of your shoulders, from the joint up to your neck.

Curve your fingers and hook them over the top of your shoulders. Feel for the area of tension, and allow your thumb to sink into it. Press firmly for 1 minute, then relax.

⬧ EXERCISE

Place a rolled towel under the affected armpit, and use the free arm to pull the elbow into the side of the body. This levers the upper arm, stretching the capsule of the shoulder joint.

✚ **PROFESSIONAL HELP**

Self-treatment of frozen shoulder is very slow, and can be greatly aided by professional help from a chiropractor.

Acupuncture is helpful in relieving pain.

The Alexander Technique will help if the problem is caused by postural problems.

••• **ORTHODOX**

Doctors generally prescribe painkillers, anti-inflammatory drugs, or the injection of steroids directly into the joint. Physiotherapy is generally recommended.

FUNGAL INFECTION

Fungal infections usually affect the skin, though they can spread to other internal organs. Common examples are athlete's foot, causing itchiness on the feet and between the toes; jock itch, affecting the skin around the groin; thrush (see **Thrush**), yeast infections of the mouth and vagina (see **Thrush, Oral; Vaginal Irritation**); ringworm, where disc-like shapes appear on the skin; and dandruff (see **Dandruff**). Nails can also be affected. The infection is caused by the multiplication and spread of common fungal organisms (usually *Candida albicans* or tinea), which commonly cause redness, inflammation, and itching. When the nails are affected, they typically turn white and crumbly. Fungal infections are more likely to occur in those whose immunity is low, particularly after taking antibiotics that kill off the natural bacteria that prevent their multiplication. They can also occur when the acid/alkali balance of the body is upset by inappropriate diet, cosmetics, hormonal imbalances, or drugs.

PREVENTION

To prevent athlete's foot, do not share or borrow shoes, socks, or towels. Change socks and towels daily. Wear cotton socks and leather shoes.

TREATMENT

■ **PRACTICAL ADVICE**

Fungal infections thrive in damp, moist environments. Wear cotton underwear to allow air to circulate, wash frequently, and dry yourself thoroughly.

Ringworm: To prevent reinfection, wash all clothes thoroughly after treatment; if scalp is infected, replace all brushes, combs, and headgear.

The infection is sometimes spread through pets: a vet can diagnose and treat infected animals.

✗ DIETARY

Enhance your immunity by eating plenty of lightly cooked green, yellow, and orange vegetables, whole-grain cereals, lean meat, or fish.

To discourage the multiplication of *Candida albicans,* avoid the following foods for at least a month: all sugar, including cakes and pastries; raw fresh fruits and dried fruits; and alcohol. Also avoid mushrooms, blue cheese, soy sauce, and other yeast-containing foods.

Incorporate plenty of olive oil into your diet; this helps fight *Candida albicans.*

Live yogurt helps restore healthy intestinal bacteria, which is essential in fighting fungal infections. Eat at least one small carton of plain, unsweetened live yogurt that contains *Lactobacillus acidophilus* daily.

Avoid coffee and tea; instead drink mineral water, rooibos tea, and other herbal teas.

Take supplements of *Lactobacillus acidophilus:* ½ teaspoon of high-potency *acidophilus* powder and ½ teaspoon of *Bifidobacteria* powder (both available from health food stores) in a glass of spring water, 2 or 3 times a day.

❀ AROMATHERAPY

Essential oil of tea tree is very effective in combating fungal infections of the skin: Add 5 drops of the oil to your bath.

To relieve itching and redness: Make a solution made up of 2 drops of essential oil of peppermint and 4 drops of German chamomile added to a basin of water. Bathe the affected area in the solution.

Dermasorb is an effective antifungal cream that contains tea tree oil but no drugs.

❧ HERBALISM

Garlic is an effective antifungal agent. Use liberally in cooking. If you do not like the taste or smell of fresh garlic, you can take garlic capsules (3 capsules, 3 times a day).

Caprylic acid, an extract of coconut, is a powerful antifungal agent available from natural foods stores: Take 3 capsules with each meal.

For athlete's foot, soak feet regularly for at least 30 minutes in a strong infusion of golden seal root: Add 1 cup of boiling water to 3 teaspoons of the powdered herb, and infuse for 15 minutes. Dry feet well and powder with arrowroot or powdered golden seal root. Use *Calendula* cream if cracks have formed.

✳ BIOCHEMIC TISSUE SALTS

Take *Silica* 6x, 4 times a day.

••• ORTHODOX

Antifungal agents are prescribed in cream, tablet, vaginal pessary, oral solution, or impregnated tampon form. Treatment is effective within a matter of days, but fungal infections have a tendency to recur. To prevent further infection, it is important to raise your immunity with the help of the treatments above.

 **_G_**

GALLSTONES

Lumps of solid matter (mainly cholesterol) found in the gallbladder. Occasionally, a stone exits from the gallbladder, blocking the flow of bile and leading to inflammation of the gallbladder; this is known as cholecystitis. Symptoms include pain in the upper-right abdomen and sometimes between the shoulder blades, nausea, indigestion, and jaundice (yellowing of the whites of the eyes, the skin, and the urine).

PREVENTION

Increase your intake of fiber, found in whole-grain cereals, fresh fruits and vegetables, oat bran, and cooked dried beans and peas.

Reduce your intake of fat (except olive oil, which may be helpful), particularly saturated fat, found in animal products.

A vegetarian diet has been shown to help prevent gallstones.

TREATMENT
✘ DIETARY

Reduce your intake of all fats except olive oil. Do not eat fried food.

A little alcohol each day (not more than two units) is thought to reduce levels of bile salts. (One unit is ½ pint of beer, a single measure of spirits, or 1 glass of wine.)

Increase your intake of bran, particularly oat bran.

Drink 6 to 8 glasses of water a day.

HERBALISM

Balmony is an ancient North American Indian remedy. When combined with fringetree, it is an effective gallstone treatment: Pour 2 cups of boiling water on 2 teaspoons of each dried herb, and infuse for 15 minutes; drink 3 times a day.

CHINESE MEDICINE

Small gallstones are dissolved with herbs such as lysimachia, pyrrosia leaf, and rhubarb.

✚ PROFESSIONAL HELP

Food allergies may contribute to gallstones. Some naturopaths recommend an elimination diet, carried out under the supervision of a practitioner.

Professional homeopathic treatment can help reduce the frequency and severity of attacks.

••• ORTHODOX

When the stones are small, drugs may be used to dissolve them.

Surgery (removal of the stones or the whole gallbladder, if necessary) is the more common treatment.

GANGLION

A cyst that develops in a joint or tendon sheath. The most common site is the back of the wrist joint, the knee, or around the ankles. It may be soft or firm, and is usually painless unless caught from time to time by the tendons that move against it.

TREATMENT

Any newly formed lump should be seen by your doctor.

◻ HOMEOPATHY

Ruta graveolens 50M: Take 1 dose and wait.

☞ MASSAGE

Using the pads of your fingers and thumb, massage over the top of and around the ganglion, using gentle pressure. This treatment, when performed every morning and every evening, will often make the ganglion disappear over time.

••• ORTHODOX

Early treatment used to be to hit a ganglion with a big family Bible, and later with a large and heavy medical textbook! While hardly a "gentle" treatment, this was often an effective way to remove the ganglion temporarily. It frequently returns, however, because the "shell" of the cyst remains behind and closes over the resulting hole. Doctors now recommend leaving ganglions alone, as they often disappear with time. Surgery is sometimes used to remove them, usually if they are cosmetically unattractive or are interfering with tendon function. A "trigger finger" is such an example: One finger gets stuck down in the bent position, and the ganglion prevents its being straightened without active help.

GANGRENE
The death of an area of flesh due to lack of sufficient blood. The flesh becomes painful, then numb, and the skin and tissue turn black. If bacterial infection sets in, it can spread to other areas, causing death to surrounding tissue. People with diabetes, arteriosclerosis, and thrombosis are more susceptible to gangrene. All treatment should be carried out in collaboration with your doctor.

TREATMENT
Treatment of gangrene consists of improving blood circulation to the affected area and preventing infection.

━ PRACTICAL ADVICE
Stop smoking. Smoking inhibits the circulation and makes the condition worse.

Keep warm. Warmth opens up the blood vessels, encouraging circulation of blood.

An area of the body vulnerable to gangrene should be in a postural position that encourages blood circulation. For example, if you have a pre-gangrenous foot, sleep with it hanging down over the side of the bed.

✗ DIETARY
Canadian research has shown good results using vitamin E to accelerate healing in difficult wounds. The study gave patients a daily dose of 800 iu of vitamin E orally, and saturated the wound with vitamin E oil.

☛ MASSAGE
Massage helps increase circulation and hence speeds the healing process. For this condition it is best carried out by a professional therapist.

••• ORTHODOX
Surgery is carried out to bypass or remove blockages in major arteries to restore circulation. Antibiotics are given to prevent infection. Diabetes must be under close supervision to prevent circulatory problems resulting in gangrene.

GAS
See **Flatulence.**

GASTRITIS

Inflammation of the delicate lining of the stomach, often due to irritation from drugs (often aspirin), alcohol, certain foods, tobacco, bacterial infection, peptic ulcers (see **Peptic Ulcer**), or stress. Acid stomach (see **Acid Stomach**) can also be a contributing factor. Symptoms include upper stomach ache, particularly after eating; nausea; and vomiting.

TREATMENT

▬ PRACTICAL ADVICE

Stop smoking.

✗ DIETARY

Reduce your intake of alcohol, caffeine (tea, coffee, cola, cocoa), carbonated drinks, and spicy food.

Increase your intake of noncitrus fruits, raw vegetables, and bland foods, such as brown rice, potatoes, and pasta, and live yogurt that contains *Lactobacillus acidophilus*.

Decrease your intake of refined carbohydrates, such as white bread and rice. These cause a rapid secretion of gastric acid, which is buffered by the protein content of whole-grain carbohydrates.

ἐ HERBALISM

Golden seal infusion is an effective tonic for irritated mucous membranes of the digestive system: Pour 1 cup of boiling water on 1 teaspoon of the powdered herb, and infuse for 10 minutes; drink 3 times a day.

▢ HOMEOPATHY

Take every 30 minutes for up to 4 doses; repeat if necessary:

Burning pains and vomiting, better temporarily with cold drinks: *Phosphorus* 6c

Stomach feels like a stone and is very sensitive to touch: *Bryonia* 6c

Stomach feels like a knot, acid reflux, and hiccups: *Nux vomica* 6c

Pain is better from eating but starts again 2 hours later: *Anacardium* 6c

～ RELAXATION TECHNIQUES

Do not eat when you are in a hurry. Try to take meals in a relaxed state and chew food thoroughly.

Biofeedback, yoga, meditation, and autogenic training can help relieve the stress associated with this condition.

Noncompetitive exercise helps relieve stress: walking, swimming, and running are all good.

Massage and aromatherapy also help with relaxation.

••• ORTHODOX

Doctors diagnose gastritis by examining the stomach lining through a gastroscope (a tube passed through the mouth into the stomach).

Acetaminophen is generally prescribed for pain relief, as aspirin can irritate the stomach lining.

Drugs may be recommended to reduce acid production and heal the stomach lining.

GASTROENTERITIS

Inflammation of the stomach and intestine, usually caused by a virus, bacteria, or toxin in contaminated food or water, or an allergic reaction. Symptoms include nausea, vomiting and diarrhea, stomach pain, and cramp, generally lasting up to forty-eight hours. In infants and the elderly, seek medical advice.

TREATMENT

✗ DIETARY

Do not eat during the attack, but drink plenty of fluids to avoid dehydration: Mix 1 quart of water with 2 scant teaspoons of sugar or honey, and 1 teaspoon of salt; drink as needed.

Once the diarrhea and vomiting have subsided, eat plain, whole-grain foods and vegetables. Bananas help settle the stomach. Live yogurt with *Lactobacillus acidophilus* helps restore protective bacteria to the stomach.

Take a supplement of high-potency *acidophilus* powder: Take ½ teaspoon of *Lactobacillus acidophilus* powder, with 1 teaspoon of *Bifidobacteria* powder, and ½ teaspoon of *Lactobacillus bulgaricus* (available from natural foods stores), in a glass of spring water, 3 times a day.

੩ HERBALISM

Meadowsweet infusion reduces acidity in the stomach, soothes the mucous membranes, and reduces nausea: Pour 1 cup of boiling water on 2 teaspoons of the dried herb, and infuse for 15 minutes; drink 3 times a day.

After the attack, decoction of slippery elm will help soothe the digestive tract: Use 1 part of the powdered bark to 8 parts of water. Mix well, bring to a boil, and simmer for 15 minutes; drink ½ cup 3 times a day.

☐ HOMEOPATHY

Take 1 dose every 10 minutes for up to 6 doses; repeat if necessary:

Profuse diarrhea accompanied by burning and colicky stomach, restlessness, anxiety, and chilliness: *Arsenicum album* 6c

Vomiting and diarrhea, with profuse cold sweats: *Veratrum album* 6c

After stimulants (coffee, alcohol, spices), alternating with fruitless urging: *Nux vomica* 6c

Burning in the rectum and anus, with involuntary evacuations: *Aloe* 6c

Greenish, painless diarrhea, with gurgling and stomach cramps, worse early morning: *Podophyllum* 6c

••• ORTHODOX

Your doctor should identify the microbiological cause of the condition. Use antibiotics only in extreme cases of infection; they are not generally recommended because they kill off healthy intestinal flora.

GERMAN MEASLES
See **Rubella.**

GIARDIASIS

An infection of the small intestine by the parasite *Giardia lamblia,* which is passed through contaminated food or water or direct hand or mouth contact. It is common in tropical countries and, more recently, in developed countries, where it spreads among people in institutions, particularly preschool children. Many seemingly clean rivers are infected with *Giardia,* which is spread by grazing animals throughout the United States. Symptoms include violent, foul-smelling diarrhea and gas, abdominal discomfort, and nausea. Children with giardiasis tend to eat poorly, and are tired, miserable, and lose weight. Stools will be loose and smelly.

PREVENTION

Always wash your hands thoroughly before handling food or eating. Dry your hands on disposable towels, with an air blower, or use your own personal towel.

In tropical countries consume only well-cooked food and bottled or boiled water.

Avoid drinking water from rivers without boiling it first.

Make sure children have a good supply of healthy intestinal bacteria to help them resist infections such as giardiasis. Children under 77 pounds can take ¼ teaspoon of *Lactobacillus acidophilus* 3 times a day, with ¼ teaspoon of *Bifidobacteria* powder, in a glass of water.

TREATMENT

Antibiotics (see Orthodox, below) are required to rid the body of the parasite. The following self-help measures complement orthodox treatment.

✗ DIETARY

To avoid dehydration (particularly important in children and the elderly), mix 1 teaspoon of salt with 1 pint of boiled water, and 2 scant teaspoons of sugar. Drink 1 pint of the mixture every hour until symptoms subside.

Grated apple left in the air to go brown helps settle the stomach.

❧ HERBALISM

Golden seal infusion helps settle the system: Pour 1 cup of boiling water on 2 teaspoons of the dried root, and infuse for 15 minutes; drink 3 times a day.

☐ HOMEOPATHY

Take 1 dose every 10 minutes for up to 6 doses; repeat if necessary:

Profuse diarrhea accompanied by burning and colicky stomach, restlessness, anxiety, and chilliness: *Arsenicum album* 6c

Vomiting and diarrhea, with profuse cold sweats: *Veratrum album* 6c

After stimulants (coffee, alcohol, spices), alternating with fruitless urging: *Nux vomica* 6c

Burning in the rectum and anus, with involuntary evacuations: *Aloe* 6c

Greenish, painless diarrhea, with gurgling and stomach cramps, worse early morning: *Podophyllum* 6c

••• ORTHODOX

Antibiotics, such as metronidazole, are given either in a single dose or over three days. Sometimes a second or third dose is necessary to rid the body of the parasite. Make sure to eat plenty of live yogurt with *Lactobacillus acidophilus* while you are taking antibiotics and afterward, to restore healthy intestinal flora that may be impaired by antibiotics. It is also advisable to take high-potency *acidophilus* powder: Take ½ teaspoon of *Lactobacillus acidophilus,* with 1 teaspoon of *Bifidobacteria* powder, and ½ teaspoon of *Lactobacillus bulgaricus* (available from natural foods stores), in a glass of spring water, 3 times a day.

GINGIVITIS

Inflammation and infection of the gums, often due to a buildup of plaque around the base of the teeth. Gums become red, swollen, and tender, and bleed easily.

TREATMENT

▬ PRACTICAL ADVICE

Good flossing and brushing is the best way to prevent and treat gingivitis. Perform the following routine morning and night: Using at least 5 inches of dental floss, wrap each end around one finger of each hand. Starting with the top right back tooth, wiggle the middle area of the floss between each tooth gently up and down several times. The aim is to remove plaque, not just bits of food caught between the teeth. Work all the way around the mouth.

Brush your teeth gently.

Brush your tongue.

Rinse your mouth several times with cold water.

Use a mouth rinse if you wish.

Be sure to brush your teeth after every meal.

✗ DIETARY

Incorporate plenty of raw fruits and vegetables into your diet.

Increase your intake of vitamin C (found in citrus fruits).

Chewing cardamom seeds has been shown to prevent gum decay.

❧ HERBALISM

For inflamed or bleeding gums, add 2 teaspoons of red sage leaves to 1 pint of water. Bring to a boil and let stand, covered, for 15 minutes; use as a mouth rinse several times a day. **Caution:** Do not use during pregnancy.

Myrrh tincture is an effective antimicrobial: Add 1 to 4 drops to 1 cup of warm water; rinse the mouth with the mixture 3 times a day.

☐ HOMEOPATHY

Take 2 times a day for up to 5 days; repeat if necessary:

Tender, bleeding gums with metallic taste and profuse salivation: *Mercurius solubilis* 6c

Gums bleed from slight touch and bleeding is slow to stop: *Phosphorus* 6c

••• ORTHODOX

Regular visits to the dentist should include professional cleaning and removal of plaque. Your dentist may recommend an antibacterial mouthwash.

GLANDULAR FEVER
See **Mononucleosis, Infectious.**

GLAUCOMA

A condition in which fluid builds up in the eye, causing an increase in pressure that can damage delicate tissues and lead to gradual vision loss. Symptoms include an aching or throbbing pain in and above the eye, gradual loss of peripheral vision, and the perception of rainbow rings around lights. Glaucoma is symptom free in the early stages; regular eye exams can help detect this problem before too much damage occurs.

TREATMENT

Treatment must be carried out in collaboration with your doctor or ophthalmologist.

✕ DIETARY

The most documented treatment of glaucoma by natural means is through supplementation with vitamin C. Since the quantities involved are larger than those contained in most supplements, you should see a naturopath for advice.

Increase your intake of bioflavonoids, which improve integrity of the blood capillaries and strengthen the tissues of the eye. Bioflavonoids are found in the skin, pith, and outer layer of fruits and vegetables, such as citrus fruits (try to obtain organic fruits if you intend to eat the peel), leafy vegetables, red onions, beetroot, and the blue or red pigment in berries.

Reduce your intake of alcohol and caffeine (tea, coffee, cola, chocolate), which can interfere with blood circulation to the eye.

Increase vitamin A–rich foods, such as liver, kidney, egg yolk, butter, cheese, dairy products, and cod liver oil.

Do not smoke.

≈ HYDROTHERAPY

To stimulate circulation to the eyes: Prepare two bowls of water, one with hot but not boiling water, one with ice-cold water. Soak a face cloth in the hot water, wring it out, place on the eyes for 2 to 3 minutes, and remove; do the same with the cold. Alternate hot and cold 3 times.

❖ REFLEXOLOGY

Massage the reflex to the eye: at the base of the second and third toes, just below where they join the sole of the left foot.

✚ PROFESSIONAL HELP

The Bates Method of eye exercises may help this condition (see **Eyesight Problems**).

••• ORTHODOX

Ophthalmologists prescribe eye drops or drugs to reduce the rate of fluid production in the eye, or to increase its outflow.

Laser surgery may be used to open up the channels through which excess fluid can be drained away.

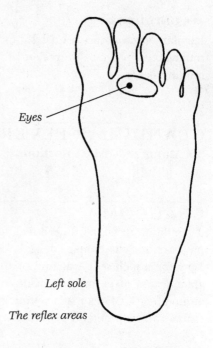

Eyes

Left sole

The reflex areas

GLUE EAR

A discharge of thick, yellow mucus from the ear, usually the result of persistent ear infections, colds, or chest complaints, which "glues up" the middle ear and restricts hearing. It may be triggered by cold weather or swimming. See also **Earache and Ear Infections.**

PREVENTION

Research shows that fewer ear infections occur in children who are breast-fed.

TREATMENT
✗ DIETARY

The buildup of mucus in the ear may result from food allergies. See **Allergies, Food,** for suggestions on testing for common allergens and how to avoid them.

Certain foods are thought to affect mucus production. Avoid cow's milk products (replace with goat's milk or soy milk), roast peanuts, and excessive sugar.

Foods that reduce mucus include garlic, onions, watercress, parsley, and celery. Try to encourage a whole-foods diet with plenty of fresh fruits and vegetables, grains, and lean meat or fish.

₰ HERBALISM

Golden seal is an effective remedy to reduce mucus: Take ¼ to ½ teaspoon of the tincture in water 3 times a day. This is a long-term treatment that could take 3 to 4 months to produce results.

☐ HOMEOPATHY

It is best to seek professional help, although the remedies listed for earache may be helpful in the short term.

❁ BACH FLOWER REMEDIES

Passion Flower and Rescue Remedy can help a child who is frightened or panicked by the pain: Give 2 drops of each under the tongue.

✴ BIOCHEMIC TISSUE SALTS

If there is thick mucus: *Kali Mur*
For intense pain: *Ferr Phos*

≈ HYDROTHERAPY

Hold a warm hot water bottle wrapped in a kitchen towel against the ear to provide relief.

✳ ACUPRESSURE

For acute pain: Gently massage down the outside of the child's arm, from the elbow to the wrist, between the two bones that make up the arm. Repeat 20 times on both arms.

✚ PROFESSIONAL HELP

Acupuncture may help improve drainage to the ear.

••• ORTHODOX

If the pressure of mucus builds up, surgery may be recommended to pierce the eardrum and allow the pus to drain out. A grommet is generally inserted to leave the hole open to drain future fluid and allow the lining of the middle ear cavity to dry out. The operation may weaken the eardrum, and you should not swim or bathe without wearing molded ear plugs.

GOITER

Enlargement of the thyroid gland at the front of the neck, which may be caused by lack of adequate dietary iodine. The gland is unable to produce enough thyroxine, and becomes enlarged in an attempt to increase production. Goiter can also develop when the gland becomes overactive or underactive (see **Hyperthyroidism; Hypothyroidism**). Symptoms include feeling hot, palpitations, irritability, weight loss, disturbed menstrual periods, and sometimes bulging eyes.

TREATMENT

Consultation with your doctor is important to determine the cause of the goiter, as treatment will vary accordingly. The recommendations below are for goiter caused by iodine deficiency. See **Hyperthyroidism** and **Hypothyroidism** for other treatments.

✗ DIETARY

Increase your intake of iodine, found in fresh saltwater shellfish and seafood, iodized salt, and foods grown on iodine-rich soil.

Some foods can inhibit your intake of iodine. If you are deficient, avoid foods such as cabbage, soybeans, turnips, mustard, cassava root, peanuts, pine nuts, and millet.

❧ HERBALISM

Bugleweed is used to treat an overactive thyroid gland, especially when symptoms include tight chest or nervous palpitations: Pour 1 cup of boiling water over 1 teaspoon of the dried herb, and infuse for 15 minutes; drink 3 times a day.

Bladderwrack, a common seaweed, has been shown to help goiter caused by an underactive thyroid gland: Pour 1 cup of boiling water onto 3 teaspoons of the dried herb, and infuse for 10 minutes; drink 3 times a day.

••• ORTHODOX

Drugs can usually correct thyroid function, but surgery may be required if individual areas of the gland are separately affected, or if a large goiter causes pressure symptoms in the neck.

GONORRHEA

See **Sexually Transmitted Diseases.**

GOUT

A buildup of uric acid crystals in the joints, especially the big toe, which becomes red, inflamed, and very painful. Gout is often an inherited condition, though it may also result from kidney malfunction, blood disorders, overindulgence in rich food and alcohol, or some drugs.

TREATMENT

✗ DIETARY

Reduce your intake of foods that stimulate the production of uric acid: fatty fish, anchovies, shellfish, meat and meat stock, and caffeine (coffee, tea, cola, chocolate).

Cherries have been found to relieve symptoms. Eat at least ½ pound every day, if available.

Take 1 gram of vitamin C a day.

Drink 6 to 8 glasses of water a day.

Avoid alcohol, which increases uric acid production.

Charcoal tablets can help reduce uric acid levels: Take 1 tablet 4 times a day.

✿ HERBALISM

Celery seed increases the elimination of uric acid: Pour 1 cup of water on 2 teaspoons of the crushed seeds, and infuse for 15 minutes; drink 3 times a day.

☐ HOMEOPATHY

To help eliminate uric acid: *Urtica urens* tincture, 3 drops in ½ glass of water, 2 times a day.

Take every 15 minutes for up to 4 doses; repeat if necessary:

- Joint feels cold but is alleviated by cold bathing, patient misanthropic: *Ledum* 6c
- Joint very painful, especially at night, patient very irritable and sensitive to rudeness: *Colchicum* 6c
- Joint feels bruised, patient terrified of being approached in case the toe is touched: *Arnica* 30c

≈ HYDROTHERAPY

Apply an ice pack to the painful area: Make an ice pack by wrapping a plastic bag full of ice cubes or a bag of frozen peas in a kitchen towel. Hold on the joint for 3 to 5 minutes, at regular intervals.

❖ REFLEXOLOGY

Massage of the area affected by gout will be painful, therefore reflexologists direct treatment at the "zone-related area," that is, a corresponding area in the body that links up to the reflexes of the affected area. In the case of gout, massage the hands and fingers on the same side as the affected foot.

••• ORTHODOX

Doctors generally prescribe nonsteroidal anti-inflammatory drugs to relieve pain and inflammation.

GRAVES' DISEASE
See **Hyperthyroidism.**

GROIN STRAIN

Pain and stiffness in the groin, due to overstretching muscles on the inside of the thigh. Groin strain is usually brought on by sudden exertion. To distinguish it from other ailments, attempt to bring the knee up to the stomach: this activates the strained muscles and intensifies the pain.

PREVENTION

The following yoga stretches are good warm-ups before exercising, and can help to prevent groin strain:

Stand with feet together, legs straight. Clasp your hands behind your back, arms straight, and bend forward from the waist. Return to standing and repeat several times.

Stand with feet together, legs straight. Clasp your hands behind your back, arms straight, and bend forward from the waist. Bend one knee slightly, straighten, then bend the other knee. Repeat several times.

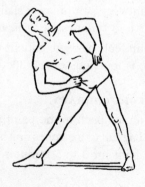

Triangle Pose: Place hands on hips, and spread the legs apart to shoulder width. Turn the right foot 90 degrees to the right and the left foot slightly inward to the right.

Keeping your body facing forward, move your trunk down toward the right leg. Hold for as long as is comfortable, then repeat on the other side.

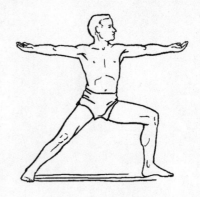

Place hands on hips, and spread the legs apart to shoulder width. Turn the right foot 90 degrees to the right and the left foot slightly inward to the right. Bend your right knee so that the thigh is parallel to the floor and the back leg is fully extended. Stretch your arms out to the side. Hold for as long as is comfortable, then repeat on the other leg.

TREATMENT

❊ AROMATHERAPY

Essential oil of sweet marjoram and rosemary help dull the pain: Add 3 drops of each to a warm bath, and soak in it.

≈ HYDROTHERAPY

Immediately after the injury, place an ice pack on the affected area: Make an ice pack by wrapping a plastic bag full of ice cubes or a bag of frozen peas in a kitchen towel. Place it on the muscle for 10 minutes; remove for 10 minutes, and repeat.

✚ PROFESSIONAL HELP

Massage or chiropractic will both help.

••• ORTHODOX

You doctor will probably recommend physiotherapy and rest.

 # H

HAIR, DRY

Some people are born with dry, brittle hair, as a result of having few oil glands in the scalp. Providing you follow the practical advice below, your hair should remain in good condition. In some cases dry hair may result from a dietary deficiency; occasionally, it is one of the first signs of thyroid problems (see **Goiter; Hyperthyroidism; Hypothyroidism**). A simple blood test to measure blood thyroxine levels can rule out this cause. Excessive cosmetic treatments and blow drying can also contribute to dry hair.

TREATMENT

■ PRACTICAL ADVICE

Avoid excessive use of cosmetics on the hair.

Use a mild shampoo, once or twice a week.

Avoid blow drying, hot rollers, or curling tongs.

Avoid excessive bleaching, tinting, and perming.

As an alternative to chemical dyes and hair tints, use natural herbal dyes such as henna, which strengthen the hair and give shine.

✗ DIETARY

Deficiencies of the following nutrients can cause dry, brittle hair:

- protein, found in lean meats, fish, cheese, cooked dried beans, and soybeans
- vitamin A, found in liver, kidney, egg yolk, butter, cheese, and milk
- vitamin B12, found in lean meats, poultry, fish, shellfish, milk, organ meats, cheese, and eggs
- vitamin C, found in fresh fruits and vegetables
- iron, found in red meat, dried fruits, dark green leafy vegetables, fish, and whole-grain breads and cereals
- zinc, found in oysters, lean meat, poultry, fish, organ meats, and whole-grain breads and cereals

Increase your intake of fatty acids, found in seeds and nuts.

Take a multivitamin and mineral supplement to help remedy any deficiencies.

••• ORTHODOX

Your doctor may refer you to a dermatologist.

HAIR, EXCESSIVE

Excessive hair growth (also referred to as hypertrichosis) is usually hereditary in origin. At times, however, it can result from a hormonal imbalance that produces growth in male patterns on the face, chest, and legs of women (also known as hirsutism). This commonly occurs at puberty or menopause, or when an adrenal gland tumor develops. Excessive hair growth can also result from taking certain drugs.

TREATMENT

○ COSMETIC

In cases where hair growth is a hereditary characteristic, treatment is purely cosmetic. The following are some of the common methods used to remove or disguise excess body hair.

Bleaching: removal of color from hair with chemical preparations. Very dark hair can be bleached using commercially prepared bleaches, or you can make your own: Mix ½ cup of 20 volume peroxide to a paste with soap flakes, and add 2 teaspoons of ammonia. Mix well, spread on hair for 10 to 15 minutes, then wash off. Repeat every few days until hairs are colorless; then repeat each month. To bleach facial hair, use a specially prepared cosmetic bleach, and test on a small area of skin first.

Shaving: removal of hair with hand razor or electric razor. Shaving leaves a hard stubble and has to be repeated at least twice a week. It is not advised on the face.

Cream depilatories: removal of hair with a chemical cream that dissolves the hair. The effect is much like shaving. It is advisable to test the cream on a small area of skin, as the products are harsh and may be problematic on sensitive skins.

Waxing: removal of hair with cold or warm wax that sticks to the hair. When the wax is pulled off, the hairs come with it, pulled out by the roots. The method can be uncomfortable (much like removing an adhesive bandage from the skin). Regrowth is slower than with shaving or depilation, and does not produce a stubble. Waxing can be done in a professional beauty salon, or with home waxing kits. It is advisable to have facial hair removed professionally, at least the first time.

Sugaring: a method similar to waxing, widely practiced in Arabic countries. A sugar paste is spread on the skin and pulled off along with the hair.

Plucking: plucking excess hair using sterilized tweezers. This method is appropriate for small areas of hair, particularly the eyebrows.

Electrolysis: removal of hair by electrical charge. This results in permanent hair removal, and is the most popular method for removing excess facial hair. A person licensed in electrolysis inserts a needle into the hair follicle; an electric current passed through the needle cauterizes the hair root. The procedure must be repeated several times to stop hair growth. It should be performed by an expert, as scarring can occur.

✚ PROFESSIONAL HELP

Homeopathic treatment can be helpful.

••• ORTHODOX

If hormonal imbalance is the cause of excessive hair growth, your doctor may prescribe anti-androgen medications.

HAIR, GREASY

Oily, greasy hair can be a result of large or numerous oil glands in the scalp, or the production of excessive oil due to hormonal disturbances (particularly during adolescence). Diet can also play a part.

TREATMENT

━ PRACTICAL ADVICE

Wash your hair often with a mild shampoo, every day if necessary.

When washing the hair, use a final rinse made up of the juice of 1 lemon in 1 pint of warm water. This helps close up the hair follicles that produce oil.

Use oil-free conditioners.

✗ DIETARY

Reduce your intake of fats and fried foods.

Increase your intake of fresh fruits and vegetable, whole-grain cereals, and low-fat protein.

Avoid coffee, tea, chocolate, and cola drinks.

HAIR, INGROWN

See **Ingrown Hair.**

HAIR LOSS

Loss or absence of hair, also known as alopecia or balding, is a hereditary and unavoidable condition in some adult men. In young people and women, temporary thinning of the hair may be a result of severe stress or shock. It may also be a side effect of medication, or the result of a dietary deficiency or hormonal imbalance.

TREATMENT

✘ DIETARY

Hair loss resulting from stress, trauma, shock, or long-term illness can be helped by the following dietary recommendations:

Increase your intake of vitamin C, found in fresh fruits and vegetables, particularly citrus fruits and juices, parsley, broccoli, green pepper, and black currants.

Take a 25-milligram vitamin B-complex supplement every day.

Take brewer's yeast: Mix 1 tablespoon in a glass of water; drink 3 times a day.

Increase your intake of protein, found in meat, fish, liver, wheat germ, dried cooked beans and peas, tofu, cheese, milk, and eggs.

▢ HOMEOPATHY

Take morning and night, for up to 1 month:

Hair loss after pregnancy: *Lycopodium* 6c

Hair loss after grief or extreme emotion, accompanied by exhaustion and indifference: *Phosphoric acid* 6c

Hair loss during menopause, with hot sweaty flushes and heavy bleeding: *Sepia* 6c

☯ CHINESE MEDICINE

Chinese doctors believe that hair is nourished by the blood, and thus influenced by the condition of the liver and kidney. Treatment is aimed at toning these organs using fleeceflower root, wolfberry fruit, or mulberry fruit.

Acupuncture may also be recommended.

✚ PROFESSIONAL HELP

Homeopathy may help.

••• ORTHODOX

If you are taking medication, ask your doctor about its potential side effects, and look for alternatives if it causes hair loss. Oral contraceptives, anticoagulants, diet pills, and thyroid medications can all contribute to hair loss.

Transplantation techniques, though limited in their ability to restore thick hair, can be performed.

HALITOSIS
See **Bad Breath.**

HANGOVER
Symptoms of headache, nausea, dizziness, and depression after drinking excessive amounts of alcohol. Many of the effects result from dehydration, and can be avoided by drinking large quantities of water before going to bed.

PREVENTION
Do not drink on an empty stomach.
Take a B-complex vitamin supplement before drinking.
Take 6 to 8 capsules of evening primrose oil before drinking.
Don't mix different drinks.
Eat while you drink.
Drink plenty of water while you drink to avoid dehydration.

TREATMENT
■ PRACTICAL ADVICE
Go out and get some fresh air.
Do not resort to the "hair of the dog." Trying to remedy a hangover with further alcohol only compounds the problem and sets up a dangerous habit of continuous drinking.

✗ DIETARY
Eating carbohydrates helps relieve the symptoms of hangover. A good remedy is a banana milkshake: In a blender, whip 1 banana, ½ glass of milk, and 2 tablespoons of honey. The banana provides potassium lost through alcohol consumption, the milk soothes the stomach, and the honey raises lowered blood sugar.

☙ HERBALISM
Willow bark is a safe, natural source of salicylates, the active ingredient found in aspirin. Take a decoction first thing to relieve a headache: Pour 1 cup of water onto 2 teaspoons of the bark, and simmer for 10 minutes. Drink hot.

☐ HOMEOPATHY
Take 1 tablet every 30 minutes, for up to 6 doses; repeat if needed:
Dizzy from bright lights, brain feels loose, nauseous but unable to vomit, angry and aggressive: *Nux vomica* 6c

Thirsty for large quantities of cold water, splitting headache aggravated by the slightest movement, wants to be left in peace: *Bryonia* 6c

Hot, sweaty, and smelly, with early-morning diarrhea: *Sulphur* 6c

---

HAY FEVER
See **Allergies, Hay Fever, and Rhinitis.**

HEARTBURN
See **Acid Stomach; Indigestion.**

HEADACHE

Pain in the head. Most headaches are due to strain and tension in the neck, facial, or head muscles, resulting from stress or poor posture. A headache can sometimes be a reaction to hunger, caffeine withdrawal, too much sleep, a stuffy room, noise, an allergy (see **Allergies, Food,** and **Allergies, Hay Fever, and Rhinitis**), sinusitis (see **Sinusitis**), low blood sugar (see **Blood Sugar, Low**), or weather changes. Persistent headaches that have no obvious cause, or headaches that wake people in the night or come and go in paroxysms, require medical investigation. See also **Migraine.**

PREVENTION

Eat regular meals.

Get enough sleep.

Take measures to avoid stress.

Get plenty of fresh air and exercise (see below).

Avoid excessive coffee or alcohol consumption.

TREATMENT

❧ AROMATHERAPY

Tension headaches respond well to aromatherapy, particularly essential oil of lavender, known for its relaxing properties. Place 1 or 2 drops of essential oil of lavender on the tips of your fingers, and massage in a circular motion across your temples, around the hollows at the sides of the eyes, behind your ears, and across the back of your neck. **Caution:** Do not let your fingers go too near your eyes.

For headaches of menstrual origin, use essential oil of sweet marjoram for the above massage.

Relax in a warm bath to which you have added 3 drops each of essential oil of sweet marjoram, Roman chamomile, and lavender.

☙ HERBALISM

Valerian infusion is a sedative that helps reduce tension and anxiety: Pour 1 cup of boiling water onto 2 teaspoons of the root, and infuse for 15 minutes; drink before going to bed.

Clinical trials have shown feverfew (*Tanacetum parthenium*) to be an effective painkiller. Use as a preventive measure: Take 2 or 3 small leaves a day, chopped up in a sandwich (a sprinkling of sugar helps to disguise the bitter taste). Feverfew tablets are available from pharmacies and natural foods stores—follow the dosage instructions on the package. You may not see results for two or three months.

☐ HOMEOPATHY

Take every 30 minutes for up to 4 doses; repeat if needed:

Throbbing and hammering, especially at the temples, sensitive to drafts on the head: *Belladonna* 6c

Pain aggravated by the smallest movement, headaches from constipation: *Bryonia* 6c

Head feels enlarged, pain eased by tight bandaging: *Argentum nitricum* 6c

Sensation of a tight band spreading from occiput to forehead, better from passing urine: *Gelsemium* 6c

Sensation of a nail boring down into the head, hypersensitive to noise: *Coffea* 6c

☛ MASSAGE

Massage can relieve tension in the muscles of the scalp, neck, and face. Using the fingertips, briskly massage the whole of the scalp, as if you were washing the hair. Then gently pull the hair all around the head.

✳ ACUPRESSURE

Massage the points illustrated on the following pages to help relieve pain.

❖ EXERCISE

Regular walking, jogging, or swimming helps prevent tension in the neck and shoulder muscles.

The following exercise sequence is a good preventive measure, and will help overcome a headache by relaxing the neck and head muscles:

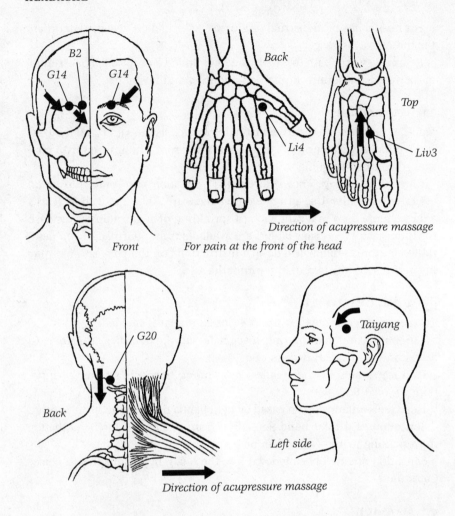

Front

Back

Li4

Top

Liv3

Direction of acupressure massage

For pain at the front of the head

Back

G20

Taiyang

Left side

Direction of acupressure massage

- While sitting, inhale and tip your head back gently, looking up at the ceiling. Don't tip it back too far—this can compress the cervical spine and make matters worse. Exhale and bring the head down so that your chin rests on your chest. Repeat 2 times.
- Exhale and turn your head to look over your right shoulder, keeping your chin level. Inhale as you turn back, looking straight ahead. Exhale as you look over the left shoulder. Inhale as you look straight ahead. Repeat twice on each side.

✚ **PROFESSIONAL HELP**

If headaches are an ongoing problem, it is worth consulting a chiropractor to investigate spinal misalignments that lead to nerve pressure or muscular tension.

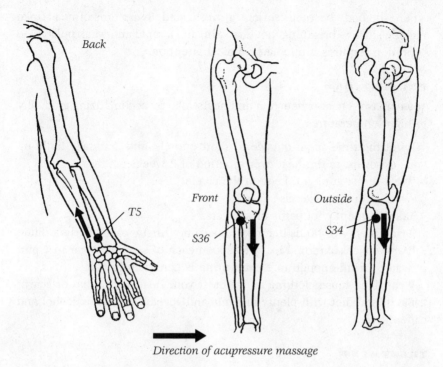

Back

T5

Front

S36

Outside

S34

Direction of acupressure massage

The Alexander Technique may be helpful for headaches related to postural problems (sitting or standing in awkward positions).

••• ORTHODOX

For single, short-term headaches, your doctor will probably recommend mild painkillers and rest.

For recurrent headaches, your doctor will want to identify the cause and treat it accordingly.

HEAT EXHAUSTION
See **Heatstroke.**

HEATSTROKE

Fatigue, fainting, dizziness, nausea, extreme sweating, and headaches resulting from extreme heat are common signs of heat exhaustion. If left untreated this can develop into heatstroke, a life-threatening illness where the body becomes seriously overheated. Symptoms of heatstroke include shallow breathing, hot, dry skin, and a rapid and weak pulse. The condition requires immediate medical attention.

PREVENTION

You can avoid heat exhaustion and heatstroke by acclimatizing gradually to high temperatures:

Limit the time spent outside to short periods, and gradually build up your exposure to the heat over a period of 2 weeks.

Avoid direct sunlight; keep to the shade.

Avoid strenuous exercise.

Take frequent cool baths or showers.

Drink plenty of fluids before you become thirsty, particularly a dilute salt and sugar solution: Mix ¼ teaspoon each of salt and sugar in 1 pint of water. Drink enough to ensure urine is consistently pale.

Wear light, loose clothing and protect your head with a hat or scarf.

Eat a light diet with plenty of fruits and vegetables; avoid alcohol and caffeine.

TREATMENT

For heat exhaustion, lie in a cool place and sip a solution of saltwater.

① **FIRST AID**

A person who does not start to recover from heat exhaustion within 30 minutes, and who has difficulty walking or becomes unconscious, requires emergency medical attention. Move the victim to a cool, shady area and remove clothing. Wrap the person in a cool, wet sheet or towel, or splash the skin with cool water. If the person is conscious, give a solution of saltwater.

▢ **HOMEOPATHY**

Take every 15 minutes for up to 4 doses; repeat if necessary:

Hot red face, throbbing headache: *Belladonna* 30c

Hot red face, throbbing headache, and loss of sense of direction: *Glonoine* 6c

••• **ORTHODOX**

Individuals with severe cases of heatstroke are admitted to the hospital for supervised oral or intravenous hydration.

HEMORRHOIDS

Swollen, protruding veins around the anus; also known as piles. They are a type of varicose vein that can lie inside the rectum or outside. Symptoms and signs include itching and pain and sometimes bleeding when bowels are moved. Hemorrhoids often occur in pregnancy or as a result of constipation or lifting a heavy object. See your doctor if you have any continuous bleeding from the anus.

PREVENTION

Hemorrhoids are rarely seen in countries where a high-fiber, unrefined diet is the norm. Increase your intake of fiber (by eating whole-grain cereals, fruits and vegetables, and low-fat protein) to help prevent hemorrhoids.

TREATMENT

▬ PRACTICAL ADVICE

Try to establish a regular routine to empty the bowels, and never resist or delay the urge to go to the toilet.

Use soft toilet paper or moist wipes to avoid irritating the hemorrhoids. Always wash and dry the area carefully after a bowel movement, finishing any wash or spray with cold water.

Hemorrhoids in pregnancy occur due to the increasing pressure of the uterus on the vessels that drain the hemorrhoidal veins. To relieve the pressure, lie on your left side for 20 minutes every 2 to 4 hours.

✖ DIETARY

The following recommendations will help relieve constipation, the major cause of hemorrhoids (for more suggestions, see **Constipation**):

Drink at least 8 glasses of water per day.

Introduce more fiber into your diet, found in bran, oats, whole-grain breads and cereals, fruits and vegetables, and cooked dried beans and peas.

Avoid coffee, strong spices, beer, and cola, as these can increase irritation.

ঽ HERBALISM

Dab the hemorrhoids with witch hazel solution (this is particularly good if they have a tendency to bleed).

Pilewort ointment: Simmer 2 tablespoons of the fresh or dried herb in seven ounces of petroleum jelly for 10 minutes, strain, and pour liquid into a container; apply to hemorrhoids at least 2 times a day. (You may like to keep an old pan specifically for herbal preparations.)

☐ **HOMEOPATHY**

Take 3 times a day, for up to 4 days; repeat if necessary:

Feels like splinters of broken glass in the rectum on passing a stool: *Ratanhia* 6c

Bruised and sore, with a congested bursting feeling: *Hamamelis* 6c

Sensation of a ball in the rectum, tendency to prolapse, worse during pregnancy: *Sepia* 6c

Hot, burning and itching, worse from getting overheated: *Sulphur* 6c

≈ **HYDROTHERAPY**

Sit in a warm bath to which you have added 4 drops each of essential oil of peppermint and cypress, and 2 tablespoons of bicarbonate of soda.

☞ **MASSAGE**

To help relieve constipation, perform the following routine first thing in the morning, before eating: Oil your hands lightly (olive oil is best). Lie down, and place one hand over the other. Keeping the fingers flat, begin by pressing down about 1 inch into the abdomen at the left corner. Make small, slow circles. Move up a little and repeat. Continue with the same procedure up the left side, across above the umbilicus (including the corners under the ribcage), and down the right side. Then make large, slow, sweeping strokes along the path just covered, but going in the reverse direction. Repeat several times.

••• **ORTHODOX**

Your doctor may prescribe rectal suppositories and creams containing corticosteroid and painkilling drugs to relieve discomfort.

Hemorrhoids are sometimes removed surgically, or may be injected with a sclerosing agent that effectively seals them off and allows them to shrivel up naturally.

HEPATITIS

Inflammation of the liver, often due to a viral infection. There are two types: hepatitis A (infectious hepatitis), which is spread by infected bowel movements passed from hand to mouth, or through infected water or food; and hepatitis B (serum hepatitis), which is spread by infected blood or body fluids. Symptoms include jaundice (yellowing of the skin), fever, severe fatigue, nausea, vomiting, headaches, and aching muscles. The condition can sometimes lead to irreversible liver damage and death, so use self-help treatments only in consultation with your doctor or other health professional.

PREVENTION

The hepatitis A vaccine is recommended for people who will have close contact with patients with the illness (such as family members and medical staff), to offer protection against outbreaks in households or institutions.

The hepatitis B vaccine is recommended for intimate contacts of sufferers of acute hepatitis B, and sexual contacts of highly infectious carriers.

TREATMENT

✗ DIETARY

Naturopaths use a number of dietary measures to treat hepatitis. Since these often require taking large doses of vitamins, it is advisable to carry out treatment under the supervision of a professional. Naturopaths may make the following recommendations:

Avoid alcohol.

Reduce your intake of saturated fats, fried food, and refined carbohydrates (white flour and sugar). Increase your intake of fiber (whole-grain cereals, fruits and vegetables, and cooked dried beans and peas), which encourage the elimination of bile acids and toxins that accumulate in the liver and gallbladder.

Some studies have shown that large doses of vitamin C improve viral hepatitis. Naturopaths recommend between 10 and 50 grams a day, or to bowel tolerance (that is, if you start to get diarrhea, lower the dose).

Vitamin B12 and folic acid have been shown to reduce recovery time. The B vitamins should be taken together in a daily 25-milligram vitamin B-complex supplement.

❧ HERBALISM

Dandelion is a well-recognized liver remedy: Put 3 teaspoons of the root into 1 cup of water, and simmer for 15 minutes; drink 3 times a day. Dandelion leaves can also be eaten raw in salad.

Milk thistle is said to promote the regeneration of diseased liver cells: Make an infusion by pouring 1 cup of water on 1 teaspoonful of the bruised seeds, and allow to stand for 10 minutes; drink 3 times a day.

Globe artichoke stimulates the elimination of bile from the body, an important factor in the treatment of hepatitis. Eat the fresh vegetable as often as possible.

☯ CHINESE MEDICINE

Practitioners of traditional Chinese medicine would treat this condition with acupuncture, and with herbs such as oriental wormwood and gardenia fruit.

••• ORTHODOX

Doctors generally recommend bed rest and abstinence from alcohol for at least 6 months. Steroid drugs may be prescribed to prevent further damage to the liver.

HERNIA

A condition in which part of an organ, usually the intestine, protrudes through a weak area of the abdominal wall. The first sign is a bulge in the abdominal wall, the groin or scrotum, the thigh, or the navel. Hernias are often a result of a congenital weakness in the abdominal wall. Sometimes they are caused by lifting or straining. If you find a tender bulge, consult your doctor. See also **Hernia, Hiatus.**

PREVENTION

▬ PRACTICAL ADVICE

Learn to lift correctly: Bend at the knees, not from the waist.

✕ DIETARY

Maintain your weight within recommended guidelines; carrying excess weight puts a strain on your entire body. (See **Obesity** for suggestions on weight loss.)

⊹ EXERCISE

Strengthen the stomach muscles with the following exercise: Lie on your back and bend your knees, leaving your feet flat on the floor. Lift your buttocks and lower back off the floor, leaving your feet and shoulders on the floor supporting the weight. Lower yourself down gently. Repeat 10 times a day.

TREATMENT

••• ORTHODOX

If you suspect a hernia, consult your doctor. He or she may try to push the hernia back, and may advise you to wear a supportive garment temporarily to hold it in place. Hernias that cannot be pushed back are removed or can be repositioned surgically. After treatment, do not lift any heavy objects for at least three months.

✻ BIOCHEMIC TISSUE SALTS

Calc Fluor 6x: Take 3 times a day to improve tissue tone.

HERNIA, HIATUS

A condition in which part of the stomach protrudes up into the chest, causing acid reflux from the stomach to the esophagus, heartburn, and pains in the chest. Hiatus hernia often occurs in people who are obese and those who smoke.

TREATMENT

▬ PRACTICAL ADVICE

To prevent regurgitation of food during the night and heartburn, raise the head of the bed slightly: place bricks or boards under the legs, or wedge the mattress using foam rubber or a bolster.

✗ DIETARY

Avoid being overweight (see **Obesity** for suggestions).

Eat small meals, slowly; do not eat late at night.

Do not lie down or bend over immediately after eating.

Avoid fatty and spicy foods, alcohol, and cigarettes.

Drink vegetable juices and herbal teas instead of coffee, tea, and cola, and do not drink during meals.

The Hay Diet improves digestion and therefore reduces reflux. It is described in several books, including *Food Combining for Health* by Doris Grant and Jean Joice (see Suggested Reading).

🍂 HERBALISM

Decoction of slippery elm: Mix 1 part of the powdered bark in 8 parts water, and simmer for 10 minutes; drink ½ cup 3 times a day.

✤ EXERCISE

Do the following exercise to strengthen stomach muscles: Lie on your back with your knees bent and feet flat on the floor. Lift your buttocks and lower back off the floor, leaving your feet and shoulders on the floor, supporting the weight. Lower yourself gently. Repeat 10 times a day.

✚ PROFESSIONAL HELP

Hiatus hernia responds well to homeopathy and chiropractic.

••• ORTHODOX

Your doctor will probably recommend antacids. In severe cases surgery may be needed to return the hernia to the stomach.

HERPES, GENITAL

A virus, usually transmitted through sexual contact, that brings an itching, burning, painful rash of small blisters in the genital area. The blisters burst, leaving small ulcers, which take around two weeks to heal. Other symptoms include swollen glands, fever, and headache. Women often find urination painful. Sometimes sores also form around the mouth. See also **Cold Sores.**

TREATMENT

The herpes virus remains in the body and may become active when you are run down or under stress. Exposure to bright sunlight, menstruation, and injury can also trigger the virus. The following treatments will help reduce the severity of the attack.

▬ PRACTICAL ADVICE

Do not have intercourse when you or your partner have an attack of herpes.

Do not share towels, sponges, or lipsticks.

Make sure to wash your hands well after touching the genital area during an attack.

To help prevent further attacks, keep your immune system healthy: eat sensibly, exercise regularly, and use stress reduction techniques (see **Stress**).

Avoid exposing the blisters to sunlight, which can activate the virus.

✗ DIETARY

The amino acids arginine and lysine have been found to influence the incidence of herpes attacks:

- Reduce your intake of arginine, found in nuts, carob, chocolate, gelatin, coconut, oats, whole-grain and white flour, peanuts, soybeans, and wheat germ.

- Increase your intake of lysine, found in fish, shrimp, prawns, chicken, lamb, milk, cheese, beans, brewer's yeast, bean sprouts, fruits, and vegetables.
- Take 1.5 grams of lysine a day as a preventive measure. Increase the dose to 3 grams a day during an attack.

Take 1 gram of vitamin C with bioflavonoids every day during an attack.

≋ HYDROTHERAPY

During an attack, take frequent warm baths to which you have added 3 tablespoons of salt.

✚ PROFESSIONAL HELP

Homeopathic treatment can help to reduce the frequency and severity of the attacks.

••• ORTHODOX

Antiviral medication, such as acyclovir, is given as a cream to reduce the duration and severity of the attack. Tablets are occasionally used to prevent recurrent attacks.

HICCUPS

A sudden contraction of the diaphragm that allows air to rush suddenly into the lungs, causing the vocal cords to close. Generally, hiccups are not serious, though they are often uncomfortable. Occasionally, prolonged hiccups can result from irritation of the diaphragm or the nerves that supply it as a result of pneumonia, stomach problems, alcoholism, or hepatitis. Prolonged attacks can be exhausting, and surgery may be recommended.

TREATMENT

Everyone has their own popular remedy for short bouts of hiccups; the following are a few of the most tried and tested ones:

Breathe into a paper bag.
Eat 1 teaspoon of sugar.
Squirt lemon juice into the back of the throat.
Suck a wedge of lemon.
For babies, give water with sugar added.

☯ CHINESE MEDICINE

Practitioners of traditional Chinese medicine commonly prescribe ginger rhubarb and berilla stems. Persistent cases are treated with acupuncture.

HIGH BLOOD PRESSURE
See **Blood Pressure, High.**

HIVES

A skin condition that brings itchy lumps (whitish with a red inflamed area around them); also known as urticaria or nettle rash. Hives are often triggered by an allergic reaction to food (see **Allergies, Food**); food additives; drugs, particularly aspirin; insect bites; or stress (see **Stress**). If the eyes, lips, or throat are affected, seek medical attention, as breathing may be impaired.

TREATMENT

Finding the cause of the hives and avoiding it is the best cure. To relieve the attack, the following remedies are helpful.

✗ DIETARY

Possible food triggers include strawberries, shellfish, tomatoes, chocolate, eggs, wheat, nuts, food additives, or milk. Try excluding each of these from your diet one by one to see if symptoms are relieved.

❧ HERBALISM

For hives brought on by anxiety or stress, try valerian infusion: Pour 1 cup of boiling water onto 2 teaspoons of the root (powder or pieces), and infuse for 10 minutes; drink during periods of stress.

Aloe vera gel soothes the rash.

☐ HOMEOPATHY

Take every 15 minutes for up to 4 doses; repeat if necessary:
Stinging, itchy rash, especially if triggered by shellfish: *Urtica urens* 6c
Burning and itching rash after getting wet: *Rhus toxicodendron* 6c
Dusky pink rash, with swelling of lips, eyelids, or throat: *Apis* 6c

≈ HYDROTHERAPY

Use one of the following:
Add 3 tablespoons of sodium bicarbonate to a bath, to relieve itching.
Add 5 tablespoons of oatmeal to the bath to soothe the rash.
Add 1 cup of vinegar to the bathwater to restore the skin's pH balance. Alternatively, apply a diluted vinegar solution to affected areas with a sterile cotton ball.

••• ORTHODOX

Your doctor will probably recommend calamine lotion to relieve itching, along with antihistamine drugs. In cases of anaphylactic shock, where the lips, tongue, and eyes are affected, and there is difficulty breathing, emergency hospital treatment is imperative.

HOUSEMAID'S KNEE

Inflammation of the pocket of tissue covering the kneecap, usually as a result of prolonged kneeling or a blow to the knee. The pocket fills with fluid and the kneecap becomes swollen, red, and painful.

TREATMENT

■ PRACTICAL ADVICE

When the knee is very painful, rest is the best treatment. Try to elevate the leg as much as possible, and do not kneel.

🌿 HERBALISM

A comfrey poultice eases the pain: Place a handful of fresh or dried comfrey leaves in a saucepan, cover with water, and bring to a boil. Remove from the heat, and place the leaves between 2 pieces of gauze. Allow to cool slightly, then place on the knee. The gauze should be hot but not burning. When the poultice cools, maintain the warmth by putting a hot water bottle wrapped in a towel on the knee.

☐ HOMEOPATHY

Take *Ruta graveolens* 6c, 3 times a day, for up to 7 days.
Apply *Ruta* cream locally.

≈ HYDROTHERAPY

Hot and cold treatment increases circulation to the area, relieves inflammation, and removes toxins. Make an ice pack by wrapping a plastic bag full of ice cubes or a bag of frozen peas in a kitchen towel. Prepare a hot water bottle, and wrap a towel around it. Place the ice pack on the knee for 10 minutes, then the hot water bottle; alternate several times. Perform this procedure morning and night.

☞ MASSAGE

Have an experienced professional massage the muscles above and below the knee joint to help encourage circulation and remove toxins from the area.

✛ EXERCISE

Once the pain and inflammation have subsided, exercise is very important to mobilize the joint. Do these exercises as often as is possible and comfortable:

Sit upright on a chair. Raise and straighten your right leg and push your heel away from you, then bend the knee fully. Repeat 5 times.

Sit upright on a chair. Raise your leg and circle it clockwise 5 times, then counterclockwise 5 times. Repeat.

Swimming is also very beneficial.

••• ORTHODOX

Your doctor will recommend rest and possibly painkillers; he or she may prescribe antibiotics if infection is present within the fluid or on the skin surface. Elastic support bandages discourage further buildup of fluid.

HYPERACTIVITY

A disorder in infants and children, manifested by abnormally overactive and restless behavior. Hyperactive babies are fidgety and cry incessantly, they often have eczema, and they eat poorly. Hyperactive children typically rock the crib, bang their heads, and are generally difficult. In school they are disruptive, unable to keep still, and have a tendency to throw things. They also exhibit short attention spans, poor coordination, and tearfulness.

✗ DIETARY

Research has shown a clear link between certain foods, additives, and hyperactivity. A strictly whole-foods diet that includes plenty of lean meat and fish and fresh fruit and vegetables is recommended for hyperactive children; zinc supplements have been shown to be beneficial. Avoid food and drink from the following list:

junk foods and processed foods

all foods and drinks with synthetic coloring, flavoring, and additives (tartrazine, E102, is especially suspect)

all aspirin preparations and artificially flavored vitamin pills and children's medicines

sugar, and foods and drinks that contain sugar

any food your child is allergic to (common allergens include milk, corn, wheat, and eggs; see **Allergies, Food**)

tap water (it can sometimes contain ingredients that cause hyperactivity, so drink only bottled spring water)

✿ HERBALISM

Research has shown that hyperactive children are often deficient in essential fatty acids. These can be replenished by supplementation with evening primrose oil. Studies have shown that 3 500-milligram capsules of evening primrose oil, taken morning and evening for 6 to 8 weeks, dropping back to 500 milligrams morning and evening, brings an improvement. Rubbing the oil into the skin can also help.

✚ PROFESSIONAL HELP

Homeopathy has been found to be helpful. Applied kinesiology can help identify specific sensitivities.

••• ORTHODOX

Some doctors recommend stimulant drugs to motivate the part of the brain that suppresses excess activity. The drugs also suppress appetite, however, thus reducing growth in children, and can cause nausea and abdominal pain. Psychotherapy and assessment for special educational needs may help you decide the best course for your child.

HYPERTENSION
See **Blood Pressure, High.**

HYPERTHYROIDISM

Overactivity of the thyroid gland and subsequent excessive production of thyroid hormones. The most common form of hyperthyroidism is Graves' disease, an autoimmune disorder in which the body produces antibodies that stimulate the production of thyroid hormones. Symptoms include weight loss, increased appetite, sweating and heat, bulging eyes, and sometimes tremors. It is most common in middle-aged women.

TREATMENT

Professional help is recommended for this condition. Some of the remedies that may be offered are listed below.

✗ DIETARY

A natural, whole-foods diet is recommended. Eat plenty of onions, seafood, and vegetables grown organically on iodine-rich soil.

?❧ HERBALISM

Bugleweed is recommended, particularly if the condition brings palpitations and tight chest: Pour 1 cup of boiling water on 1 teaspoon of the herb, and infuse for 15 minutes; drink 3 times a day.

☯ CHINESE MEDICINE

Hyperthyroidism is thought to be caused by heat in the liver. Marine plants and seaweed are prescribed. Acupuncture can be helpful.

✚ PROFESSIONAL HELP

Professional homeopathic treatment may be helpful.

••• ORTHODOX

Your doctor will recommend drugs to inhibit the production of thyroid hormones. Surgery may be needed to remove part of the thyroid gland.

HYPOGLYCEMIA
See **Blood Sugar, Low.**

HYPOTHERMIA

An abnormal fall in body temperature to 95° F or below. Symptoms include shivering, slow pulse, pallor, lack of energy, drowsiness, and confusion, which may lead to lowered heart rate and breathing rate and loss of consciousness. The condition is common in elderly people living alone in poorly heated homes. Hypothermia requires immediate medical attention.

PREVENTION

To prevent hypothermia in the elderly, make sure the living area is heated to at least 65° F. They should wear warm clothing (including a hat, if temperatures are low). It is important to eat hot food and drink warm drinks several times a day.

When walking or climbing in cold, isolated locations, always carry a survival bag that includes a space blanket.

TREATMENT

① FIRST AID

Cover the victim's head. Give warm drinks, but no alcohol. Do not rub the skin or expose the victim to direct heat (for example, do not use hot water), as this may cause death. Instead, gradually warm the victim by moving him or her to a warm place, if possible, covering with blankets, and giving hot drinks. Contact a doctor immediately, or call for emergency medical help. If you are outside, get into a sleeping bag with the person to transfer your body heat.

••• ORTHODOX

Treatment varies depending on the age of the victim. Gradual warming with heat-reflecting materials is used. In severe cases patients are admitted to intensive care, where their blood can be warmed.

HYPOTHYROIDISM

Underactivity of the thyroid gland, leading to insufficient production of thyroid hormones, which regulate metabolism. Symptoms include lack of energy, muscle weakness, dry skin and hair, weight gain, and recurrent infections. Sometimes the thyroid gland enlarges, producing a lump at the front of the neck (known as goiter; see **Goiter**). Hypothyroidism in children results in delayed development. Medical diagnosis is made through a blood test. You can also make a diagnosis by taking your temperature for three consecutive mornings: if it is below 97.6° F, consult your doctor.

TREATMENT

Professional help is recommended for this condition. Some of the remedies you may encounter are listed below.

✗ DIETARY

Treatment consists of supplementing the diet with natural thyroid hormones fabricated from iodine and the amino acid tyrosine:

Increase your intake of iodine, found in seafood, shellfish, seaweed, and kelp. Use iodized salt.

Avoid foods that inhibit the uptake of iodine, such as turnips, cabbage, soybeans, peanuts, pine nuts, and mustard.

Take supplements of the amino acid tyrosine: 250 milligrams a day.

Increase your intake of the following nutrients:

- vitamin A, found in liver, kidney, egg yolk, butter, fortified margarine, cheese and cream, cod liver oil
- vitamin C, found in fresh fruits and vegetables
- vitamin E, found in seeds and seed oils, nuts, and wheat germ

- riboflavin, found in milk products, liver, green leafy vegetables, and mushrooms
- niacin, found in lean meat, chicken, fish, and dried cooked beans
- pyridoxine, found in lean meat, wheat germ, brewer's yeast
- zinc, found in lean meat, oysters, poultry, fish, organ meats, and whole-grain cereals

❧ HERBALISM

Bladderwrack helps regulate thyroid function. Take it in tablet form, or as an infusion: Pour 1 cup of boiling water on 2 teaspoons of the herb, and infuse for 10 minutes; drink 3 times a day.

❖ EXERCISE

Aerobic exercise stimulates the production of thyroid hormones. Try brisk walking, running, swimming, or bicycling for least 15 minutes a day.

••• ORTHODOX

Treatment consists of replacing the deficient hormones with thyroxine, usually for the patient's entire life. A goiter may be surgically removed.

 *I*

IMPETIGO

A contagious bacterial skin infection common in children. Symptoms include reddened skin and blisters that burst, leaving a yellow, crusty appearance, usually around the nose and mouth. When babies are affected, seek medical attention.

TREATMENT

■ PRACTICAL ADVICE

Change bed linen daily; do not share towels, face cloths, or clothes that may spread infection.

✗ DIETARY

Avoid all fruit and sugar, eat plenty of raw and cooked green, yellow, and orange vegetables, whole-grain breads and cereals, vegetable protein, or fish and poultry.

❋ AROMATHERAPY

Essential oil of tea tree, as an oil or ointment, is an effective antibacterial agent. Apply at night.

₹ HERBALISM

Bathe the blisters with marigold solution to resist infection and aid healing: Add 5 drops of marigold tincture to ½ pint of cooled boiled water.

☐ HOMEOPATHY

Take 3 times a day for 3 days; repeat if necessary:

Cracked and scabby nostrils, yellow crust on the chin, whitewashed tongue: *Antimonium crudum* 6c

Thick brown crusts on the face with thick yellow discharge from the eyes: *Dulcamara* 6c

When the rash is on the scalp, and blisters ooze pus: *Mezereum* 6c

••• ORTHODOX

Doctors usually prescribe antibiotic tablets and ointment. Children should stay away from others until the infection clears.

IMPOTENCE

The inability to achieve or maintain an erection, which can result from a number of causes: stress, fatigue, anxiety, guilt, depression, drugs, or alcohol. About 10 percent of cases are caused by physical or structural problems, such as diabetes or spinal cord disorders. An erection may take longer to achieve or occur less frequently as men get older, due to changes in circulation or lowered levels of the male sex hormone, testosterone.

TREATMENT

✗ DIETARY

Avoid alcohol, nicotine, and caffeine. These constrict the blood vessels and inhibit blood flow, needed to achieve an erection.

✲ AROMATHERAPY

Essential oils of clary sage, sandalwood, and ylang ylang are renowned for encouraging relaxation and feelings of sensuality. Try adding 2 drops of each to 4 teaspoons of your massage oil, or to a warm bath.

☯ CHINESE MEDICINE

Practitioners of traditional Chinese medicine believe that too much anxiety can bring an energy stagnation in the liver. Treatment varies depending on the patient, but Sextone and cibot root are often prescribed.

☛ MASSAGE

Learning how to massage each other can be pleasurable and erotic for sexual partners. It is relaxing for the giver and the receiver, slows down lovemaking, and helps open up both partners to communication.

✳ ACUPRESSURE

Acupressure massage of the points shown in the figure on the facing page can be useful in some cases.

♣ EXERCISE

Moderate exercise helps you to relax while boosting energy levels; it also increases physical awareness and stimulates sexuality.

If you are already exercising, don't overdo it. Too much activity can leave you exhausted and reduce stimulation; moderation is the key.

～ RELAXATION TECHNIQUES

General stress and anxiety often inhibit sex drive. Feeling tense about daily activities or events, or nervous about your sexual performance, diverts blood away from the sexual organs.

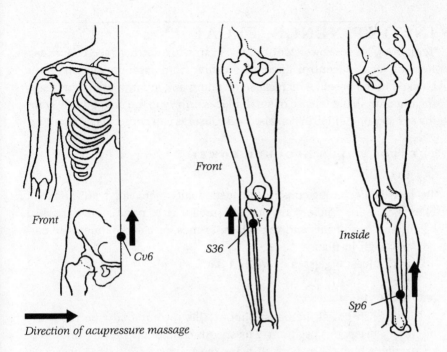

Front

Cv6

Front

S36

Inside

Sp6

Direction of acupressure massage

A yoga or meditation class may help you learn to unwind and relax. Exercise is also a good method, as it usually energizes at the same time as it relieves stress. Aromatherapy and massage are good methods of relaxation. Self-hypnosis and relaxation tapes can also help. Using one of these techniques before you go to bed will help clear your mind of concerns.

You may be able to resolve anxiety about relationships or sex by talking with your partner at a time when you are not trying to "perform." Explaining your concerns honestly without feeling guilty helps dispel anxiety.

Sexual anxiety that is not relieved by the above suggestions may be helped by psychosexual counseling. This is usually carried out with both partners, who are encouraged to relearn their sexual experience together, and explore what is causing the stress in their sexual relationship. Specific exercises may be recommended to break the vicious circle of performance-related anxiety.

••• ORTHODOX

Some medications inhibit erection, so discuss this problem with your doctor if you are taking drugs.

Sex therapy is sometimes offered for psychologically induced impotence.

Penile implants can help men whose impotence is caused by structural problems or disease.

INCONTINENCE, FECAL

Temporary loss of bowel control may occur with diarrhea (see **Diarrhea**). Regular lack of control generally results from fecal impaction—feces blocked in the bowel, which cause irritation and inflammation leading to the uncontrollable release of small pieces. Injury to the anal muscles during surgery or childbirth can also be a cause, as can dementia or paralysis.

TREATMENT FOR BLOCKED BOWEL

DIETARY

Try to avoid becoming constipated by gradually increasing your intake of fiber. Eat more whole-grain cereals (bread, rice, pasta), dried cooked beans, and fresh fruits and vegetables. Prunes, figs, and oatmeal are particularly high in fiber.

Drink at least 6 glasses of water a day.

HERBALISM

For a sluggish bowel, herbalist Simon Mills recommends the following mixture: 4 teaspoons psyllium, 2 teaspoons chamomile flowers, and 1 teaspoon alder buckthorn bark. Powder the mixture and take 1 teaspoon a day.

Decoction of senna is a powerful laxative, to be used only on a short-term basis: Put 1 teaspoon of the dried bark (powdered or broken up) into a saucepan (not aluminum), add 1 cup of water, bring to a boil, and simmer for 15 minutes; strain, and drink 3 times a day.

HOMEOPATHY

Take 3 times a day for 4 days; repeat if needed:

Involuntary evacuation after coughing or sneezing with loss of sensation in the rectum: *Causticum* 6c

Involuntary evacuation when passing urine or flatus: *Aloe* 6c

ACUPRESSURE

Lie on your back, with your knees bent. Place all fingertips on the midpoint of the chest, where the ribs meet. Press firmly down for 30 seconds, breathing deeply; then move the hand down halfway to the navel, and press for 30 seconds, breathing deeply; then move down to midway between the navel and the pubic bone, and press down firmly for a further 30 seconds, breathing deeply.

EXERCISE

Take a 30-minute walk each day, or jog or swim 3 times a week.

✳ YOGA

Rapid abdominal breathing helps activate the digestive system: Exhale forcibly, using the abdomen; then inhale by relaxing the abdomen. Repeat 10 times, allowing the abdomen to go in and out rhythmically; then relax for 20 seconds and do 10 more.

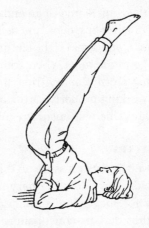

You can make this breathing more effective by doing it while in the Half Shoulder Stand: Lie on your back with your legs straight, and raise your legs as you inhale. Exhale, bringing your hips off the ground. Bend your knees if you want to, and place your hands under your hips to support yourself. While in this position, take 10 breaths quickly in and out, letting your abdomen move in and out rhythmically with the breathing. Bend your knees, and slowly lower your feet and hips to the ground.

••• ORTHODOX

Your doctor may recommend glycerin or laxative suppositories to relieve constipation.

Enemas may be advised to empty the bowel.

INCONTINENCE, URINARY

The inability to control urination can be due to injury, disease, or weakness of the muscles controlling the bladder. In men it may also be a symptom of prostate problems (see **Prostate, Enlarged**). Early signs include leaking urine when coughing, lifting, or laughing. Lack of urinary control may occur after childbirth as a result of weakened pelvic floor muscles.

TREATMENT

▬ PRACTICAL ADVICE

Some drugs affect bladder control, particularly those prescribed for high blood pressure. Ask your doctor about the potential effects of any drugs you may be taking. If they are causing incontinence, ask for alternatives.

Women who are also affected by stinging or burning sensations during urination may have cystitis, which can be easily treated (see **Cystitis**).

Keep the genital area clean and dry. Wash after going to the toilet. Avoid using scented soaps, talcs, and deodorants in the genital area. Wear cotton underwear, and avoid tight clothing and nylon.

Only go to the toilet when your bladder is full. Do not get into a habit of making precautionary trips; this will prevent the bladder from filling up and working properly. Drink at least 2 quarts of fluid over the course of the day. This will ensure regular use of the bladder muscles.

✕ DIETARY

Excess weight puts pressure on the muscles controlling the bladder. It will be difficult to overcome urinary incontinence if you are overweight. See **Obesity** for suggestions on how to lose the extra pounds.

Straining due to constipation weakens bladder muscles. Introduce more fiber into your diet, and follow the recommendations listed under **Constipation.**

☐ HOMEOPATHY

Take 3 times a day for 4 days; repeat if needed:

Involuntary urination from coughing, sneezing, or laughing, or after forcible retention: *Causticum* 6c

Involuntary urination when lying down or after getting the feet wet: *Pulsatilla* 6c

☯ CHINESE MEDICINE

Practitioners of traditional Chinese medicine generally recommend golden lock tea for this condition.

✳ ACUPRESSURE

Massaging the points illustrated in the figure on the facing page several times a week may be helpful.

⁙ EXERCISE

For women: Do the following exercise to strengthen the pelvic floor muscles, which control urination: To locate the muscles, try stopping the flow when you urinate. Then try tightening (contracting) and relaxing the muscles when you are not urinating. Every day, practice tightening and relaxing these muscles (when not urinating). At first they will feel weak, so start with just a few contractions, but do them frequently (at least 5 contractions, 10 times a day); gradually, build up to 10 contractions, 10 times a day or more. You can contract and relax your pelvic floor muscles while sitting, lying, or standing, while working, cooking, or watching

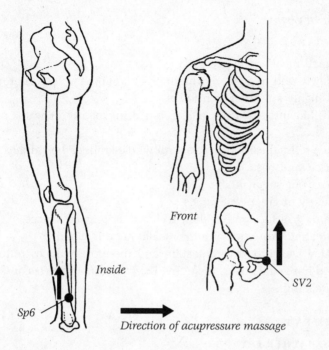

Front

Inside

Sp6

SV2

Direction of acupressure massage

television. Progress will be slow, but if you follow this routine regularly, the muscles will strengthen. Once or twice a week, check your progress by stopping the flow when you urinate: after six or eight weeks of exercise, you should find it easier to stop the flow.

••• ORTHODOX

Your doctor may recommend hormone replacement therapy if the bladder outlet muscle has weakened as a result of menopause.

Physiotherapy may also be advised. The therapist may use mild electrical stimulation to produce pelvic floor contractions, or may suggest internal weight training—holding weighted balls in the vagina to strengthen and tone the muscles.

INDIGESTION

A general term for discomfort brought by eating. Symptoms include stomach pain, acid in the stomach (see **Acid Stomach**), nausea, and gas. It is often caused by eating too much or too quickly, or by eating rich or spicy food. Stress may also be a contributing factor.

PREVENTION

✗ DIETARY

Eat small meals regularly.

Eat slowly and in a relaxed manner, and chew the food thoroughly.

Avoid highly spiced or rich foods.

Limit fluid intake during meals, but drink plenty of water between meals.

Replace refined carbohydrates with whole-grain carbohydrates (bread, brown rice, and pasta).

Reduce your sugar intake.

Eat plenty of green vegetables.

Steam or grill food rather than frying it, and avoid sauces.

Avoid eating fruit with or after meals. Keep it separate.

The Hay Diet improves digestion and therefore reduces reflux. It is described in several books, including *Food Combining for Health* (see Suggested Reading).

TREATMENT

❄ AROMATHERAPY

Lie or sit and massage the abdomen with 1 teaspoon of a carrier oil containing 1 drop of essential oil of peppermint or ginger (or 2 drops in 2 teaspoons). Always massage in a clockwise direction.

❧ HERBALISM

Meadowsweet infusion protects and soothes the mucous membranes of the stomach, reduces acidity, and relieves nausea: Pour 1 cup of boiling water onto 2 teaspoons of the dried herb, and infuse for 15 minutes; drink 3 times a day.

▢ HOMEOPATHY

Take 1 tablet every 15 minutes for up to 4 doses; repeat if needed:

After rich foods, with gas and rancid belching: *Carbo vegetabilis* 6c

After spicy food, stimulants, alcohol: *Nux vomica* 6c

Burning pain, worse in the small hours of the morning: *Arsenicum album* 6c

Stomach keeps filling up with gas, explosive belching and flatulence, worse from sweets and nervousness: *Argentum nitricum* 6c

Intolerant of legumes (peas, beans, and lentils), onions, and garlic, and large meals in general, flatulence gets obstructed and becomes painful: *Lycopodium* 6c

☯ CHINESE MEDICINE

Sprouted hawthorn berry, wheat berry, and rice can relieve discomfort.

～ RELAXATION TECHNIQUES

Set aside a regular time for eating. Try to clear your mind of concerns before you sit down. Do not read or watch television while eating, and try not to think about or discuss problems or worries; concentrate on thoroughly chewing and enjoying your meal.

Try to find time for the following routine once a day: Find a quiet place where you won't be disturbed. Lie on a firm surface, close your eyes, allow your breathing to slow, and begin to be aware of how your body feels. Consciously try to relax every part of your body in turn. Begin with your face (your eyes, your forehead, your jaw), and work down to your toes. The whole procedure should take at least 10 minutes.

❖ REFLEXOLOGY

Massage the area relating to the stomach, found on both soles of the feet, above the midline in the arch.

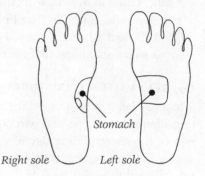

Stomach

Right sole   Left sole

••• ORTHODOX

Doctors recommend antacids for temporary relief, but they should not be used long term. If indigestion lasts for more than a few days, and especially if you feel generally unwell, consult your doctor.

INFECTION

A wide range of symptoms and illnesses caused by bacteria, viruses, or fungi that invade and spread through the body. Signs of infection, which include inflammation, fever, joint aches, redness, and pus, are a natural manifestation of the immune system's fight against the disease.

TREATMENT

▬ PRACTICAL ADVICE

Take as few drugs as possible. Drugs often suppress the formation of white blood cells, which are vital for fighting infection. Antibiotics alter the natural flora of the body, making it more susceptible to infection.

Limit your intake of alcohol, nicotine, chemicals, and food additives, which also impair immunity.

Get plenty of rest.

✕ DIETARY

The following antioxidants help boost immunity and resist infection:

- vitamin C, found in black currants, parsley, broccoli, green peppers, strawberries, oranges, and tomatoes
- vitamin E, found in wheat germ, seeds and seed oils, margarine, and egg yolk
- beta-carotene, found in green leafy vegetables and yellow vegetables and fruits
- vitamin B-complex: 1 25-milligram supplement a day
- selenium, found in whole-grain flour, mackerel, pork, eggs, and cheese
- zinc, found in oysters, liver, meat, Cheddar cheese, beans, and lentils
- magnesium, found in Brazil nuts, whole-grain flour, plain chocolate, lentils, and parsley

Avoid sugar, including that found in fruits and fruit juices.

～ RELAXATION TECHNIQUES

Stress has been shown to reduce the body's immunity to infection. Getting adequate exercise, and participating in yoga or meditation, can help reduce the stress of everyday life. If you are anxious or stressed for reasons that seem beyond your control, you may want to seek help from a mental health professional.

••• ORTHODOX

Any fever produced by infection requires an explanation. The cause could be anything—a common cold, a chest infection, malaria, or AIDS. Any unexplained fever that lasts longer than one or two days should be assessed by a doctor.

INFERTILITY

You or your partner may be considered infertile if you have been having unprotected intercourse for a year and have not been able to conceive. This does not necessarily mean you cannot have a child, but it may mean you need help in establishing optimal conditions for fertilization. The most common causes of infertility are inadequate healthy sperm production by the man, or failure to ovulate in the woman. However, there are a number of other possible causes, and finding the reason for infertility is the first step to treatment.

TREATMENT

■ PRACTICAL ADVICE

The most likely days or nights you will conceive are the thirteenth, fourteenth, and fifteenth days before your next menstrual period. Make a record of the dates of your period, and try to time intercourse during the fertile period.

Abstaining from intercourse for a day or two before these dates ensures a healthy sperm count during the fertile period.

Sperm need to be kept cool, so men should avoid tight clothing and underwear, hot baths, and whirlpool baths.

The best position in which to conceive is with the man on top. After ejaculation, the woman should remain lying down for at least 30 minutes.

Do not use KY jelly, as this may inhibit sperm movement. Egg white, which encourages sperm movement, is a good alternative lubricant.

Do not douche after intercourse.

✕ DIETARY

Eat a balanced diet of whole-grain cereals, fresh fruits and vegetables, lean protein, cooked dried beans and peas, and vegetable oils.

Increase your intake of vitamin E, found in wheat germ, nuts, vegetable oils, and seeds.

Stop smoking and drinking caffeine (coffee, tea, chocolate, cola), as these can interfere with ovulation and sperm production.

Avoid alcohol completely, since even small amounts can render susceptible males infertile.

Try to maintain your normal weight. Being underweight or overweight can sometimes interfere with conception. Eat sensibly, however; this is not the time to crash diet. See **Obesity** for suggestions on losing weight.

Supplementation with vitamin B6 has been shown to reduce birth defects. The recommended daily intake for women who would like to conceive is 0.4 milligrams.

❖ EXERCISE

Do not overexercise. Studies show that intensive training can reduce sperm count in men and suppress ovulation in women. Reduce your schedule, and change your activities to more gentle, relaxing exercise.

∼ RELAXATION TECHNIQUES

Stress can affect the ability to conceive in one or both partners. Try one or more of the following suggestions to relax:

Attend a relaxation, yoga, or meditation class.

Have a regular massage, acupressure, or aromatherapy session.

Take up a hobby or sport that you enjoy, and which engages your whole attention, but avoid overdoing it.

Take time out to do nothing in particular (read, take a bath, go for a walk, listen to music).

If problems are bothering you, talk about them. A counselor or psychotherapist may be able to help if you are unable to discuss problems with friends or family.

Do not take on additional responsibilities at this time. Learn how to say no.

✚ PROFESSIONAL HELP

Chinese medicine and professional homeopathy treatment are known to be effective.

••• ORTHODOX

If the above recommendations do not lead to a pregnancy, your doctor may want to examine both partners to rule out any physical causes of infertility.

Men who produce inadequate sperm may want to consider artificial insemination by a donor.

For women, drugs may be given to stimulate ovulation, or surgery may be carried out to clear blocked fallopian tubes.

If none of these results in conception, in vitro fertilization may be the final option.

INFLAMMATORY BOWEL DISEASE

A general term for inflammatory disorders affecting the small and large intestine. Crohn's disease and colitis (see **Colitis; Crohn's Disease**) are examples of inflammatory bowel disease. The cause of these diseases is unknown, but many suspect they are triggered by food allergies. Symptoms include diarrhea, stomach pain, and sometimes blood and mucus in the stools.

TREATMENT

✕ DIETARY

The most common food allergens are milk products, cereals (wheat, oats, barley, rye, corn), and caffeine (coffee, tea, cola, chocolate). For suggestions on pinpointing a food allergy, see **Allergies, Food.**

Increase your intake of fiber, found in whole-grain cereals; if you are allergic to cereals, eat plenty of fruits and raw vegetables.

Eat plenty of live yogurt with *Lactobacillus acidophilus* to promote the growth of healthy intestinal flora, essential for good digestion. Supplements of *Lactobacillus acidophilus* will activate bowel bacteria: Take ½ teaspoon of *Lactobacillus acidophilus,* with 1 teaspoon of *Bifidobacteria* powder, and ½ teaspoon of *Lactobacillus bulgaricus* (available from natural foods stores), in a glass of spring water, 3 times a day.

🐾 HERBALISM

Garlic supports the growth of natural beneficial bacteria in the colon, and kills infection. Use garlic copiously in cooking. You can take garlic capsules (3 capsules, 3 times a day) if you do not like the taste or smell of fresh garlic.

☐ HOMEOPATHY

Take every 15 minutes for 4 doses; repeat if necessary:

Sudden spasms with ineffectual urge to move bowels: *Nux vomica* 6c

Colic with exhausting diarrhea and much gas; voiding gas provides little relief: *China* 6c

Colic, bending double and hard massage brings relief: *Colocynth* 6c

Rumbling and gurgling after rich food: *Pulsatilla* 6c

••• ORTHODOX

Your doctor may prescribe anti-inflammatory drugs to relieve the swelling.

INFLUENZA
See **Flu.**

INGROWN HAIR

Sometimes hairs grow down under the skin, causing inflammation and pimples. This often occurs in people with very curly hair, and is more common on areas that are shaved, particularly facial or pubic hair.

PREVENTION

The major cause of ingrown hairs is shaving; allowing the hair to grow may discourage ingrown hairs.

For women who want to remove facial or leg hair, waxing is an alternative to shaving that tends not to produce ingrown hairs. See **Hair, Excessive,** for information on hair removal.

Ingrown hair often results from shaving too closely. Using an electric razor does not give as close a shave, but it may prevent ingrown hairs. If you prefer a wet shave, gently brush the skin with a wet loofah first to remove dead cells. Soak the area to be shaved in water for at least 10 minutes to soften the hair. Place shaving foam or gel on the area and leave it on for a few minutes to soak in. Use a single-bladed razor and do not shave too closely. Place a hot washcloth over the area for a few minutes after shaving. Finish off with a creamy lotion or aftershave, to keep the hairs soft.

TREATMENT

■ **PRACTICAL ADVICE**

If a hair is obviously ingrown, place a hot face cloth over the area for 5 minutes, and ease out the hair with tweezers that have been sterilized in boiling water for 1 minute. Dab the open pore with hydrogen peroxide or essential oil of tea tree to prevent infection. If you cannot see the hair, keep the hot cloth on the area until it emerges.

••• **ORTHODOX**

Your doctor would ease out the hair with the above method.

INGROWN TOENAIL

The edges of one or both sides of the toenail (usually that of the big toe) press into the adjacent flesh, leading to pain, infection, and inflammation.

PREVENTION

Ingrown toenails often result from incorrect nail cutting, stubbing your toe, or dropping something on it.

When you cut your toenails, soak the feet first to soften the nails. Cut the nail straight across—never in an oval shape. Do not cut it too short; your nail should cover the toe to protect it. File down sharp edges with an emery board.

Wear protective shoes when you walk on rough ground or lift heavy objects.

TREATMENT

■ PRACTICAL ADVICE

Soak the foot in a warm solution of water and antiseptic or a warm marigold solution (5 drops of marigold tincture to 1 quart of water) to soften and cleanse the nail. Dry and insert a thin strand of sterile cotton in between the nail and the flesh. This will lift the nail away from the flesh and help it to grow out. Change the cotton every day.

Wear open-toed sandals, or soft, comfortable shoes. Tight or pointed shoes will press the nail in further.

••• ORTHODOX

Most doctors will prescribe antibiotics to treat the infection.

Minor surgery under local anesthetic removes the edge or all of the nail, enabling the inflamed skin to settle down and heal before the new nail grows in (this takes about nine months). This is often the only way to allow healing, since inflammation cannot be relieved while pressure from the nail is present.

INSECT BITES AND STINGS

Insect bites, such as fly and mosquito bites, can spread infection and disease, as well as being itchy and tiresome. Bee and wasp stings are painful and can cause allergic reactions in some people.

PREVENTION

■ PRACTICAL ADVICE

Mosquitoes often come out at night. If you are sitting out in the evening, wear light clothing that covers the skin, particularly the wrists, arms, and ankles. Place mosquito screens over windows, and use a mosquito net around your bed. Insect repellents, such as sprays or slow-release coils, help keep the mosquitoes away.

Do not wear scented toiletries outside.

Wear light clothes; dark ones attract insects.

Cider vinegar rubbed on the skin is an effective insect repellent.

✗ DIETARY

Take thiamine (vitamin B1) to prevent bites. Large amounts of thiamine are excreted through the body and give off an odor that repels insects. Take a 100-milligram tablet 3 times a day.

Daily doses of zinc help repel insects. Take at least 60 milligrams a day.

Garlic helps repel insects. If you do not like the taste or smell of fresh garlic, you can take garlic capsules (3 capsules, 3 times a day).

✽ AROMATHERAPY

Essential oil of eucalyptus is a natural insect repellent. Make up a solution by adding 5 drops of the essential oil to 1 cup of water, and dab on the exposed areas of the body.

Essential oil of citronella is also an effective insect repellent: Dab sparingly on exposed areas of skin.

☐ HOMEOPATHY

Take *Ledum* 6c, 2 times a day, to help prevent mosquito bites.

TREATMENT

▬ PRACTICAL ADVICE

A bee leaves its stinger in the flesh; gently scrape it out with a sterile knife or needle. Take care not to push it further in, and do not suck it out. If the sting is in the mouth or throat, rinse the mouth with ice water, suck ice cubes, and seek medical help immediately.

Bee stings are acidic and can be neutralized by dabbing a solution of 2 teaspoons of bicarbonate of soda mixed with 1 cup water on the sting.

Wasp stings are alkaline. Neutralize them by dabbing vinegar or lemon juice on the sting.

Wash insect bites thoroughly with soap and water. Try not to scratch, as this may cause them to become infected.

To relieve the itching, dissolve 1 teaspoon of baking soda in 1 cup of water, soak a piece of cloth in the solution, and bathe the bites.

✽ AROMATHERAPY

Rub 1 drop each of essential oil of tea tree or lavender on the bites; repeat every hour until the irritation stops.

❧ HERBALISM

Dab tincture of witch hazel on mosquito bites.

☐ HOMEOPATHY

Dab *Pyrethrum* tincture on the sting.

When an allergic reaction to a bee sting occurs, take *Apis* 6c every 10 minutes until professional help can be obtained.

✿ **BACH FLOWER REMEDIES**

Rescue Remedy is useful, especially for children.

✳ **BIOCHEMIC TISSUE SALTS**

Take *Nat Mur* 6x: Crush the tablet and apply locally.

••• **ORTHODOX**

Calamine lotion is a harmless remedy that will soothe the skin and relieve itching.

For those who experience large swellings after being bitten, some doctors recommend wetting the skin and rubbing an aspirin over the bite to control inflammation.

Antihistamine drugs are recommended for an allergic reaction.

Antibiotics are given for infected bites.

In the case of severe allergic reaction—swelling of the lips, tongue, and throat, accompanied by breathing problems—call for emergency medical help immediately.

INSOMNIA

Difficulty sleeping. Most people with insomnia have problems getting to sleep or staying asleep. The cause is often anxiety, though insomnia can also result from illness, pain, depression, environmental factors, lack of exercise, and drugs.

TREATMENT

▬ **PRACTICAL ADVICE**

Establish a bedtime and a rising time and stick to it. Do not oversleep in the morning.

Avoid daytime and evening napping. Do not allow yourself to sleep until you get to bed.

Do evening activities that allow you to relax without falling asleep: an evening walk, talking with someone, playing a game, or doing gentle household chores are good; television may send you to sleep before bedtime.

Make sure your sleeping conditions are comfortable and quiet. Make sure the bedroom is adequately heated and ventilated.

Try to resolve problems before going to sleep. If you are lying awake worrying, put the light on and write down what is worrying you. Promise yourself that you will deal with the issues in the morning, when you are fresh.

✗ DIETARY

Eat your evening meal at least 2 hours before retiring.

Avoid caffeine (coffee, tea, chocolate, cola), tobacco, and alcohol.

✿ AROMATHERAPY

Lavender is known to help relaxation. Add 5 drops of essential oil of lavender to a bath, and soak in it before retiring.

Put 3 drops of lavender on a handkerchief or tissue to inhale.

⁊ HERBALISM

Valerian tea is a natural sedative: Pour 1 cup of boiling water over 2 teaspoons of the root, and infuse for 15 minutes; drink before going to bed.

Passiflora is also excellent. If you are buying supplements over the counter, follow the instructions on the package; otherwise, consult a naturopath or nutritionist.

☐ HOMEOPATHY

When feeling hyped up, wide awake, or sensitive to every little noise: *Coffea* 6c, every 30 minutes

When unable to sleep through overexhaustion: *Arnica* 6c, every 30 minutes

☯ CHINESE MEDICINE

Practitioners of traditional Chinese medicine often recommend fleece-flower stem, poria, and wild jujube seeds, which do not sedate, but have a beneficial effect on the nervous system.

⁙ EXERCISE

Regular aerobic exercise (walking, jogging, or swimming) helps relieve tension and anxiety, and relaxes the body, permitting better sleep. Be sure not to exercise strenuously close to bedtime—this can keep you awake.

✳ ACUPRESSURE

Regular massage of the points illustrated in the figure on the facing page can be very helpful in treating insomnia.

～ RELAXATION TECHNIQUES

Do the following routine before retiring, or once you are in bed: Lie on a firm surface, close your eyes, allow your breathing to slow, and begin to be aware of how your body feels. Consciously try to relax every part of your body in turn. Begin with your face (your eyes, your forehead, your jaw), and work down to your toes. The whole procedure should take at least 10 minutes.

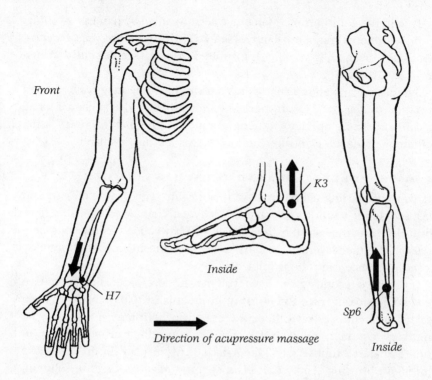

Front

K3

Inside

H7

Sp6

Direction of acupressure massage

Inside

••• ORTHODOX

Solving the problem that is causing insomnia is the first step. Doctors may prescribe sleeping pills or tranquilizers as a short-term measure, but only for severe cases, and as a last resort, as they can be addictive.

INTERCOURSE, PAINFUL

Pain during sexual intercourse affects both men and women. The pain may be around the external genitals, or, in the case of women, internal. Sometimes soreness in either partner can be due to anxiety, inadequate foreplay, lack of lubrication, or too forceful penetration. Taking more time to make love, and discussing sexual practices and problems openly with your partner, can help overcome problems. Sexual counseling may be useful to facilitate such discussion.

CAUSES, PREVENTION, AND TREATMENT: MEN

A burning sensation on ejaculation or urination suggests urethritis or prostatitis (see **Prostatitis; Urinary Tract Infection;** and Nonspecific Urethritis under **Sexually Transmitted Diseases**).

Pain in the penis during intercourse accompanied by redness, swelling, lumps, or sores may be balanitis (see **Balanitis**), herpes (see **Herpes, Genital**), or another sexually transmitted disease (see **Sexually Transmitted Diseases**).

Soreness or irritation of the penis after intercourse may result from a reaction to a spermicide or lubrication, or an allergy to rubber if using a condom. There are many different brands on the market, so try using different products. Hypoallergenic condoms are also available.

CAUSES, PREVENTION, AND TREATMENT: WOMEN

If you are starting a first or new relationship, you may feel sore and bruised. Using a lubricant such as KY jelly can help avoid this. To relieve bruising, soak in a warm bath to which you have added 5 drops of essential oil of either lavender or clary sage. Take the homeopathic remedy *Arnica* 6c once every hour for 1 day.

If you have recently given birth, you may be sore, especially if you have had an episiotomy (see **Episiotomy**). Wait at least 10 days before having sexual intercourse. Pelvic floor exercises can help tone up the vaginal muscles: contract and relax the muscles controlling urination 5 or 10 times, at least 3 times a day. Take *Arnica* 6c twice a day for up to 2 weeks to relieve bruising. Apply *Calendula* cream, *Calendula* tincture solution, or vitamin E oil to the stitches to promote healing.

Pain, itching, and irritation accompanied by unusual vaginal discharge may be a sign of thrush or of trichomoniasis (see **Thrush; Trichomoniasis**).

If you are urinating more often than usual, or experiencing a burning feeling when you urinate, an inflamed bladder may be contributing to the discomfort (see **Cystitis**).

If you have reached the age of menopause, hormonal changes may make your vagina tighter and drier than before (see **Menopausal Problems**). Using a lubricant, such as KY jelly, could solve this problem.

If intercourse and the use of tampons are difficult or impossible, the cause may be a spasm of the muscles surrounding the vaginal entrance (see **Vaginismus**).

If you feel internal shooting pain during penetration and your periods have become more painful, you may have endometriosis (see **Endometriosis**) or cervical erosion (see **Cervical Erosion**). Experimenting with different positions for intercourse may lead to more comfortable sex. Consult your doctor if you suspect one of these may be the cause of pain.

INTERMITTENT CLAUDICATION

Pain in the calves, resulting from a blockage of blood flow in the arteries due to atherosclerosis (see **Atherosclerosis**). The pain often starts after walking a short distance, forcing you to stop frequently for rests. In extreme cases blood clots form in the arteries, leading to death of an area of tissue, gangrene, and possible amputation. If you suspect you have intermittent claudication, consult your doctor.

TREATMENT

▬ PRACTICAL ADVICE

Stop smoking. This is the most effective way to prevent or halt this condition.

Excess weight may contribute to the ailment, so try to maintain your normal weight (see **Obesity** for weight loss recommendations).

✗ DIETARY

Studies have shown great improvement by combining walking with supplementation: Take 300 to 400 iu of vitamin E a day.

Intermittent claudication is a sign of arterial disease. Avoid foods high in cholesterol, such as red meat and dairy products, and increase your intake of high-fiber, whole-grain cereals, and fresh fruits and vegetables.

Increase your intake of magnesium, found in nuts, cooked dried beans and peas, whole-grain breads and cereals, soybeans, dark green leafy vegetables, milk, and seafood.

ɀ HERBALISM

Hawthorn infusion is a good tonic for the circulatory system: Pour 1 cup of boiling water on 2 teaspoons of the berries, and infuse for 20 minutes; drink 3 times a day.

▢ HOMEOPATHY

Baryta muriatica 6c: Take 3 times a day for 3 weeks.
Proteus 30c: Take as needed during acute attacks.

❖ EXERCISE

Walking is the best exercise for this condition. Try to walk at least 1 hour a day. Walk until you feel moderate discomfort in the legs, then stop for a rest. Keep repeating the walk-pain-rest cycle. After two or three months of daily exercise, bypass blood vessels develop in the legs to overcome blocked ones, relieving pain.

If the weather does not permit walking, stationary indoor bicycling is an alternative. Follow the same routine as above. Always consult your doctor before beginning any exercise routine.

••• ORTHODOX

Arterial reconstruction using various synthetic grafts, used in about one-third of cases, can be very effective and durable. The feet must be stringently cared for to avoid infection or injury, as infection or trauma can lead to gangrene.

IRRITABLE BLADDER

An irritable bladder manifests with the sudden uncontrollable urge to urinate. It is often a result of a bladder infection (see **Cystitis**), a bladder stones (see **Bladder Stones**), or obstruction to the outflow of urine by an enlarged prostate gland (see **Prostate, Enlarged**). In many cases the cause cannot be found, but the following treatments may help.

TREATMENT

▬ PRACTICAL ADVICE

Drink at least 2 quarts of water a day.

Consult your doctor to see if you have a urinary tract infection (see **Urinary Tract Infection**).

Make sure to empty the bladder completely each time you urinate.

Women should always wipe from front to back after going to the toilet, to avoid spreading germs from the anus to the vagina.

Empty the bladder after intercourse.

Wear cotton underwear.

☐ HOMEOPATHY

Take every 15 minutes for 4 doses during acute attacks:

Urge to urinate, but nothing comes: *Nux vomica* 6c

Pain that is relieved if urination is postponed: *Equisetum* 6c

Urine feels like scalding water; violently painful: *Cantharis* 6c

Burning pain at the end of urination and afterward: *Sarsaparilla* 6c

Stinging pains better from cold bathing: *Apis* 6c

⬧ EXERCISE

For women: The muscles that control urination may need to be strengthened. During the day, contract and relax these pelvic floor muscles when you are not urinating. The more often you do it, the stronger the muscles will become (for details, see Exercise under **Incontinence, Urinary**).

••• ORTHODOX

Your doctor may suggest a urodynamic study to measure the flow and volume of urine passed through the bladder. This study can diagnose problems in the bladder and in the urethra—the tube that leads from the bladder to the outside—so that accurate and precise treatment can be planned. Treatment may include drugs to suppress the nervous impulse to the bladder, or to relax the bladder muscles.

IRRITABLE BOWEL SYNDROME

A condition whose symptoms include cramp-like stomach pains, swollen abdomen, and alternating phases of constipation, hard stools, and diarrhea, often accompanied by gas; also known as spastic colon. The cause is not fully understood, but symptoms are thought to result from improper functioning of the muscular contractions of the large intestine; stress may contribute to the severity of the illness. Women are more susceptible to it than men.

TREATMENT

✗ DIETARY

Studies show that increasing the intake of fiber is one of the most effective cures for this condition. Fruits, vegetables, oat bran, and cooked dried beans and peas are good sources of fiber. The effect is not immediate, and symptoms may worsen during the first 2 weeks of treatment. However, you should see an improvement within four months of increasing your fiber intake.

Some people with irritable bowel syndrome have a lactose intolerance, which prevents them from digesting milk. Try abstaining from all dairy products for 2 weeks to see if symptoms are relieved. See **Lactose Intolerance** for more details.

Different foods and food combinations bring irritable bowel syndrome in different people. To find out what is upsetting you, try keeping a diary and noting everything you eat, including the circumstances in which you eat and your mood.

Eat plenty of natural, unsweetened live yogurt with *Lactobacillus acidophilus* (one large carton a day) to ensure a supply of the healthy bacteria that are essential to digestion.

If you cannot tolerate yogurt, take nondairy supplements of *Lactoba-cillus acidophilus*. Take ½ teaspoon of *Lactobacillus acidophilus,* 1 teaspoon of *Bifidobacteria* powder, and ½ teaspoon of *Lactobacillus bulgaricus* (available from natural foods stores), in a glass of spring water, 3 times a day.

❅ AROMATHERAPY

Massage the abdomen with relaxing and antispasmodic essential oils to help to relax any tension in the muscles and enhance digestion. Mix 3 drops each of essential oil of peppermint and black pepper with 4 tea-spoons of carrier oil or lotion, and massage the abdomen very gently: Put one hand over the other and gently knead the stomach, using small circular motions. Start at the right bottom corner, moving upward to the right of the lower ribs, across the abdomen to the left lower ribs, down to the left bottom corner, and back across to the right.

🦐 HERBALISM

Peppermint infusion relieves intestinal spasm and gas: Pour 1 cup of boiling water onto 1 heaping teaspoon of the dried herb, and infuse for 10 minutes; drink as needed. Try to replace tea, coffee, and carbonated beverages with peppermint infusion.

☐ HOMEOPATHY

Take every 15 minutes for 4 doses; repeat if necessary:

Sudden spasms with ineffectual urge to move bowels: *Nux vomica* 6c

Colic with exhausting diarrhea and much gas; voiding gas provides little relief: *China* 6c

Profuse diarrhea accompanied by burning and colicky stomach, restlessness, anxiety, and chilliness: *Arsenicum album* 6c

Burning in the rectum and anus with involuntary evacuations: *Aloe* 6c

Greenish, painless diarrhea with gurgling and stomach cramps, worse early morning: *Podophyllum* 6c

☯ CHINESE MEDICINE

Practitioners of traditional Chinese medicine may recommend dandelion, along with magnolia bark, to ease the bloated sensation. Rhubarb and Chinese angelica prevent constipation, while poria aids diarrhea.

∿ RELAXATION TECHNIQUES

Stress contributes to the severity of this condition. Yoga, meditation, or biofeedback have been seen to reduce symptoms. For more information, see **Stress.**

••• ORTHODOX

Your doctor may prescribe antispasmodic drugs to relieve stomach pain, and antidiarrheal drugs to prevent long-term diarrhea.

ITCHING

Intense irritation or tickling that may be felt all over the body, or in one particular place. It may be a sign of skin disease, such as dandruff, eczema, or psoriasis (see **Dandruff; Eczema; Psoriasis**). Anal itching may be caused by hemorrhoids (see **Anal Itching; Hemorrhoids**). Vaginal itching may be due to a yeast infection (see **Thrush**). More generalized itching, which affects the whole body, may be a sign of diabetes (see **Diabetes**). Often itching is caused by cosmetics, bath products, detergents, too much washing, or rough clothing. It is particularly common in the elderly. The following treatments are for itching that has no apparent underlying disease.

TREATMENT

■ PRACTICAL ADVICE

Try not to scratch, as this aggravates the irritation. Keep your nails short, so that you cannot break the skin and infect it. Apply a cool, wet compress to the area when the urge to scratch occurs.

Soap irritates itchy skin, so use as little as possible. Substitute mild cleansing lotions for soap, or simply use water and a face cloth to wash.

Avoid talcs and scented bath products.

Wear loose, soft clothing, and cotton underwear. Avoid itchy fabrics.

🐾 HERBALISM

To relieve itchy skin, add a strong infusion of chickweed to your bathwater: Pour 3 cups of boiling water on 10 teaspoons of the dried herb, and infuse for 15 minutes.

☯ CHINESE MEDICINE

Practitioners of traditional Chinese medicine may recommend dittnay bark or broom cypress fruit.

≈ HYDROTHERAPY

Ground oatmeal is a soothing agent. Add 2 cups to a warm bath and soak in it.

••• ORTHODOX

Your doctor may recommend antihistamines, and also soothing lotions, creams, or ointments; calamine is effective, and probably the safest to use. Hydrocortisone or stronger steroid creams may be used in severe cases, under your doctor's supervision.

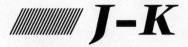 # *J-K*

JAUNDICE

Yellowing of the skin and whites of the eyes as a result of an underlying liver disorder that leads to an accumulation of bile products in the body. This may be due to hepatitis (see **Hepatitis**); cirrhosis (see **Cirrhosis**); blockage of the bile duct by a stone or tumor; or the abnormal destruction of red blood cells, which leads to the release of large quantities of red pigment into the blood.

TREATMENT

Consult your doctor before you begin any treatment.

✗ DIETARY

Eat plenty of fruits and raw vegetables, along with vegetable protein (soy, cooked dried beans, peas, whole-grain cereals).

Drink lemon juice and carrot juice every day.

Reduce your intake of all fats, including nuts and seeds.

Avoid alcohol, caffeine, and smoking.

⅔ HERBALISM

Dandelion-root decoction is a gentle liver tonic: Put 3 teaspoons of the chopped dried root into 1 cup of water, bring to a boil, and simmer for 10 minutes; drink 3 times a day.

☐ HOMEOPATHY

Persistent jaundice in newborns: *Chamomilla* 6c, 2 times a day

If *Chamomilla* doesn't help within 48 hours: *Lycopodium* 6c, 2 times a day, for up to 3 days

☯ CHINESE MEDICINE

Traditional Chinese medicine relates jaundice to dampness in the liver and gallbladder. Oriental wormwood and gardenia fruit or corktree bark may be recommended to clear the dampness.

✚ PROFESSIONAL HELP

Professional homeopathic treatment may be helpful for jaundice caused by hemolytic anemia (when the red blood cells are broken down more quickly than they are replaced).

••• ORTHODOX

A blood test is necessary to confirm diagnosis. Treatment is aimed at clearing up the underlying cause of jaundice.

JELLYFISH STINGS

Jellyfish stings generally result in a mildly itchy or painful rash. Occasionally, they may cause more severe symptoms of vomiting, sweating, and breathing difficulties, which require immediate medical attention.

TREATMENT

① FIRST AID

Do not rub the sting. Rinse it immediately with saltwater.

If fragments of the tentacle remain in the skin, apply vinegar or alcohol to inactivate them. Do not touch them, but try to scrape them off using a knife, a razor, the edge of a credit card, a towel, or sand.

Keep the affected skin cool.

☐ HOMEOPATHY

Medusa 30c (a remedy prepared from jellyfish sting): Take 1 dose as soon as possible, and then hourly for as long as necessary.

••• ORTHODOX

Your doctor may prescribe painkillers, antihistamines, or hydrocortisone cream to reduce the inflammation. A tetanus injection may be recommended.

JET LAG

Disruption of normal sleep and wake cycles caused by flying across different time zones. Symptoms include fatigue, irritability, lack of concentration, disorientation, and sleep and appetite disturbances.

TREATMENT

▬ PRACTICAL ADVICE

Get plenty of sleep in the few days before the flight.

Try to arrange to fly by day and arrive in the evening or at night.

Avoid alcohol during the flight, but drink plenty of other fluids to prevent dehydration.

Eat light meals during the flight.

✗ DIETARY

The following jet lag diet, devised by Dr. Charles Ehret, has been shown to help reset the body clock and prevent symptoms of jet lag. First, determine your breakfast time at destination on your day of arrival. Three days before departure day, keep to the following routine:

- Day 1: Eat a high-protein breakfast and lunch, and a carbohydrate dinner. No coffee, tea, or cola except between 3 P.M. and 5 P.M.
- Day 2: Fast on light meals of salads, soups, fruits, and juices. No coffee, tea, or cola except between 3 P.M. and 5 P.M.
- Day 3: Do the same as day 1.
- Day 4: Fast on light meals; if you drink coffee, drink only in the morning when traveling west; or in the evening when traveling east. Do not drink alcohol during the flight; sleep until breakfast time if possible. Break the fast at destination breakfast time, and eat a high-protein meal. Stay awake and active, and continue meals according to the mealtimes at the destination.

Another possibility is the following: For 1 week before departure and for 2 days after arrival, take Aminoplex amino acids, 2 capsules a day, and magnesium ascorbate vitamin C, 2 grams a day.

❀ AROMATHERAPY

Some airlines are now using aromatherapy to help relax travelers. Lavender is recommended to encourage relaxation, rosemary or lemon to refresh and keep you alert.

▢ HOMEOPATHY

Arnica 6c: Take every 3 hours during the flight, and then 2 times a day for 3 days after landing.

Cocculus 6c: Take 3 times a day for 3 days after landing, where there has been a significant change of time zones.

JOCK ITCH
See **Fungal Infection.**

KIDNEY STONES

Hard deposits of salts that collect in the kidney ducts or pass into the ureter, the tube leading down to the bladder; also known as urinary tract calculi. Stones that remain in the kidney may give mild pain in the back above the waist on one side. Stones that get stuck in the ureter produce excruciating and unmistakable pains that cause you to double up and render you helpless. Mild cases of this condition can be helped by the recommendations below, though it is advisable to consult a health professional.

TREATMENT

✗ DIETARY

Drink at least 3 quarts of water a day.

Reduce your intake of animal protein; increase your intake of vegetables and whole-grain cereals.

Kidney stones are generally an accumulation of excess deposits of calcium phosphate or calcium oxalate. To prevent stones, reduce your intake of calcium-rich foods (milk, cheese, butter, and other dairy products); reduce your intake of oxalate-rich foods (chocolate, celery, grapes, green peppers, beans, parsley, spinach, strawberries, blueberries, beetroot, tea).

Increase your intake of vitamin A, essential to the health of the lining of the urinary system. Vitamin A–rich foods include liver, kidney, egg yolk, fortified margarine, cod liver oil, and dark green, yellow, and orange vegetables (broccoli, carrots, sweet potatoes).

Daily supplements of vitamin B6 (10 milligrams a day) and magnesium (not magnesium carbonate) (300 milligrams a day) have been shown to prevent recurrence of kidney stones.

Use 2 tablespoons of extra-virgin olive oil daily in cooking or salad dressings.

Increase your intake of magnesium-rich foods (nuts, cooked dried beans and peas, whole-grain breads and cereals, soybeans, dark green leafy vegetables, milk, and seafood).

⅔ HERBALISM

Some herbal remedies are thought to help ease the stones out of the system. Herbalist David Hoffman recommends a combination of stone root, parsley piert, gravel root, and pellitory-of-the-wall. Put 1 teaspoon of each herb in 1 cup of water and simmer for 15 minutes; drink 3 times a day.

Decoction of stone root alone is also effective: Put 3 teaspoons of the dried root in 1 cup of water, and simmer for 15 minutes; drink 3 times a day.

Aloe vera juice helps reduce the size of stones.

⊹ EXERCISE

Physical activity helps move calcium to the bones, which need it. Inactivity tends to keep it in the kidney, where it forms stones. Regular walking, swimming, running, or cycling will help prevent kidney stones.

••• ORTHODOX

Small, gravelly stones may pass through the system on their own. Doctors may break up larger stones in the ureter or bladder using an extracorporeal shock-wave lithotriptor, which disintegrates the stones with a shock wave from outside the body, or ultrasonic lithotripsy, in which stones are broken up by an ultrasonic probe passed into the body through a telescopic tube.

KNEE PAIN

Knee pain can arise from a number of different conditions that may affect the bones themselves, the joint structures inside, or the muscles, ligaments, and tendons outside. Knees are weight-bearing joints susceptible to a large amount of wear and tear and are a common site of pain. See also **Housemaid's Knee.**

PREVENTION

Do at least 15 minutes of warm-up stretches prior to exercising.

Buy new, well-fitting running shoes regularly.

Run on a soft surface rather than hard ground or cement, if possible.

TREATMENT: FOR PAIN CAUSED BY EXERCISE OR STRAIN

✂ DIETARY

If you are overweight, you are putting more stress on the knees. Try to bring your weight down to the optimum level for your height (see **Obesity** for suggestions).

Take 6 500-milligram capsules of evening primrose oil a day.

≈ HYDROTHERAPY

Ease pain and swelling by applying an ice pack or hot and cold treatments. Hot and cold packs encourage the circulation of blood through the knee, flushing out toxins and bringing fresh blood to promote healing. It is an extremely effective treatment for this condition: Prepare an ice pack by wrapping ice cubes or a bag of frozen peas in a kitchen towel. Prepare a hot water bottle and wrap it in a towel. Elevate the leg. Place the ice pack on the knee for 10 minutes, then do the same with the hot water bottle. Repeat the procedure 3 times, several times a day.

☞ MASSAGE

Massage has a similar effect to hot and cold treatment: it increases circulation to the knee and helps flush out toxins. It also relaxes tense muscles and ligaments. Get regular massage from a professional therapist, or try the following routine: Sit with your knee bent. Place your thumbs on the outside of your leg, and rest your fingers and palms on the sides of your legs. Run your thumbs down the muscles, slowly exerting pressure until you reach the ankle bone. (This is called stripping the muscle.) Move your hands around to the inside of the ankle and massage up the inside leg. Finally, put your thumbs in front of and below the knee and your hands around the calf, with your fingers behind the knee, and strip down the back of the calf with your fingers.

✳ ACUPRESSURE

Massage of the points illustrated may be useful in many cases of knee pain.

⁜ EXERCISE

The following exercises will help strengthen the muscles supporting the knee. Do them *only* if they do not produce any pain in the knee. Try to do the exercises at least 2 times a day.

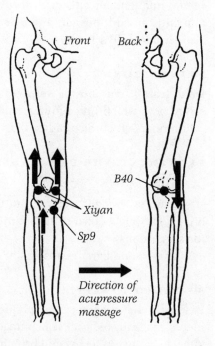

Sit on the floor with your legs stretched out in front of you. Place a rolled towel under the sore knee Tighten the muscles in your leg without moving the knee, hold for 30 seconds, then relax. Repeat 20 times.

Sit with your back against a wall, legs stretched out in front. Raise the leg with the sore knee a few inches off the ground, hold for 5 seconds, then release. Do 20 lifts, then rest, then do another 20.

Lie on your stomach on the floor. Place the strap of a weighted bag over your ankles and bend your knees, lifting your legs and the bag 20 times. Rest and repeat.

Swimming and rowing are good activities because they put no pressure on the knees, and help strengthen leg muscles.

✚ PROFESSIONAL HELP

A chiropractor would recommend massage, ultrasound treatment, exercises, and possibly manipulation.

Acupuncture may be helpful in relieving pain.

••• ORTHODOX

Treatment depends on the cause of pain. It may range from ice treatment (as above) to the prescription of anti-inflammatory drugs, physiotherapy, or surgery.

 **L**

LABOR PAINS

Pain before and during childbirth, experienced by most women who give birth. In the months before delivery, women should consider the many different ways to deal with labor pain.

■ PRACTICAL ADVICE

Many women find that lying down increases the pain of contractions. Walking around has been found to increase the efficiency of contractions and shorten labor. Kneeling, standing, or squatting often brings pain relief.

Undergoing labor in the presence of people you know and trust helps create an atmosphere of security, allowing you to relax, which in turn reduces pain.

❋ AROMATHERAPY

Essential oils of lavender and clary sage are the oils most commonly used in childbirth: Add between 4 and 6 drops to the bath, or use in combination with a carrier oil or lotion for massage during labor (see below).

▢ HOMEOPATHY

There are numerous remedies to help with labor pains, of which the following are the most common. Repeat dosage as often as the situation demands:

Sudden, spasmodic pains with anger and impatience, wants to open the bowels with every contraction: *Nux vomica* 6c

Hypersensitivity to all external stimuli—touch, light, slightest noise: *Coffea* 6c

Hot and stuffy, weepy, and needing reassurance: *Pulsatilla* 6c

Frightened and panicky, chews her fist from the pain: *Aconite* 6c

≈ HYDROTHERAPY

Floating in warm water helps; some women also choose to deliver in water. Birthing pools are available in some hospitals, or you may be able to rent one privately. Delivery in water should only be done in the presence of experts and with specialized birthing equipment.

☛ MASSAGE

Massage to the back and the buttocks can be helpful during labor. When performing the following massage, use talc rather than oil as a lubricant. Listen to the woman in labor and do what she says:

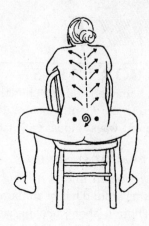

The mother-to-be can be squatting, supported over a large beanbag, or sitting, facing the back of a chair with a pillow as support. She can have her head in her arms.

Between contractions, place the flat of your hands on her back and lean toward her, performing slow, firm strokes from the center of the lower back out to the sides. Alternate with right and left hands, or work with both together, moving gradually up the back. Gentle neck stroking also helps.

During contractions, do feather-light circular massage on the sacral triangle, or just lean both hands gently across the lower spine and wait. Listen to the woman and do as she says.

✳ ACUPRESSURE

Learn these points before the delivery:

Bend your leg, and place your thumb between your inner anklebone and the Achilles tendon. Massage deeply with the thumb for 1 minute, and repeat on the other side. Hold both points simultaneously if you wish.

Use the nail of your index finger to scratch the outside of the nail of the little toe for 30 seconds. Repeat on the other side.

◯ TRANSCUTANEOUS ELECTRICAL NERVE STIMULATION (TENS)

This technique is used more and more in delivery rooms. An adaption of traditional acupuncture techniques, it consists of a small battery-powered unit that sends out electrical stimuli to two electrodes attached to the skin. This "blocks" the transmission of pain sensation along the nerves between the electrodes, reducing the pain sensation. It works immediately, is completely safe, and provides a moderate degree of pain relief.

••• ORTHODOX

Breathing nitrous oxide gas and air (entonox) through a mouthpiece brings some pain relief. It may also make you lightheaded and sleepy. It does enter the baby's system, though the effects are unknown.

Epidural: a local anesthetic, injected into the space between the spinal cord and the lumbar region of the backbone. It can give complete pain relief; though it does enter the baby's system, it is less harmful than pethidine.

Pethidine: a powerful painkilling narcotic drug, injected into a vein or into the buttock muscle. It gives effective pain relief within 10 minutes, along with drowsiness, nausea, and a drunken high. These effects are sometimes seen in the baby, who is floppy, less responsive, and likely to encounter breathing problems on delivery.

Other drugs that are less harmful may be available to you. Consult your doctor in this regard before you go into labor.

LACTOSE INTOLERANCE

The inability to digest one of the sugars found in milk can lead to symptoms of bloating, gas, stomach cramps, vomiting, and frothy diarrhea. Symptoms often resemble colitis (see **Colitis**), and are sometimes mistaken for it. Lactose intolerance is especially common among those of African, Mediterranean, or Asian origin.

TREATMENT

✗ DIETARY

If you think you may be unable to digest milk, test your tolerance level by giving up all milk products and foods containing milk for at least 2 weeks. If your symptoms disappear, it is likely you have a lactose intolerance. You may find, however, that you are able to tolerate small quantities of milk. Introduce dairy products back into your diet gradually, in small quantities, noticing how much it takes to set off a reaction. Organize your diet according to what you can tolerate.

Milk contains important sources of calcium. If you reduce your intake of milk or give it up altogether, make sure you eat plenty of other calcium-rich foods, such as canned fish (sardines or salmon), tofu, dark green leafy vegetables, cooked dried beans, dried apricots, and sesame seed products.

You may find you can eat live yogurt; it contains *Lactobacillus acidophilus,* the enzyme needed to digest milk, and is rich in calcium.

Replace milk-based drinks with soy milk or dairy-free milk. Buttermilk or goat's milk may be more digestible than ordinary cow's milk.

Lactase, the enzyme that digests milk in the stomach, is available from natural foods stores. A few drops of lactase put in milk and left overnight digests the lactose, and the milk will no longer cause digestive problems.

••• ORTHODOX

Doctors advise replacing lactose-containing products with soy-based products. Often a child grows out of lactose intolerance and can resume dairy products by the age of ten or twelve.

LARYNGITIS

Inflammation of the larynx (voice box) generally caused by a virus or bacteria, or by straining the voice. Symptoms include pain, coughing, and hoarseness. In children, laryngitis may manifest as croup (see **Croup**). Consult your doctor if voice loss persists for more than two weeks.

TREATMENT

━ PRACTICAL ADVICE

Avoid alcohol.
Stop smoking.

❋ AROMATHERAPY

Essential oils of sandalwood and lavender are soothing. To use in a gargle: Add 1 drop of each to ½ glass of warm water; add 2 drops of essential oil of lemon or peppermint if you have an infection.

⁇ HERBALISM

Decoction of echinacea is effective against viral and bacterial attacks of laryngitis: Put 2 teaspoons of the powdered root in 1 cup of water, bring to a boil, and simmer for 15 minutes; drink 3 times a day.

▢ HOMEOPATHY

Take 1 dose every hour for 4 doses; repeat if necessary:

Barking cough, with burning and irritation in the larynx, after getting chilled: *Aconite* 6c

Stringy yellow catarrh, metallic-sounding cough, and husky voice with raw pain: *Kali bichromicum* 6c

Burning pain, tightness in the chest, and hoarseness eased by eating ice cream: *Phosphorus* 30c

Laryngitis from overuse of the voice, splinter-like pains on swallowing: *Argentum nitricum* 6c

CHINESE MEDICINE

Practitioners of traditional Chinese medicine believe this condition results from heat and poison in the lungs. Treatment would be with honeysuckle flowers, peppermint, and licorice.

≋ **HYDROTHERAPY**

Steam inhalations will help soothe inflamed mucous membranes in the larynx. Fill a basin with boiling water. Sit or stand with your head over the basin, and a towel over your head to trap the steam. Inhale deeply. **Caution:** If you suffer from asthma, avoid steam inhalations.

••• **ORTHODOX**

Most doctors recommend antibiotics to reduce infection, and steam inhalations, as above. If you have been hoarse for more than four weeks, you should be examined by a specialist to rule out more serious abnormalities.

LEAD POISONING

Swallowing or inhaling lead can cause impaired mental development in children, anemia, and damage to the nervous and digestive systems. It can also bring subtle symptoms of weakness, lethargy, and lack of coordination. The most common sources of lead poisoning are licking or eating old paint with high lead content, inhaling traffic exhaust fumes, drinking water from old lead pipes, or storing food in lead-glazed pottery.

PREVENTION

Avoid canned food; lead solder is often used in canning.

Do not eat food grown in industrial or urban areas exposed to exhaust fumes.

Do not buy fruits and vegetables from roadside vendors.

If you live in an old building, check your plumbing to make sure that lead is not used in the system. If in doubt, always run the water for a few minutes before drinking; if possible, arrange an alternative drinking water supply, or install a water filter that is capable of filtering out lead.

Pregnant women should avoid exposure to heavy traffic fumes; children should not play near busy roads.

TREATMENT

✗ DIETARY

Calcium prevents the accumulation of lead in the body. Increase your intake of low-fat dairy products, canned sardines and salmon, green leafy vegetables, and sesame seed products (tahini, halvah, hummus).

Vitamin C helps to neutralize lead. Increase your intake of fresh fruits and vegetables, particularly citrus fruits, or take supplements.

Zinc and magnesium also help in the removal of lead. If you are buying supplements over the counter, follow the instructions on the package; otherwise, consult a naturopath or nutritionist for the correct dosage.

Kelp contains sodium alginate, which combines with lead, allowing it to be excreted from the body. Take kelp tablets, or sprinkle kelp powder on your food. Use dried seaweed in cooking.

The amino acid glutathione is effective in removing lead from the body: Take 1 to 3 grams a day.

✿ AROMATHERAPY

To help the lethargy, weakness, and lack of coordination: Add 2 drops each of grapefruit, rosemary, and lemon essential oils to your daily bath.

••• ORTHODOX

Most doctors diagnose lead poisoning through a blood test. Calcium EDTA or dimercaprol is given to remove excess lead from the body.

LEG ULCER

A sore on the leg that fails to heal; also known as a varicose ulcer. It often occurs in elderly people with poor circulation or varicose veins, which prevent the supply of fresh blood from reaching the wound and allowing it to heal. Leg ulcers are typically pale and weepy in the center and red and itchy around the edge.

TREATMENT

✗ DIETARY

Daily oral supplements of vitamin E (400 to 800 iu) and zinc (30 milligrams) stimulate the circulation and encourage healing.

✿ AROMATHERAPY

Bathe the ulcer with a solution of 1 cup of distilled water and 2 drops each of essential oil of clove and geranium.

☐ HOMEOPATHY

Gunpowder 6x is a wonderful blood purifier, and will assist healing by internal cleansing.

••• ORTHODOX

Treatment consists of eradicating the infection (which prevents healing) and improving circulation. Your doctor may recommend dressings, leg elevation, and removal of varicose veins.

LICE

Infestation with blood-sucking parasites that live in the hair, causing itching and redness of the scalp. You may be able to diagnose lice through the sight of white or yellowish eggs (nits) attached to the hair. The parasites are often passed between schoolchildren. For pubic lice, see **Sexually Transmitted Diseases.**

PREVENTION

▬ PRACTICAL ADVICE

Regularly check the hair for nits or lice.

❋ AROMATHERAPY

Use the following rinse if there is an outbreak of lice at your child's school, or exposure in some other way: Comb the hair with a comb that has been left in a mug of water with 10 drops of red thyme between combings.

☐ HOMEOPATHY

Psorinum 30c: 1 dose for children who are recurrently prone to lice.

TREATMENT

▬ PRACTICAL ADVICE

If a child has lice, the entire family should be treated and school authorities should be alerted. Using a special shampoo or scalp lotion that contains malathion is the best way to kill the lice. After using the product, comb the hair with a fine-toothed comb. Wash clothing, towels, and all brushes and combs. Inspect the hair with a fine-toothed comb every day to make sure there is no reinfestation.

❋ AROMATHERAPY

After shampooing, rinse the hair slowly with 1 pint of water containing 6 drops each of sweet thyme and rosemary, stirring well before use. Towel dry and allow to finish drying naturally. Comb with a fine-toothed comb.

LOW BLOOD SUGAR
See **Blood Sugar, Low.**

LOWER BACK PAIN

Pain in the lower back that can result from an exaggerated inward curvature of the lower spine, known as lordosis or swayback; more commonly known as lumbago. It may also be caused by poor posture, muscle strain from lifting, being overweight, having weak stomach muscles, or arthritis. Lower back pain can also result from degenerative diseases such as arthritis, or from an infection in the bones themselves. It is advisable to consult a professional before attempting self-help treatment.

TREATMENT

The following treatments are for lower back pain resulting from lordosis or muscular strain.

❋ BACH FLOWER REMEDIES

Difficulty relaxing and sleeping: Agrimony
Weariness of mind and body: Hornbeam

☛ MASSAGE

General back massage, concentrating particularly on the lower back and the buttock muscles, helps reduce muscle tension and pain, and restore lost mobility. Do not massage over the vertebrae, but to either side, working upward and outward with stroking movements. Spend a little more time on areas of tension or "knots," using small, circular movements to relax the muscles.

✳ ACUPRESSURE

Massage the points illustrated in the figure on the facing page using deep thumb pressure for at least 1 minute.

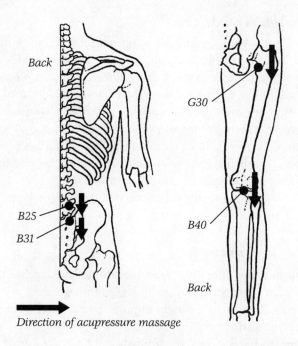

Back

G30

B25

B31

B40

Back

Direction of acupressure massage

✦ EXERCISE

The following exercises help strengthen the stomach muscles, taking strain off the lower back. Stop if they produce pain.

Pelvic Tilt: Lie on your back on the floor, place one hand under the small of the back, then try to squash the hand by pressing the small of the back down to the floor. Hold for 10 seconds, then relax. Repeat 15 times.

Abdominal Scrunches: Lie on your back with your knees bent, and slowly raise your head and chest a couple of inches off the floor, pointing your outstretched hands toward your knees. Hold for 3 seconds and relax. Repeat 10 times.

Lumbar Stretch: Lie on your back, draw both knees up to your chest, and clasp your hands around them, pulling them inward to your chest. Hold for 5 to 10 seconds, relax, and repeat 10 times.

Lumbar Stretch 2: Bring your legs inward to your chest as in Lumbar Stretch, above, but this time make a wide circle with the tops of the knees. Repeat 5 times clockwise, 5 times counterclockwise.

Lumbar Roll: Lie on your back, and bend your knees so that your feet rest near to the buttocks. Keeping the knees together, let them fall over to the left side, while keeping your shoulders and feet flat on the floor. Repeat 3 times in each direction.

~ RELAXATION TECHNIQUES

Tension exacerbates pain, so the following relaxation routine may help reduce the pain. Lie on your back, and support the knees with a pillow or bolster. It may also help to put a thin pillow or rolled-up hand towel under the small of the back. Experiment with the position until you are comfortable. Now try to let go of your pain: Close your eyes, allow your breathing to slow, and begin to be aware of how your body feels. Consciously try to relax every part of your body in turn. Begin with your face (your eyes, your forehead, your jaw), and work down to your toes. The whole procedure should take at least 10 minutes.

If you are unable to relax, try using relaxation tapes, or learn meditation or biofeedback.

+ PROFESSIONAL HELP

Chiropractic provides effective treatment through massage, ultrasound, and manipulation. Exercises may also be recommended.

The Alexander Technique will help improve posture, and is highly recommended for this condition.

Acupuncture is effective in reducing pain.

••• ORTHODOX

Your doctor will probably recommend anti-inflammatory drugs and muscle relaxants, along with physiotherapy.

LUMBAGO
See **Lower Back Pain.**

LUPUS ERYTHEMATOSUS

An autoimmune disorder in which the white blood cells, which usually attack foreign invaders, instead turn on the body's connective tissue, causing severe inflammation; a red, blotchy rash that appears on the cheeks and bridge of the nose; nausea; fatigue; fever; joint pain; and weight loss. Sometimes lupus can lead to problems with internal organs, such as the lungs, liver, and heart; therefore all treatment should be carried out in collaboration with a doctor.

TREATMENT

▬ PRACTICAL ADVICE

Some drugs can trigger lupus. Talk to your doctor if you are taking medication.

✗ DIETARY

A change in dietary fat intake and type has been shown to reduce inflammation caused by lupus. Instead of meat and dairy products, eat more fish, particularly herring, mackerel, sardines, and salmon. The vital ingredient found in fish is called eicosapentaenoic acid (EPA), which you can also take in supplement form, available at natural foods stores.

Studies have shown that vitamin E supplements can help relieve this disorder. Take up to 800 iu daily in supplement form. Apply vitamin E oil or cream to the rash.

Increased intake of vitamin B5 (pantothenic acid) helps this condition. The vitamin is found in its natural form in liver, fish, chicken, cheese, whole-grain breads and cereals, avocados, cauliflower, cooked dried peas and beans, nuts, dates, and potatoes.

People with lupus often find they have food allergies or sensitivities. See **Allergies, Food.**

Increase your intake of selenium, found in whole wheat, brown rice, oatmeal, poultry, lean meat, organ meats, and fish.

••• ORTHODOX

Doctors generally prescribe nonsteroidal anti-inflammatory drugs to relieve joint pain, antimalarial drugs for the rash, and corticosteroid drugs for fever.

LYME DISEASE

A disease that is transmitted by tick bites. Often there is no sign of a bite; then an area of redness develops surrounding the bite, followed by fever, headache, lethargy, muscle aches, and swollen joints. If the disease is not treated early, the heart and nervous system can also be affected.

PREVENTION

Cover yourself up when outside in grass, woodland, scrub, or caves. Wear shoes, socks, long pants, a shirt, and a hat.

Use an insect repellent, particularly around the ankles.

Check yourself for ticks before going inside. Wearing light clothing will help you see them—brush them off your clothing.

Indoors, inspect the skin, scalp, and pubic hair area for ticks, tiny specks that cling to the skin. Inspect children daily during the summer.

Check your pets for ticks daily to keep them from bringing ticks into the house. Tick collars and sprays can be of some help.

TREATMENT

If you find a tick on your body, *do not* try to pull it out or scrub it off, as its mouthpart may remain in your flesh. Specialized kits are available in camping supply stores and pharmacies for pulling ticks out completely; consult your doctor about proper methods. Once the tick is out, wash the bite with soap and water.

Keep an eye on the bite in the next few weeks. If you see redness developing around the area, consult your doctor immediately.

••• ORTHODOX

Lyme disease can be difficult to diagnose. If you strongly suspect Lyme disease, you may want to repeat a test that comes back negative.

A specific course of antibiotics will arrest (but not reverse) Lyme disease that is diagnosed before joint swelling occurs.

If inflammation has set in, your doctor will recommend nonsteroidal anti-inflammatory drugs and sometimes corticosteroids.

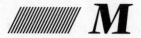 **M**

MANIC DEPRESSION

A mental disorder characterized by extreme mood swings. These may be recurrent periods of depression, or alternating phases of mania and depression. During the "high" or manic phase, the sufferer may be overly enthusiastic, self-confident, hyperactive, and sometimes reckless. During the "low" or depressive phase, the sufferer is unable to see the positive side of life, and is consumed by anxiety and guilt. Treatment should be in consultation with a doctor.

TREATMENT

■ PRACTICAL ADVICE

Talking therapies, such as counseling, psychotherapy, or psychoanalysis, are extremely helpful in dealing with the symptoms and implications of this illness.

Support and help from others in a similar situation can also help.

✗ DIETARY

A number of nutritional imbalances have been shown to contribute to depression. Your diet should balance whole-grain cereals with plenty of fresh fruits and vegetables (raw, if possible), and low-fat meat, fish, and dairy products.

The following dietary supplements may help:

* vitamin C: 1 gram a day
* vitamin B-complex: 25 milligrams a day
* magnesium: 500 milligrams a day
* amino acids: DLPA (D,L-phenylalanine) 400 milligrams a day, or L-phenylalanine 100 to 500 milligrams a day. **Caution**: Do not take if you suffer from high blood pressure.

Oral contraceptives can interfere with nutrient absorption, so naturopaths recommend finding an alternative means of contraception.

Avoid caffeine (tea, coffee, chocolate, cola) and alcohol.

Some naturopaths carry out biochemical tests to determine mineral deficiencies that may contribute to depression.

🌿 HERBALISM

St. John's wort has been shown to relieve symptoms of anxiety, depression, and low self-esteem. It also helps improve quality of sleep: Take ¼ to ¾ teaspoon of the tincture in water, 3 times a day.

❖ EXERCISE

Studies have shown that exercise can have a tremendously beneficial effect on mood disorders, particularly in alleviating depression. A regular exercise program of at least 30 minutes of aerobic activity, 3 times a week, is recommended.

∼ RELAXATION TECHNIQUES

Techniques to reduce stress, such as massage, yoga, meditation, aromatherapy, and acupressure, are helpful in alleviating the anxiety common to this illness. See **Stress** for suggestions.

✚ PROFESSIONAL HELP

Hypnosis can sometimes relieve tension and anxiety.
Professional homeopathic treatment can also help.

••• ORTHODOX

Depression is generally treated with antidepressant drugs. Mania is often controlled with lithium, a specific antimanic drug that reduces nervous activity in the brain. Long-term use produces side effects, including stomach upsets, tremor, drowsiness, and sometimes kidney damage.

MASTITIS

Painful inflammation of one or both breasts, with fever and flu-like symptoms; sometimes occurs while breast-feeding. Bacteria may enter cracked or sore nipples, leading to infection and the development of an abscess.

PREVENTION

Mastitis often develops as a result of painful breast-feeding. According to La Leche League, this can be prevented by positioning your baby correctly. The baby should be facing you, the head should be in the crook of your elbow, the buttocks in your hand. Support your breast with the other hand. Make sure the baby has your nipple deep inside his or her mouth, so that the nipple does not move and get irritated and sore.

When you begin feeding, limit the time on each nipple to avoid soreness.

Be sure to insert your finger into the baby's mouth to break the suction before removing the nipple.

Avoid using soap on your nipples, as this will dry out the skin.

Make sure you dry your nipples well (a hair dryer will help to remove all moisture) before covering them.

Rubbing a little of your own milk into sore nipples will help them to heal.

TREATMENT

▬ **PRACTICAL ADVICE**

Expelling excess milk brings relief: Hold a warm cloth on the breasts to encourage the flow of milk.

Apply vitamin E cream to heal cracked nipples.

☐ **HOMEOPATHY**

Take every 15 minutes for 4 doses; repeat if needed:

When there is excessive milk production and high fever, with red streaks on breasts: *Belladonna* 6c

When breasts are hot, hard, and painful: *Bryonia* 6c

Nipple cracked and infected: *Silicea* 6c

When pain radiates all over the body and the breast is engorged and purple: *Phytolacca* 6c

👁 **CHINESE MEDICINE**

A poultice made from powdered dried rhubarb root mixed with olive oil is applied to the breasts to ease pain. Madder root, peony bark, and dandelion are also prescribed.

••• **ORTHODOX**

Barrier sprays and antiseptic solutions are sometimes used to protect and prepare the nipples for lactation.

Once mastitis has set in, most doctors recommend antibiotic drugs, along with painkillers.

If there is no infection, breast-feeding can continue. If an abscess occurs, it will be drained (see **Abscess**).

ME (MYALGIC ENCEPHALOMYELITIS)
See **Chronic Fatigue Syndrome.**

MEASLES
A viral illness that generally occurs around the age of one to three years. The first signs are cold-like symptoms, followed by a rash behind the ears, spreading over the body; the eyes are often red and sensitive to light. The

child may have a high fever, and a cough. Stomach pains, vomiting, and diarrhea may also occur. In some complicated cases of measles, chest and ear infections can develop, and in rare cases, inflammation of the brain tissue.

TREATMENT

▬ PRACTICAL ADVICE

Put the child to bed in a dimmed room. Try not to let the child watch television or read. Instead, spend time with the child, keeping him or her calm.

✘ DIETARY

During the fever stage, give the child plenty of fluids, including fruit and vegetable juices.

Once the fever has gone down, introduce simple foods, such as cereals and vegetable soup.

❧ HERBALISM

Yarrow infusion helps reduce the fever. Use it during the first stages of the illness: Pour 1 cup of boiling water over 2 teaspoons of the dried herb, and infuse for 15 minutes; drink hot 3 times a day.

Echinacea decoction will combat the virus, ease out the rash, and help clear mucus. Use it once the fever has started to come down: Put 2 teaspoons of the root in 1 cup of water, and simmer for 15 minutes; drink 3 times a day.

☐ HOMEOPATHY

Seek professional homeopathic advice *immediately* if the rash is slow to develop or suddenly disappears.

Take 1 tablet every hour, for up to 4 doses; repeat if needed:

- Sudden onset with fever, restlessness, and intense dislike of light: *Aconite* 6c
- Burning bright red skin, hot head, and cold extremities, feverish and delirious: *Belladonna* 6c
- Mildly feverish, weepy and clingy, creamy yellow discharge from the eyes and nose: *Pulsatilla* 6c
- Hot, acrid discharge from the eyes with a bland discharge from the nose: *Euphrasia* 6c

☯ CHINESE MEDICINE

The body is encouraged to detoxify and the rash to come out by giving safflowers, peppermint, and honeysuckle.

≋ **HYDROTHERAPY**

To soothe the rash, soak in a warm bath to which you have added 3 tablespoons of baking soda.

••• **ORTHODOX**

Many doctors recommend immunization of children against the measles virus. In the United States, proof of immunization is required before the child can attend school. The vaccine should not be given to children under the age of one, nor to those who have a family history of seizures or epilepsy.

MEASLES, GERMAN
See **Rubella.**

MEMORY PROBLEMS

Memory loss, also known as amnesia, is the inability to recall or memorize information. Short-term memory loss is certainly part of the aging process. It can also result from anxiety, depression, stress, poor nutrition, inadequate sleep, or lack of brain stimulation. Memory loss accompanied by confusion, lack of concentration, or a change in behavior is usually an indication of a medical disorder and requires professional help.

TREATMENT

▬ **PRACTICAL ADVICE**

Some drugs can sometimes cause memory problems. If you are taking medication, discuss alternatives with your doctor.

The more you exercise your brain, the longer and the better it will serve you. Try to do activities that stimulate the brain: reading, crossword puzzles, games, and classes that require mental concentration and learning. From time to time, test your memory by trying to memorize poetry or lines from a novel or play.

If you find you are forgetting a name, a date, an event, or a word, try to make associations that will bring it back. For example, if you forget people's names, try to remember what they look like, where you met them, what they were wearing, and so on. In your mind, try to find everything you can associate with the forgotten issue; eventually, the links will lead you to remember what you have forgotten.

If you find you are constantly losing things, take mental photographs when you put things down. Sometimes even holding up an imaginary camera and taking a picture will help you to remember.

Writing things down can help improve your memory. Make lists of things you have to remember. If you are likely to forget to look at the list, put up notes in prominent places.

✗ DIETARY

Nerve cells require acetylcholine for healthy functioning. Acetylcholine is formed in the body from lecithin, found in eggs, sunflower oil, and soybean oil. Lecithin can also be bought in granule form from most natural foods stores. To be effective it must contain phosphatidyl choline. Studies have shown that taking supplements of up to 70 grams of lecithin a day can improve memory skills.

Increase your intake of protein: The amino acids present in protein are vital to brain functioning. You could also take a supplement that combines all 22 free-form amino acids.

Make sure your diet is high in whole-grain cereals, fruits and vegetables, and low-fat protein. Take a multivitamin and mineral supplement once a day to ensure adequate intake of other nutrients essential to good mental functioning.

☯ CHINESE MEDICINE

Practitioners of traditional Chinese medicine treat memory loss caused by stress or fatigue with herbs such as Chinese wolfberry, Chinese fleeceflower root, and black ginger seed. Acupuncture would also be recommended.

••• ORTHODOX

You doctor will investigate the cause of severe memory loss, particularly if there are signs of other mental problems. Treatment will depend on the diagnosis.

MÉNIÈRE'S DISEASE

A disorder of the inner ear where an increase in the fluids of the inner canals leads to hearing and balance problems. Typical symptoms are ringing or buzzing in one or both ears, bouts of nausea, hearing loss, and dizziness.

TREATMENT

■ PRACTICAL ADVICE

Stop smoking.

✗ DIETARY

Naturopaths recommend a salt-free, whole-foods diet, high in raw and cooked vegetables, seaweed, seeds, nuts, beans, low-fat yogurt, and fish. Avoid caffeine (coffee, tea, cola, chocolate), fried foods, alcohol, and food additives and preservatives.

Reduce your intake of fluids, except water, which helps to detoxify the system.

❋ AROMATHERAPY

Add essential oils of lavender, geranium, or sandalwood to a bath to help relieve stress.

☐ HOMEOPATHY

Ménière's disease responds well to professional homeopathic treatment.

⊹ EXERCISE

Exercise daily to increase blood circulation. Walking, swimming, cycling, and jogging are all suitable activities.

∼ RELAXATION TECHNIQUES

Stress and tension play a large part in triggering attacks of Ménière's disease. Try one or more of the following suggestions to relieve stress:

Meet other Ménière's sufferers by joining a support group.

Attend a yoga class, or learn to meditate.

Have a regular massage from a professional therapist, or exchange massages with a friend or family member.

Allow yourself to do things you enjoy. You may develop a hobby or a sport, or simply take some time off to do nothing in particular (have a bath, read a magazine, listen to music, and so on).

If you are unable to determine the cause of stress, or have problems you are unable to resolve, talking to a counselor or psychotherapist may help.

♣ REFLEXOLOGY

Massage the ear point, located where the little toe joins the sole of the left foot (see figure on the following page).

Massage the eustachian tube area, located in between the third and fourth toes, where they join the sole of the left foot.

Massage the sinuses, located on the pad of all toes except the big one.

••• ORTHODOX

Your doctor may prescribe anti-nausea drugs.

Surgery results in hearing loss, so it should be your last resort.

Ultrasonic radiation may enable vertigo to be treated without permanent hearing loss.

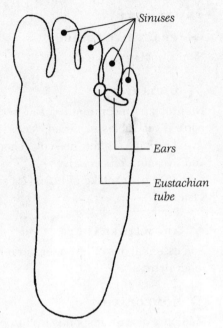

The reflex areas

MENOPAUSAL PROBLEMS

Menopause literally means the end of menstrual periods. It typically occurs during the late forties and fifties. Although many women sail through menopause without any problems, some experience varying degrees of symptoms:

hot flushes
night sweats, often leading to sleep disturbance
vaginal dryness, which results in painful sexual intercourse
dry skin (see **Skin, Dry**) and brittle hair
psychological problems, including poor concentration, anxiety, depression, tearfulness
brittle bones (see **Osteoporosis**), leading to frequent fractures that may be slow to heal
varicose veins (see **Varicose Veins**)
rheumatic symptoms (see **Rheumatoid Arthritis**)
constipation (see **Constipation**)
irregular bleeding

TREATMENT

Treatments for many of the symptoms listed above are described in detail in other sections of this book. The following recommendations are general treatments to ease you through menopause.

✖ DIETARY

Sound nutrition throughout life is one of the best ways to prevent problems with menopause. Dietary changes made at the onset of symptoms can also help.

Eat whole-grain cereals, plenty of fruits and vegetables, and low-fat protein. Avoid coffee, alcohol, sugar, chocolate, and refined or processed foods.

Research has shown that increased intake of vitamin E relieves many of the symptoms of menopause. Vitamin E is found in vegetable oils, seeds, wheat germ and nuts, avocados, peaches, whole-grain cereals, spinach, broccoli, asparagus, and dried prunes. It can also be taken as a supplement: 400 iu a day is the recommended dosage, and this can be built up gradually to 800 iu. If you are diabetic or suffer from high blood pressure or rheumatic heart disease, consult a professional before increasing your intake of vitamin E.

Psychological problems associated with menopause are often helped by increasing your intake of the B vitamins. The richest natural source of vitamin B-complex is wheat germ. Eat 2 tablespoons a day with fruit and cereal, and take one B-complex supplement a day.

Calcium is a vital nutrient, both before and during menopause, to counteract brittle bones. It is also said to reduce stress and nervous disorders, and may help relieve hot flushes. To ensure adequate intake of calcium, eat at least 3 servings of calcium-rich foods daily. These include low-fat milk, cheese, or yogurt, dark green leafy vegetables, cooked dried beans, and whole-grain cereals. If you do not eat dairy products, it is essential to eat dark green leafy vegetables such as broccoli, kale, and mustard greens every day.

🌿 HERBALISM

Ginseng contains substances with the ability to regulate hormones. Clinical trials have shown that 400 to 1,200 milligrams of Siberian ginseng daily relieved hot flushes, vaginal dryness, sweats, and anxiety.

☯ CHINESE MEDICINE

Acupuncture can help. Commonly recommended herbs include Chinese angelica, romania, peony root, and thorowax root.

✛ EXERCISE

Studies have shown that regular exercise is highly beneficial in counteracting menopausal problems. Aerobic exercise, which also includes stretching, muscle strengthening, and relaxation, is the best. Walking, jogging, swimming, or aerobics classes are suitable. Combine one of these with a weekly yoga class to aid relaxation.

••• ORTHODOX

Hormone replacement therapy (HRT) is often offered to women with menopausal problems. It provides estrogen and progesterone in the form of vaginal cream, pills, skin implants, or a slow-release skin patch. It relieves hot flushes and vaginal dryness, and prevents brittle bones. However, the side effects of long-term use of hormone therapy are not clear, and some studies suggest it may increase the likelihood of developing breast or endometrial cancer.

MIGRAINE

A throbbing headache usually on one side of the head, accompanied by visual problems and sometimes nausea or vomiting. A migraine can be an individual attack or a recurrent problem triggered by anxiety, anger, excitement, depression, shock, overexertion, or changes in diet, climate, or routine. An attack can last for anywhere between two hours and two days.

TREATMENT

✗ DIETARY

Migraine is sometimes triggered by low blood sugar (see **Blood Sugar, Low**).

Specific foods thought to trigger migraines in children include cow's milk, egg, chocolate, orange, wheat, cheese, tomato, rye, benzoic acid, tartrazine, fish, beef, pork, soy, bacon, coffee, yeast, and peanuts. Foods that trigger migraines in adults include cheese, red wine, monosodium glutamate, nitrates, and chocolate. To identify foods that may be a problem, check labels on foods scrupulously and keep a record of everything you eat, noting also any symptoms that appear. After a few months, you may become aware which foods trigger a migraine. If you think you have identified a trigger, avoid the food for at least 1 month. During this time note down your symptoms, along with other foods eaten. If the migraine symptoms decrease, avoid the food group for another 3 months. After this, you may find you can tolerate small amounts of it (once or twice a week only). However, if symptoms return, avoid the food altogether. You may have to carry out this process with many different foods to find the culprit.

❀ AROMATHERAPY

Try inhalations, baths, or massages using essential oil of true melissa or rosemary and sweet marjoram. An aromatherapy massage is very relaxing.

❧ HERBALISM

Medical studies have shown that feverfew (*Tanacetum parthenium*) is an effective remedy for reducing the intensity and frequency of migraine attacks. Take 2 or 3 small leaves of feverfew a day, chopped up in a sandwich (a sprinkling of sugar helps to disguise the bitter taste). Feverfew tablets are available from pharmacies and natural foods stores—follow the dosage instructions on the package. The results may take two to 3 months to become apparent.

☐ HOMEOPATHY

Take every 15 minutes for up to 6 doses; repeat if needed:

For hammering pain that comes and goes with the sun, accompanied by visual disturbances and preceded by numbness and tingling in the lips: *Natrum muriaticum* 6c

Visual disturbances with vomiting and burning in the gut: *Iris versicolor* 6c

Preceded by visual disturbances that ease as the headache begins: *Kali bichromicum* 6c.

Pain spreads from the occiput to the right eye, accompanied by flushes of heat: *Sanguinaria* 6c

Severe pain round the left eye and down the left side of the face, with tears from the affected eye, and severely aggravated by tobacco smoke: *Spigelia* 6c

☯ CHINESE MEDICINE

Professional acupressure and acupuncture treatments can be very effective.

✳ ACUPRESSURE

Massage your head as if you were shampooing your hair.

Place your thumbs underneath the base of the skull on either side of the spinal column. Tilt your head back slightly and press upward for 2 minutes while breathing deeply.

It can be very helpful to massage the points illustrated in the figure on the following page. Use deep thumb pressure for at least 1 minute.

❖ EXERCISE

Regular aerobic exercise has been shown to reduce attacks of migraine. Swimming, walking, or running for 30 minutes, 3 times a week, is recommended. Yoga stretches help ease mental and physical tension.

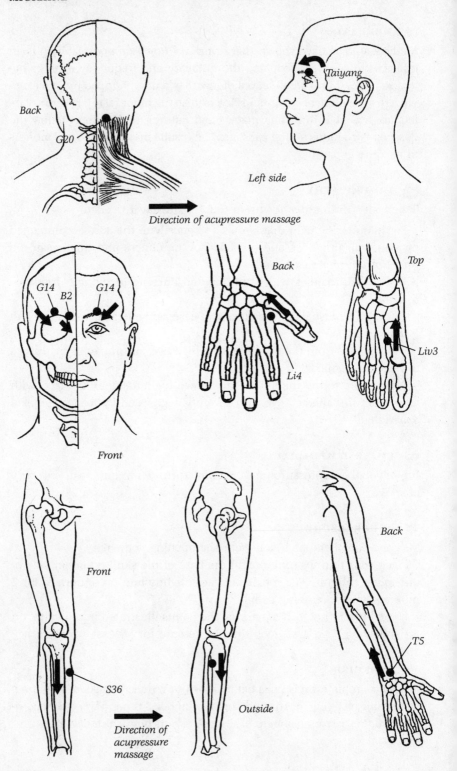

Back

G20

Taiyang

Left side

Direction of acupressure massage

G14 B2 G14

Front

Back

Li4

Top

Liv3

Front

S36

Outside

Direction of acupressure massage

Back

T5

～ RELAXATION TECHNIQUES

Migraine is often triggered by stress. Learning how to anticipate and deal with stressful situations may reduce attacks:

Learn to identify your fears and concerns; making a list can sometimes help.

Learn to deal with these problems one by one; try talking to a friend, relative, or health care practitioner, counselor, or psychotherapist.

Avoid creating unnecessary stress; for example, always give yourself plenty of time, so that you don't have to rush to appointments; try not to take on more work or activities than you can handle; learn to say no.

Attend a yoga or meditation class, take regular exercise, or develop a hobby to help you relax.

❖ REFLEXOLOGY

Massage the area relating to the head; this includes all the toes, particularly the big toes.

Massage the neck area, located where the toes join the sole of the foot.

✚ PROFESSIONAL HELP

Applied kinesiology is used to detect allergies.

Chiropractic can help when the migraine is related to a spinal misalignment.

A dentist or orthodontist may be able to help when the migraine is related to a jaw misalignment (see **Temporomandibular Joint Syndrome**).

••• ORTHODOX

If you are taking oral contraceptives, your doctor would probably recommend an alternative method of contraception.

Painkillers may also be prescribed, along with drugs that have a stabilizing effect on the blood vessels of the head.

MISCARRIAGE

Loss of the baby before the pregnancy has come to term. Miscarriage is relatively common: one in six pregnancies ends in miscarriage. There is often no specific cause; however, most miscarriages are believed to result from fetal abnormalities, hormonal imbalances, structural problems in the uterus, weak cervical muscles, industrial or environmental toxins, or a fall. Signs of a miscarriage include lower abdominal cramps, bleeding, or staining. Contact your doctor immediately if any of these symptoms occur.

TREATMENT AFTER A MISCARRIAGE

If you have had a miscarriage, it is advisable to delay the subsequent conception for 3 months. Spend this time bringing your health up to peak with the following guidelines.

✗ DIETARY

Eat 2 to 4 servings a day of protein-rich foods (fish, poultry, eggs, beans, peas, nuts, seeds).

Eat plenty of whole-grain cereals (bread, rice, pasta).

Eat 5 to 7 portions a day of fruits or vegetables.

Eat a minimum of 3 portions of calcium-rich foods: dairy products or green leafy vegetables.

Drink spring water, fruit juices, herbal teas, and milk drinks; avoid caffeine (coffee, chocolate, tea, cola), alcohol, and cigarettes.

Avoid raw meat and fish, and uncooked vegetables that you have not thoroughly washed yourself.

☐ HOMEOPATHY

Take every 15 minutes for 6 doses:

Where there is a risk of miscarriage after an accident or shock: *Arnica 6c*

Where there is a risk of a miscarriage caused by amniocentesis: *Hypericum 6c*

✿ BACH FLOWER REMEDIES

Take Rock Rose, 4 times a day.

⁘ EXERCISE

Gentle stretching, swimming, or yoga helps strengthen the body in preparation for childbirth. It also relaxes the mind and alleviates stress.

✚ PROFESSIONAL HELP

Chiropractic may help to minimize structural stress on supporting ligaments in the pelvic area and improve blood circulation and mobility.

Professional homeopathic treatment after a miscarriage is often helpful, particularly where there is a history of recurrent miscarriages.

••• ORTHODOX

Consult your doctor if you have any bleeding in pregnancy. If your doctor does diagnose a threatened miscarriage, it does not necessarily mean that miscarriage will follow. Bed rest may be recommended, though there is no hard evidence that this prevents miscarriage.

If you do miscarry, your doctor may want to perform a dilatation and curettage (D and C) to remove any fragments from the uterus that might get infected or cause irregular bleeding or pain.

In cases of recurrent miscarriage (three or more), a new type of treatment known as immunotherapy is available in some hospitals.

MONONUCLEOSIS, INFECTIOUS

A condition caused by the Epstein-Barr virus. Symptoms include exhaustion, fever, sore throat, muscular aches and pains, and swollen lymph glands, particularly in the neck; also known as glandular fever. It is common in people aged ten through twenty-five, and is generally transmitted through saliva; hence it is also known as the "kissing disease."

TREATMENT

■ PRACTICAL ADVICE

Rest is very important in treating this condition. You may feel tired for two or three months after recovery, so take it easy to prevent a relapse.

Avoid alcohol and smoking.

✗ DIETARY

A whole-foods diet with plenty of fresh fruits and vegetables is vital to build resistance. If you cannot eat easily, try freshly squeezed fruit juices and vegetable soups.

Take 500 milligrams of vitamin C, 3 times a day.

Take a 50-milligram vitamin B-complex supplement, 3 times a day.

To boost immunity after an attack, eat a whole-foods diet rich in fruits and vegetables, with a high intake of foods rich in the following nutrients:

- vitamin A, found in liver, kidney, egg yolk, low-fat dairy products, and cod liver oil
- beta-carotene, found in dark green, yellow, and orange vegetables and fruits
- vitamin E, found in vegetable oils, seeds, wheat germ, and nuts
- vitamin C, found in fruits and vegetables
- the B vitamins, particularly vitamin B6, found in lean meat, wheat germ, brewer's yeast, fish, soybeans, peas, and peanuts
- copper, iron, zinc, and selenium, found in lean meats, poultry, fish, whole wheat bread, brown rice, and oatmeal

﹩ HERBALISM

Tincture of myrrh helps fight infection: Take ¼ to ¾ teaspoon of the tincture in 1 cup of warm water, 3 times a day.

☐ HOMEOPATHY

Take 3 times a day for up to 7 days; repeat if needed:

- Sleepy and stupefied, dark mottled rash, purplish throat with ulcers on the tonsils: *Ailanthus* 6c
- Profuse offensive sweats, painfully swollen neck glands, exhausted and shaky: *Mercurius* 6c
- Sensation of a hot ball in the throat, with pain darting into the ears on swallowing, generalized aching: *Phytolacca* 6c

A number of remedies are extremely helpful for patients who experience a permanent impairment in their level of health or general energy after recovering from the acute phase. Consult a professional homeopath.

☯ CHINESE MEDICINE

Practitioners of traditional Chinese medicine treat this condition by eliminating heat in the blood, liver, and stomach. Red peony, dyers' woad leaf, honeysuckle, forsythia fruit, chrysanthemum flowers, and dandelions would be prescribed. Individual treatment is recommended.

••• ORTHODOX

Doctors recommend rest and plenty of warm drinks. Most people recover after four to six weeks, without medication.

MORNING SICKNESS

Nausea and vomiting in early pregnancy as a result of changing hormonal levels, experienced by about 50 percent of pregnant women. Despite its name, morning sickness commonly occurs at any time of the day or night; and despite the discomfort, this is not usually a sign of an unhealthy pregnancy.

TREATMENT

✗ DIETARY

Start the day with herbal tea, such as chamomile, and a few dry crackers.
Avoid fried and fatty foods.
Pineapple (juice or fruit) relieves nausea.

Eat small meals often. If you do not feel like eating, maintain your blood-sugar level with orange juice, fruit, milk drinks, soup, or nuts.

Keep some nourishing snacks to nibble on: almonds are particularly nutritious.

❧ AROMATHERAPY

Add essential oils of mandarin and lavender to your bath.

Put 2 drops each of peppermint and sandalwood oil on a tissue or handkerchief and inhale.

Add 2 drops each of peppermint and sandalwood oil to 2 teaspoons of a carrier oil, and massage into the chest and stomach in a clockwise direction.

ぐ HERBALISM

Ginger is effective in reducing nausea: Pour 1 cup of boiling water on 1 teaspoon of the freshly grated root, and infuse for 5 minutes; drink when needed.

☐ HOMEOPATHY

Take every hour for up to 4 doses; repeat if needed:

Feeling nauseous at the thought or smell of food or from traveling, but better after eating: *Sepia* 6c

Nausea made better by vomiting: *Nux vomica* 6c

Nausea relieved by eating with profuse salivation and a history of anemia: *Lactic acid* 6c

Nausea and vomiting relieved by keeping the abdomen uncovered: *Tabacum* 6c

☯ CHINESE MEDICINE

Practitioners of traditional Chinese medicine generally recommend "hot" foods, such as ginger, green and red peppers, chicken, cinnamon twigs, and onions. "Cold" foods, such as bananas, grapefruit, lettuce, and watermelon, should be avoided.

✳ ACUPRESSURE

Place your right thumb on the inside of your left wrist, two thumbbreadths from the center of the wrist joint toward the elbow. Massage with the thumb, using a deep circular motion, for 1 minute, while taking deep breaths. Do the same on the other wrist.

••• ORTHODOX

Generally, doctors avoid giving drugs during pregnancy. However, if you are vomiting all your food, and are at risk of dehydration, antacids and certain antihistamines may be prescribed.

MOSQUITO BITES
See **Insect Bites and Stings.**

MOTION SICKNESS
A feeling of uneasiness, headache, sweating and salivation, pallor, nausea, and vomiting while traveling by car, bus, boat, or rail. It is caused by the effect of movement on the organs of balance in the inner ear. Anxiety, lack of oxygen, a full stomach, the sight of food, reading, or focusing on nearby objects often makes symptoms worse.

PREVENTION

○ SEA TRAVEL

Try to stay outside on deck, where you can see the horizon. Enclosed spaces increase feelings of nausea.

Avoid heavy meals while traveling, though a light snack may help.

Lie down, if possible.

Don't read or play games that require focusing on moving objects or words.

Stay in the midline of the boat, as this part oscillates less than the sides.

○ ROAD/RAIL TRAVEL

Try to travel in the front seat; focusing on the road ahead helps stabilize the balance system.

Do not eat or drink just before traveling.

Do not allow smoking in the car.

Sit still.

Do not read or play games that require focusing on moving objects or words or stationary objects inside the car.

TREATMENT

❀ AROMATHERAPY

Add 4 drops each of essential oil of peppermint and ginger to a carrier oil or lotion, and massage into the chest before traveling. Sprinkle a little of the same mixture on a handkerchief, and sniff it if you feel nauseous.

ᏅᎾ HERBALISM

Ginger root absorbs stomach acid and prevents sickness: Take 2 ginger root capsules 30 minutes before traveling, or chew a piece of fresh, peeled ginger root.

☐ HOMEOPATHY

Take every hour, as soon as symptoms begin:

Nausea made worse by the smell of food, made better by eating: *Sepia* 6c

Nausea with a metallic taste in the mouth and feeling very giddy: *Cocculus* 6c

When overtired and irritable: *Arnica* 30c

Chilly, with the sensation you would feel better for vomiting: *Nux vomica* 30c

Angry and frustrated: *Staphysagria* 30c

✿ BACH FLOWER REMEDIES

Scleranthus and Rescue Remedy are recommended before and during traveling, as needed.

✳ ACUPRESSURE

Place your right thumb on the inside of your left wrist, 3 finger-widths from the center of the wrist crease. Massage with the thumb, using a deep circular motion, for 1 minute, while taking deep breaths. Then do the same on the other side.

The same treatment can be obtained by wearing acupressure wrist bands, available in many pharmacies, supermarkets, and travel goods shops. The bands have a small ball attached. When placed on the pressure point described above, the ball exerts continuous pressure while the band is worn.

••• ORTHODOX

Doctors may recommend taking antihistamine drugs such as dimenhydrinate or cinnarizine 30 minutes to 1 hour before traveling. Myoscine is useful too, and can be used in the form of a skin patch giving a slow-release formulation.

MOUNTAIN SICKNESS
See **Altitude Sickness.**

MOUTH ULCERS

White, gray, or yellow spots, which occur singly or in clusters in the mouth. Often they are inflamed, with a red border, and are extremely painful. Sometimes mouth ulcers result from injury (biting the side of the mouth or being cut by sharp braces, for example); they can be a sign of digestive disorders, or a physical response to stress or a virus. Consult your doctor about any ulcer that fails to heal within three or four weeks.

TREATMENT

✗ DIETARY

Naturopaths recommend a purifying diet of fruit juices, fruits, and vegetables for 2 days. Follow this with a whole-grain diet with plenty of raw and cooked vegetables (if your mouth is too sore to eat rough food, liquefy the vegetables). Avoid foods that may cause allergies (see **Allergies, Food**).

Take daily supplements of vitamin A (750 micrograms), vitamin E (250 milligrams), and vitamin B2 (10 milligrams).

Apply vitamin E oil (squeezed from a pierced capsule) directly to the ulcers.

❀ AROMATHERAPY

Mix 1 drop of essential oil of geranium and lavender to ½ cup of water. Use as a mouthwash 3 or 4 times a day.

❧ HERBALISM

Myrrh is an effective antimicrobial agent, recommended specifically for mouth ulcers: Add ⅕ teaspoon of the tincture to 1 cup of warm water, and use as a mouthwash 3 times a day.

You can also use the tincture undiluted as a mouthwash. It will sting a little, but is effective.

If the ulcers result from injury, rub a little aloe vera gel on them.

▢ HOMEOPATHY

Take every 2 hours on the first day, and 3 times a day for 2 to 3 days:

When ulcers are on the edges of the tongue, with burning pain: *Arsenicum album* 6c

Yellowish indented ulcers that feel firm and thick, with stinging pain: *Kali bichromicum* 6c

Ulcers on the palate or tongue, yellowish and spongy, with gums that bleed easily: *Mercurius solubilis* 30c

••• ORTHODOX

Use antiseptic mouth rinses on a short-term basis. Soluble hydrocortisone pellets or oral pastes are also prescribed for mouth ulcers.

MULTIPLE SCLEROSIS (MS)

A disease of the central nervous system, where the myelin sheaths covering nerve fibers in the brain and spinal cord are gradually destroyed. The wide range of symptoms includes tingling, pins and needles or numbness, difficulty walking, foot dragging, loss of coordination, distorted sensation, blurred vision, slurred speech, fatigue, and incontinence.

TREATMENT

✗ DIETARY

Avoid foods high in saturated fat: meat, dairy products, hard fats, and store-bought pastries and snacks. (You can make your own pastries from whole-grain flour and polyunsaturated margarine.)

Increase your intake of essential fatty acids, found in polyunsaturated margarines and oils (sunflower, safflower, soy, sesame, cottonseed, corn, rapeseed), nuts and beans (avoid coconuts and peanuts), liver, and green leafy vegetables.

Food sensitivities may enhance your symptoms (see **Allergies, Food**). Milk is a common allergen in MS sufferers. Applied kinesiology can be useful in detecting food sensitivities.

Avoid junk foods and processed foods, and avoid sugar.

Eat whole-grain cereals, and plenty of fresh fruits and vegetables.

The following daily dietary supplements have been shown to be helpful:

- 500 milligrams evening primrose oil (3 capsules, 3 times a day), with meals
- 1,000 milligrams fish oil, in capsules or cod liver oil supplement
- 100 iu vitamin E (3 times a day)
- 1 25-milligram vitamin B-complex tablet a day
- 50 milligrams vitamin B6
- 1 gram vitamin C (3 times a day)
- 15 milligrams elemental zinc
- 50 milligrams magnesium

☞ MASSAGE

Regular massage increases blood circulation, prevents stiffness, enhances mobility, and improves general well-being. Learn to do massage by attending a class, or exchanging treatments with a friend or family member.

ⵜ EXERCISE

Gentle daily swimming, dancing, walking, trampolining, and gentle stretching and aerobics are all helpful in maintaining mobility. However, do not allow yourself to become fatigued by exercise. Consult your doctor before you begin any exercise program.

✳ YOGA

Studies have shown that regular yoga helps prevent deterioration. Some areas have special classes for people with MS.

✚ PROFESSIONAL HELP

The Alexander Technique helps postural problems, coordination, and movement.

Homeopathic treatment helps in some cases.

••• ORTHODOX

Physiotherapy is very important to maintain the use of limbs.

Hyperbaric oxygen treatment, where pressurized oxygen is introduced into the body, has been shown to help some people.

Short courses of steroids are prescribed for acute attacks.

MUMPS

A viral illness that causes infection and swelling of the glands, particularly the salivary glands and the parotids, situated below and in front of the ears. The infection, which is highly contagious, usually occurs in children between the ages of three and ten. Symptoms include mild sickness and discomfort and swelling in each of the glands in turn. Fever, headache, and difficulty swallowing may follow. Mumps in male teenagers and adults can cause inflammation of the testes.

TREATMENT

▬ PRACTICAL ADVICE

Children do not have to stay in bed unless the fever is high, but should be kept warm and quiet. They may be infectious to others until the swelling totally subsides.

✗ DIETARY

Eat light foods, such as soups, juices, fruits, and vegetables.
Avoid dairy products, eggs, sugar, and red meat.
Drink plenty of fluids.

❧ HERBALISM

Poke root decoction is effective in detoxifying the glands and removing phlegm: Put ¼ teaspoon of the root in 1 cup of water, and simmer gently for 10 minutes; drink 3 times a day.

☐ HOMEOPATHY

Take 3 times a day for 3 to 4 days:

Child is flushed and hot, with throbbing pain in the glands, worse on the right side: *Belladonna* 6c

Pain worse on the left side, with difficulty in swallowing liquids, and intolerance of any covering of the throat: *Lachesis* 6c

Stiff neck from swollen glands, profuse and offensive salivation: *Mercurius solubilis* 6c

••• ORTHODOX

A child in great pain will probably be given painkillers.

In male adolescents or men, corticosteroid drugs will be given to reduce inflammation in the testes, which can lead to infertility.

A mumps vaccination is available, and is usually given in combination with measles and rubella vaccines. It should not be given to children under a year old.

 *N*

NAIL PROBLEMS

Healthy nails should be strong, smooth, and flesh-colored. Common problems include nail biting, nails that split or flake, the development of ridges, fungal infections (see **Fungal Infection**), and stunted nail growth. See also **Ingrown Toenail.**

TREATMENT

■ PRACTICAL ADVICE

Keep nails well manicured: File down any rough points or edges that you may be tempted to bite. Keep the cuticles soft, and ease them back every time you wash your hands.

For bitten nails: Paint fingernails with bitter aloes, available from most herbalists. It makes the nails taste unpleasant and discourages biting.

For fragile nails: Damaged nails and cuticles can stunt growth: Keep the nails in shape by gentle filing with an emery board. Keep cuticles pushed back by gentle massaging with cream after a bath or shower—use your fingertips to do this, never use anything sharp.

✗ DIETARY

Iron deficiency (see **Anemia**) can lead to nail problems. The most common sign is nails that grow to be spoon-shaped. Iron deficiency also causes brittle nails that crack easily. Increase your iron intake with red meats, fish and poultry, and green leafy vegetables. Vitamin C increases iron absorption, so incorporate oranges, grapefruits, or their juice into your meals. Avoid drinking tea before, during, or after a meal, as this inhibits iron absorption.

Splitting and breaking nails can also be caused by lack of vitamin A and protein. Incorporate liver, cod liver oil, and carrot juice into your daily diet.

Fungal infections and infections of the skin fold at the base of the nail (paronychia) can be helped by increasing your intake of the B-complex vitamins, found in brewer's yeast (take ½ teaspoon in a drink 3 times a day). Eat plenty of live yogurt with *Lactobacillus acidophilus* every day, or take supplements of *Lactobacillus acidophilus.* Take ½ teaspoon of *Lactobacillus acidophilus,* 1 teaspoon of *Bifidobacteria* powder, and ½ teaspoon of *Lactobacillus bulgaricus* (available from natural foods stores) in a glass of spring water, 3 times a day.

White spots on the nails may be a sign of zinc and vitamin B6 deficiency. Remedy this by increasing your intake of poultry and fish, whole-grain cereals, brewer's yeast, and wheat germ.

❋ BIOCHEMIC TISSUE SALTS
Silica 6x up to 4 times a day will encourage healthy nail growth.

⁘ EXERCISE
Exercising the fingers (typing, playing the piano, doing craft work) speeds up the growth of nail tissue. Regular massaging to keep the cuticles back will also help.

••• ORTHODOX
Treatment consists of correction of any underlying nutritional deficiency, or any causative medical disorder, such as a fungal infection, psoriasis, thyroid disease, or respiratory condition.

NAUSEA
Feeling sick, with or without vomiting. Nausea can result from eating rich foods (see **Indigestion**); drinking too much alcohol (see **Hangover**); food poisoning (see **Food Poisoning**); shock; experiencing unpleasant smells, sights, or tastes; migraine (see **Migraine**); stress (see **Stress**); as a reaction to a mild or serious disease; motion (see **Motion Sickness**); as a side effect of some drugs; and pregnancy (see **Morning Sickness**).

TREATMENT
✗ DIETARY
For food-induced nausea:

If you are able to eat, take easily digestible whole-grain cereals, vegetable soups, or steamed vegetables.

Drink plenty of fluids, particularly water.

Nibbling dry biscuits can help relieve nausea.

❋ AROMATHERAPY
Nausea caused by stress or emotional disturbances is best treated with essential oils of sandalwood or lavender: Add 4 drops of each to a warm bath.

🐌 HERBALISM

Black horehound infusion is an effective remedy for nausea caused by stress or nervousness: Pour 1 cup of boiling water on 2 teaspoons of the dried herb, and infuse for 10 minutes; drink 3 times a day.

Chamomile infusion soothes the stomach. Tea bags are widely available.

Ginger is an effective remedy for most types of nausea: Place 1 teaspoon of the fresh grated root in 1 cup of boiling water, infuse for 5 minutes, and strain; drink when needed.

▢ HOMEOPATHY

Feeling nauseous at the thought or smell of food or from traveling, but better after eating: *Sepia* 6c

Nausea made better by vomiting: *Nux vomica* 6c

Nausea relieved by eating, with profuse salivation and a history of anemia: *Lactic acid* 6c

Nausea and vomiting relieved by keeping the abdomen uncovered: *Tabacum* 6c

✳ ACUPRESSURE

Place your right thumb on the inside of your wrist at the point three finger-widths down your arm from the wrist crease. Press firmly for 1 minute. Then move the thumb to the point two finger-widths from the crease, and press for 1 more minute. Repeat on the other wrist.

••• ORTHODOX

Consult your doctor about persistent and unexplained nausea lasting more than 48 hours. Once the cause has been established, antiemetic drugs that relieve nausea by suppressing the vomiting reflex in the brain may be prescribed.

NEARSIGHTEDNESS
See **Eyesight Problems.**

NECK PAIN AND STIFFNESS

Usually, neck pain is a result of muscle spasm originating in fatigue, tension, bad posture, long hours spent at a desk, or driving. It can also result from a strain or injury (see **Whiplash Injury**). Consult your doctor about neck pain accompanied by a severe headache, nausea, and intolerance of light. See also **Fibrositis; Torticollis.**

PREVENTION

■ PRACTICAL ADVICE

To reduce neck pain caused by bad posture:

Make sure your chair is the right height for your desk: your feet should be flat on the ground, and your back upright. You should not have to hunch to do your work.

Do not hold the phone between your shoulder and ear.

Get up and walk around every hour or so to change position. Go out for a walk at lunchtime and get some exercise before or after work.

Try to sleep on your back or side, not your stomach.

✳ YOGA

You can practice these postures at any time. Use them as a preventive measure, or to relieve neck pain and strain. Do each movement at least 3 times, twice a day.

Let your head slowly drop forward as far as it will go toward your chest. Hold this position for 20 seconds. Lift your head and let it fall back as far as it will go; hold for 30 seconds.

Turn your head to the right as far as it will go without straining; hold for 20 seconds. Turn back to center and drop your chin to your chest. Lift your chin and turn the head to the left as far as you can go; hold for 20 seconds. Bring the head back to center and drop forward again.

Let your head fall to the side so that your ear approaches your shoulder (do not bring your shoulder to your ear); hold for 20 seconds. Repeat on the other side.

If the neck and shoulder muscles are stiff, stand facing a wall with your feet about 3 feet from the base. Place your hands flat on the wall, above your head and at shoulder width. Keeping your arms and legs straight, let your head and shoulders fall between your arms toward the wall. Hold the position for up to 20 seconds.

TREATMENT

≈ HYDROTHERAPY

To reduce neck pain and inflammation, try hot and cold treatments. Make an ice pack by wrapping a plastic bag full of ice cubes or a bag of frozen peas in a kitchen towel. Also prepare a hot water bottle wrapped in a towel. Apply the ice pack to the painful area for 10 minutes, then apply the hot water bottle for 10 minutes. Repeat the procedure, and carry out morning and night.

☞ MASSAGE

Turn your head to the left side, and place the ends of the fingers of your right hand at the top of the large muscle which runs from the back of the right-hand side of your head to the collar bone (sternocleidomastoid muscle). Massage the length of the muscle with firm stripping movements. Do the same on the other side.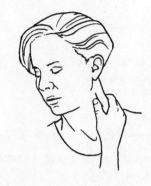

Hook the fingers of both hands over your shoulders, and squeeze the muscles lying between the neck and the shoulder joints.

If you regularly suffer neck pain, it is worth having a regular massage from a therapist. You can also learn to do massage with a friend and exchange treatments.

✳ ACUPRESSURE

Massage the points illustrated with deep thumb pressure for 1 minute.

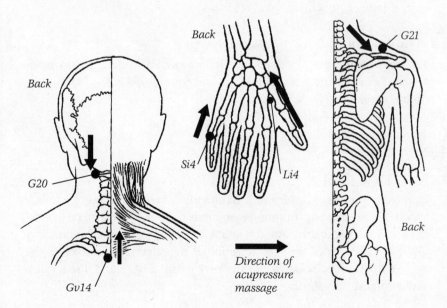

Back

Back

G21

Back

G20

Si4

Li4

Gv14

Back

Direction of
acupressure
massage

～ RELAXATION TECHNIQUES

Neck pain is often a sign of fatigue or stress. Try to recognize its onset and adjust your schedule to allow less tension and more sleep (see **Stress**).

Make a neck rest by putting 2 tennis balls in a sock and tying the end. Lie down on the floor, putting the sock under your neck. The balls should be on either side of the spine. Relax in this position for between 5 and 10 minutes a day.

✤ REFLEXOLOGY

If the neck is too sensitive to move or massage, reflexology can help.

Massage the neck area, located where the big toe joins the foot on the sole of the left foot.

Massage the cervical spine area, located along the inner side of both feet, along the joint of the big toe.

Rotate the big toe.

✚ PROFESSIONAL HELP

If symptoms persist, consult a chiropractor; treatment usually consists of massage and gentle manipulation. If there is underlying disease, you will be referred to a general practitioner, or to a specialist for an X-ray.

The Alexander Technique is very useful in correcting postural problems relating to neck pain and stiffness.

••• ORTHODOX

For less severe cases, try deep heat lotions, available over the counter.

Your doctor may prescribe painkillers and nonsteroidal anti-inflammatory agents if your case is severe.

NEURALGIA

Pain caused by nerve injury or inflammation. Symptoms may include a shooting pain, tingling, numbness, or bouts of pain. It can also be a burning sensation that occurs after an attack of herpes or shingles. It typically affects the nerves of the face (trigeminal neuralgia); the nerves at the back of the leg (see **Sciatica**); or the back of the tongue and throat (glossopharyngeal neuralgia).

TREATMENT

✗ DIETARY

B vitamins are important for the normal functioning of nerve cells:

Increase your intake of vitamin B1, found in pork, green peas, oranges, dried beans and peas, wheat germ, and brewer's yeast.

Increase your intake of vitamin B2, found in milk, green leafy vegetables, mushrooms, asparagus, avocados, and broccoli.

Increase your intake of vitamin B7 (biotin), found in liver, oatmeal, egg yolk, soybeans, mushrooms, bananas, peanuts, and brewer's yeast.

Take a vitamin B-complex supplement daily.

❋ AROMATHERAPY

Add 2 drops each of essential oil of lavender and basil to inhalations, baths, or massage oils to relax the nervous system. One drop of valerian will enhance the effectiveness.

❧ HERBALISM

St. John's wort has sedating and painkilling properties. To make an infusion: Pour 1 cup of boiling water on 2 teaspoons of the dried herb, and infuse for 10 minutes; drink 3 times a day.

Valerian infusion reduces tension and aids sleep: Add 1 cup of boiling water to 2 teaspoons of the root, and infuse for 15 minutes; drink when needed.

☐ HOMEOPATHY

Take every 15 minutes for up to 4 doses; repeat if necessary:

Pain after exposure to cold wind: *Aconite* 6c

Shooting pain after an injury or spinal injection: *Hypericum* 6c

≈ HYDROTHERAPY

Make an ice pack by wrapping a plastic bag full of ice cubes or a bag of frozen peas in a kitchen towel. Hold the ice pack to the affected area for 10 minutes. Wait 10 minutes, then apply again for a further 10 minutes. Do this 2 times a day.

✚ PROFESSIONAL HELP

Chiropractic should be your first step in seeking therapy.

Practitioners of traditional Chinese medicine would use acupuncture and herbs to treat this condition.

Hypnotherapy can be useful in treating this condition.

Transcutaneous electrical nerve stimulation (TENS), available in many hospitals, works in the same way as acupuncture without using needles: electrodes block electrical pain impulses to the brain and stimulate the release of endorphins, the body's own pain relief hormones.

••• ORTHODOX

Your doctor would try to identify and resolve the source of nerve irritation. This may involve surgery. If the problem cannot be resolved, pain relief and nerve tissue stabilizers, such as carbamazepine, are often recommended.

NIGHTMARES/NIGHT TERROR

Vivid and unpleasant dreams that often bring a sense of suffocation. Nightmares are common in children aged eight to ten, particularly if the child is unwell or anxious. In adults, anxiety, trauma, or drugs are often the cause of bad dreams and night terror. Night terror is more common in children aged four to seven. They do not wake up, but become agitated and start screaming, often within the first three hours of falling asleep, and are unable to recognize familiar faces. The child usually calms down after a while and does not remember the event the next day.

TREATMENT

■ PRACTICAL ADVICE

Limit evening television watching in children: some of the programs may be unsuitable and cause fright; the flickering screen may also stimulate the child.

☐ HOMEOPATHY

Take at night, every 5 minutes until calmed:
  With a terrible fear of the dark: *Stramonium* 30c
  Hallucinations during sleep, wakes glassy eyed: *Belladonna* 30c
  Highly impressionable and imaginative, frightened of ghosts and thunderstorms: *Phosphorus* 6c

✿ BACH FLOWER REMEDIES

Nightmares, for those who wake in fear and panic, afraid to go back to sleep: Take Aspen.

  A child who wakes screaming from a nightmare: Sip Rock Rose in water.

••• ORTHODOX

No medication is given; in fact, drugs could make the problem worse. Doctors advise parents to give gentle reassurance to children who wake up with nightmares. It is not necessary to talk about the content of the nightmare, but better to distract the child onto a more comfortable topic.

NITS
See **Lice.**

NONSPECIFIC URETHRITIS
See **Sexually Transmitted Diseases.**

NOSEBLEED

Nosebleeds are common in children, and are not generally a cause for concern. They sometimes occur as a result of something hitting the nose, which damages delicate blood vessels, or during or after a cold or nasal infection. If a nosebleed occurs after a head injury, and is accompanied by drowsiness, vomiting, or headache, or if the bleeding does not stop within 10 minutes, seek emergency help.

TREATMENT

▬ PRACTICAL ADVICE

Sit up. Do not lie down, as this forces the blood down the throat.

Blow your nose once to remove the clot that may be keeping the blood vessels open.

Pinch the nose with thumb and forefinger along the sides of the bony prominence in the middle of the nose; hold the pinch until the bleeding stops.

Wet a piece of sterile cotton with cold water, and plug up the bleeding nostril.

✗ DIETARY

For persistent nosebleeds, take 2 grams of vitamin C complex a day, and/ or beetroot concentrate—this is rich in bioflavonoids, which strengthen blood vessels. Also increase your intake of foods rich in vitamin C and bioflavonoids, especially citrus fruits.

❧ HERBALISM

Take nettle infusion if nosebleeds occur frequently for no apparent reason: Pour 1 cup of boiling water onto 3 teaspoons of the dried herb, and infuse for 10 minutes; drink 3 times a day.

☐ HOMEOPATHY

Take every 10 minutes for 4 doses; repeat if necessary:

When nosebleed results from a blow or injury or washing the face: *Arnica* 6c

Bright red blood that is slow to clot: *Phosphorus* 6c

Nosebleeds during sleep: *Sulphur* 6c

Dark, black, and stringy discharge during the summer: *Crocus sativa* 6c

✳ BIOCHEMIC TISSUE SALTS

Ferr Phos 6x: Place 1 tablet up each nostril.

✳ ACUPRESSURE

Press the spot between the tip of the nose and the lip for 30 to 60 seconds.

••• ORTHODOX

If heavy bleeding continues after 10 minutes, or if blood is being swallowed down the back of the throat, then it is advisable to seek emergency help at a hospital. In severe cases doctors will use pressure packs within the nose, or diathermy, a procedure to shrivel up the bleeding blood vessels.

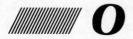 # *O*

OBESITY

Obesity is generally defined as being at least 20 percent over the optimum desired weight for one's height. The reasons for obesity are unclear, and may be due to a variety of causes, including heredity. Often obesity is due to unconscious overeating and lack of activity, which may be combined with emotional conflicts and problems. Some believe that obese people have an unusually slow metabolism; hormonal imbalances may also play a role.

TREATMENT

■ PRACTICAL ADVICE

Keep a record of what, when, and where you eat. This will make you more aware of your eating habits and how much you consume.

Always sit at a table to eat, and be conscious of what you are doing. Don't eat while walking, reading, talking on the phone, watching television, and so on.

Eat slowly and chew the food well.

When you go grocery shopping, buy only whole-grain cereals, low-fat protein and dairy products, and fruits and vegetables. By limiting yourself to these foods, you will avoid the temptation of foods that have higher calories and less nutrition.

If you have a tendency to use food as a way to reward or comfort yourself, try to think of other ways you can do this: For example, an occasional massage or aromatherapy session can provide a real treat and give more long-term physical and mental enjoyment than the temporary pleasure and subsequent guilt and remorse brought by overeating.

It is always easier to make dietary and lifestyle changes if you are motivated by others engaged in the same struggle. Join a group where you can compare notes to make weight loss easier and more enjoyable.

✗ DIETARY

Crash dieting may bring temporary weight loss, but it rarely has a permanent effect. Moreover, it often leads to nutritional deficiencies, demoralization, and unhealthy eating habits, and has been shown to be detrimental to health. The following guidelines help establish long-term balanced eating habits that will help you maintain your optimum weight.

Gradually replace all refined foods with whole-grain foods (whole-grain bread, rice, pasta, oatmeal) and fresh fruits and vegetables. You will find you need less of this food to satisfy your appetite than if you eat refined foods.

Eat moderate amounts of low-fat protein (chicken with skin removed, and fish) and vegetable protein, such as soy products, and dried cooked beans and peas.

Eat moderate amounts of low-fat dairy products.

Avoid all junk and snack food, sugar, and sugar-containing foods.

Limit your intake of alcohol.

Eat 4 small meals a day.

Try not to eat between meals, but if you are hungry, eat a fruit or vegetable.

Drink at least 6 glasses of water a day.

Bee pollen, available in natural foods stores, is said to stimulate the metabolism and suppress the appetite. Start with a few granules (to make sure you are not allergic to it), and gradually build up to 1 teaspoon a day.

Brewer's yeast is helpful in reducing the craving for sweet foods. Take 1 to 2 teaspoons in fruit juice before each meal.

The amino acid phenylalanine has been shown to help weight reduction: The recommended dosage is 100 to 500 milligrams a day, taken at night on an empty stomach.

The Hay Diet has helped many people—the basic premise is not eating starch and protein at the same meal. *The Food Combining Diet* by Kathryn Marsden is based on an adaptation of the Hay Diet for the purposes of weight loss.

◻ HOMEOPATHY

Phytolacca berry tincture, 3 drops in water, 3 times a day, regulates appetite.

Fucus 3x, 3 times a day, when obesity may be thyroid-related.

✛ EXERCISE

Exercise is essential to any weight-loss program. It helps speed up metabolism and burn calories, and in most cases it also reduces appetite. Start off slowly, and gradually increase the exertion and time spent exercising; avoid excess strain, fatigue, and stiffness. Engage in moderate aerobic activity (sufficient to bring mild breathlessness and an increased pulse rate) for at least 20 minutes, 3 times a week. Walking, running, skipping, cycling, aerobics, dancing, and swimming are all suitable. Consult your doctor before you begin any exercise program.

✚ **PROFESSIONAL HELP**

Chinese medicine considers obesity to result from problems in the spleen and kidney. Acupuncture and herbal treatment are used to strengthen these organs.

Counseling or psychotherapy may help resolve emotional conflicts and problems.

••• **ORTHODOX**

Treatment of obesity is very controversial. Some physicians recommend dietary changes and exercise. Others suggest appetite-suppressant drugs under close supervision; however, these often have significant and unpleasant side effects. Taking diuretics, thyroid hormones, and amphetamines is potentially dangerous. Surgery is sometimes suggested, and ranges from jaw wiring to stomach stapling. Undoubtedly, natural means of weight loss are far superior to any of these techniques.

ORAL THRUSH
See **Thrush, Oral.**

OSTEOARTHRITIS

The most common type of arthritis, resulting from general wear and tear on the joints. The cartilage lining the joints typically degenerates, and bony outgrowths may form. Symptoms include pain, stiffness, inflammation, and sometimes loss of function.

TREATMENT

 DIETARY

Osteoarthritis has been seen to improve with increased intake of the following nutrients:

- Magnesium: found in Brazil nuts, whole-grain flour, plain chocolate, lentils, and parsley
- Selenium: found in whole-grain cereals (whole-grain bread, rice, oatmeal), poultry, lean meat, and fish
- Zinc: found in lean meat, poultry, fish, liver, and whole-grain cereals
- Vitamin E: the best source is wheat germ, which can be liberally sprinkled over food

Excess weight increases the discomfort of osteoarthritis. If you are overweight, try following the recommendations under **Obesity.**

A vegetarian diet has been seen to help osteoarthritis, and can also help in weight reduction.

Increase your intake of oily fish, such as mackerel and herring.

☯ CHINESE MEDICINE

If osteoarthritis is treated in the early stages, warming herbs can help: pubescent angelica root, ledebouriellua root, timospora stem, and cinnamon twigs are recommended. Acupuncture may also be recommended.

≈ HYDROTHERAPY

Providing your general health and circulation are good, you can use a cold compress to relieve pain and inflammation: Soak a piece of cotton material large enough to wrap around the joint in cold water. Wring it out, place over the joint, and cover it with two thicknesses of flannel or woolen material, pinned in place. Leave the compress on for 4 to 8 hours. It will draw the heat out of the joint and become warm. Use the compress on alternate days.

Swimming is an excellent way to loosen stiff joints and to stop muscles becoming weak. Many hospitals or physiotherapy units have specially heated pools where you can swim regularly in a safe environment.

☞ MASSAGE

Massaging the osteoarthritic joint will improve circulation and reduce swelling and pain. With a little cream or oil as a lubricant, lightly stroke the muscles and flesh around the joints in the direction of the heart, using your fingertips or the heel of your hand. If you can't use your hands, roll a clean tennis ball over the area to provide a similar effect.

••• ORTHODOX

Your doctor will probably prescribe painkillers to reduce discomfort, and nonsteroidal anti-inflammatory drugs to reduce swelling.

Physical therapy is recommended, including exercises and heat treatment.

Joint replacement surgery is carried out in severe cases.

OSTEOMALACIA

Softening and subsequent weakening of the bones due to calcium or vitamin D deficiency. In children, the disease is known as rickets. Early symptoms include pain in the bones, particularly the neck, legs, hips, and ribs. Children with rickets typically have bowed legs or knock knees, malformed teeth, and in babies, an enlarged head.

TREATMENT

Osteomalacia is rare in people who are well nourished, active, and get plenty of fresh air and sunlight. It is generally found in malnourished children, women who have multiple pregnancies, people who have poor diets, or elderly people who tend not to go outside (sunshine is an important source of vitamin D).

TREATMENT

✗ DIETARY

Increase your intake of calcium, found in low-fat dairy products: milk, yogurt, green leafy vegetables, and sesame seed products, such as tahini and halvah.

Increase your intake of vitamin D: Get outside for moderate periods of sunshine, eat plenty of vitamin D–rich food (milk, lean meats, chicken, and fish).

Take a multivitamin and mineral supplement that contains vitamin D and calcium.

✻ BIOCHEMIC TISSUE SALTS

Calc Phos 6x, taken 4 times daily, promotes the absorption of calcium and phosphorus from the diet.

••• ORTHODOX

If kidney disease or resistance to vitamin D is a problem, higher doses of vitamin D are recommended. Childhood rickets results in permanent bone deformity or lack of growth, which cannot be remedied.

OSTEOPOROSIS

Thinning of the bones and loss of bone density as a result of loss of calcium. The bones become fragile and brittle, causing frequent fractures. Women who have reached menopause are more susceptible to osteoporosis because their bodies stop producing estrogen, which helps maintain bone mass.

PREVENTION

Little can be done once the bone tissue is lost, but much can be done early in life to prevent osteoporosis.

▬ PRACTICAL ADVICE

Stop smoking. Nicotine interferes with calcium absorption.

✗ DIETARY

Make sure you are getting adequate calcium. The best sources are low-fat milk, yogurt, canned fish, green leafy vegetables, and dried, cooked beans and peas. You should have at least 3 daily servings of dairy products, along with a variety of other calcium-rich foods throughout the day. If you do not eat dairy products, increase your intake of dark green leafy vegetables, such as mustard greens, beet greens, kale, and broccoli, and calcium-fortified soy milk.

Vitamin D is essential to calcium absorption. It is found in enriched dairy products and fish oil. It is also processed in the skin on exposure to sunlight.

Eating complex carbohydrates (foods such as bread, rice, pasta, and potatoes) is thought to help prevent osteoporosis. Try always to eat whole-grain cereals.

The following daily supplements help prevent osteoporosis and are useful if you have a low-calcium diet:

- calcium citrate: 1 gram
- magnesium citrate: 500 milligrams
- vitamin B6: 100 milligrams
- folic acid: 1 milligram

Reduce your intake of caffeine, which inhibits absorption of calcium. Reduce your intake of alcohol, which accelerates bone loss.

☯ CHINESE MEDICINE

Herbal treatment can help this condition if it is caught in the early stages. Practitioners of traditional Chinese medicine generally recommend Angelica sinensiseucomia bark, Chinese licorice, cibot rhizome, and eucomia bark.

⚜ EXERCISE

Bone loss occurs more rapidly if you do not exercise. Weight-bearing exercise increases and sustains calcium content in the bones. Walking, running, aerobics, and racquet sports are the best types of activities. Exercise for 30 minutes, at least 3 times a week.

••• ORTHODOX

Hormone replacement therapy (HRT) is prescribed for menopausal women to substitute reduced estrogen production. However, it does have side effects (see **Menopausal Problems**).

Disodium etifronate has been shown to reverse osteoporotic changes in menopausal women and may help reduce the likelihood of fractures.

OVARIAN CYST

Fluid-filled or solid sacs of tissue that grow on or near the ovaries. Usually cysts bring no symptoms, though they may sometimes disrupt menstrual cycles; large cysts may press on another structure, causing pain, discomfort, or swelling.

TREATMENT

DIETARY

Some research points to the fact that women with ovarian cysts frequently suffer from thyroid deficiency (see **Hypothyroidism**). You can find out if this is the case by taking your temperature first thing every morning; if on average you have a temperature lower than 97.6°F, you are likely to be thyroid deficient. The following recommendations will help resolve this:

- Increase your intake of fresh saltwater fish and shellfish, and use iodized salt.
- Take a thyroid gland extract, available in natural foods stores.
- Vitamin E is helpful in eliminating cysts. The best natural sources are vegetable oils, seeds, wheat germ, and nuts. A daily supplement of 800 iu is recommended.

Some naturopaths believe that cysts are the body's mechanism for ridding itself of toxins. To aid the purification process, they advise following a diet based on the following guidelines:

- Drink at least 8 glasses of spring water a day.
- Eat organically produced food and free-range meat.
- Eliminate sugar, coffee, tea, carbonated drinks, and refined foods.
- Vitamin B-complex is helpful in detoxifying the body: Take 50 to 100 milligrams a day.

☐ HOMEOPATHY

Take 1 tablet, 3 times a day, for up to 2 weeks:

Left ovary gives pain, worse in morning, less during menstrual period: *Lachesis* 6c

Right ovary gives stinging pain, with painful periods: *Apis* 6c

✜ EXERCISE

Vigorous exercise is a good way to increase circulation and elimination.

••• ORTHODOX

Small, benign cysts that result from changes occurring during the menstrual cycle are usually left alone. Large cysts are usually surgically removed, sometimes along with the ovary.

OVULATION PAIN

In menstruating women, the reproductive system releases an egg between the tenth and seventeenth day of the cycle. This is known as ovulation, and is felt by some women as a cramp or pain, which can occur on one side of the lower abdomen or both.

PREVENTION

✿ AROMATHERAPY

Massage. 4 drops each of essential oil of basil, sweet marjoram, and lavender in 2 tablespoons of a carrier oil or lotion into the abdomen, in a clockwise direction, on the eighth to twelfth day of your cycle.

TREATMENT

✗ DIETARY

Daily, throughout the month, take evening primrose oil, 6 500-milligram capsules, and 1 25-milligram B-complex tablet.

❧ HERBALISM

Pennyroyal infusion helps promote the menstrual process and strengthen uterine contractions: Add 2 teaspoons of the dried herb to 1 cup of cold water, and let sit for 15 minutes; drink 3 times a day. **Caution:** Do not take if you are trying to conceive.

▢ HOMEOPATHY

Take every 15 minutes for up to 4 doses; repeat if needed:

Pain relieved by warmth and doubling up, often more on left side: *Colocynth* 6c

Pain made better for stretching back: *Dioscorea* 6c

✻ BIOCHEMIC TISSUE SALTS

Mag Phos 6x: Dissolve 2 tablets in a little warm water and sip frequently.

≈ HYDROTHERAPY

Place a warm hot water bottle, wrapped in a towel, on the area of pain.

Take a warm bath to which you have added 4 drops each of essential oil of sweet marjoram and clary sage.

✳ ACUPRESSURE

Massage the points illustrated, using deep thumb pressure, for at least 1 minute.

••• ORTHODOX

The pain of ovulation is usually mild and represents a normal physiological process. Doctors recommend only mild painkillers, if anything.

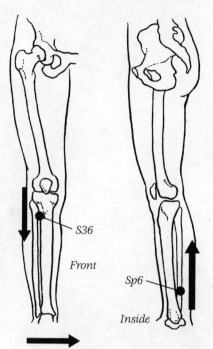

S36

Front

Sp6

Inside

Direction of acupressure massage

 **P**

PAIN

A sensation that can range from mild discomfort to an excruciating experience. Initially, pain acts as a warning signal that something is wrong and requires treatment. Ongoing chronic pain is defined as pain that lasts, despite treatment, for more than six months.

TREATMENT FOR ONGOING CHRONIC PAIN

■ PRACTICAL ADVICE

It can be difficult to identify and accept pain that does not have a specific cause or reason. One of the first steps in treatment is to come to terms with the fact that your pain really exists as a condition, and that you are taking control in dealing with it. Accepting your pain allows you to negotiate a realistic future that offers happier and healthier options.

Join a support group. Shared experience can help you understand and accept pain.

Try to continue with activities or hobbies you did before the pain set in; develop other new interests too.

Really try to talk and think less about your pain.

✗ DIETARY

Research has shown that the amino acid D,L-phenylalanine (DLPA) provides significant pain relief. The recommended dosage is 2 375-milligram tablets, 3 times a day, prior to meals. If there is no improvement, double the dose. If there is still no improvement, discontinue the treatment. Relief is usually apparent within seven days; after this you can gradually reduce the dosage until you achieve a minimum maintenance dose.

Where the pain results from inflammation, 6 500-milligram capsules of evening primrose oil and 1 25-milligram B-complex tablet a day may help.

❀ AROMATHERAPY

Aromatherapy massage promotes relaxation. You can also use essential oils yourself to help you relax. Lavender has been shown to have relaxing and sedating properties. Soak in a bath in which you have put a few drops of essential oil of lavender, or put a few drops on a handkerchief and sniff regularly.

☛ MASSAGE

Getting a massage from a friend, a family member, or a massage therapist promotes deep relaxation. It is extremely beneficial for many types of pain. However, consult your doctor first to make sure that the treatment is appropriate for your condition.

✳ ACUPRESSURE

For general pain relief, use deep pressure on the points illustrated, preferably with the thumb, for at least 1 minute.

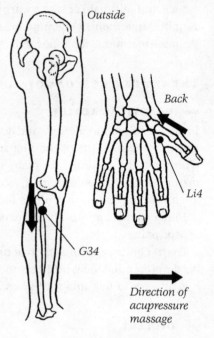

Outside

Back

Li4

G34

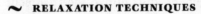

Direction of acupressure massage

✥ EXERCISE

Exercise helps release endorphins, the body's natural painkillers, as well as providing distraction from the pain. Consult your doctor before you begin any of the following programs.

Daily walking on flat ground: Go as far as is comfortable for the first week. If you experience a flare-up of pain, cut back the exercise until the pain settles. Increase your walking gradually.

Swimming: Swimming often provides all-around pain relief, while exercising the muscles. Special hydrotherapy pools at physiotherapy units are specially heated for pain sufferers.

∿ RELAXATION TECHNIQUES

Relaxation promotes the release of stress-reducing endorphins, which in turn relieves pain.

Set aside a period of time each day to rest. Sit or lie in a comfortable position, do not answer the phone or door, and tell others not to disturb you. Listen to music or a relaxation tape.

If your mind is constantly going over concerns and anxieties, make two lists: In one column, list the problems in their order of priority; in the other column, list the potential solutions. Take two minutes for each problem, then put the paper aside and start your relaxation.

Try the following routine to help achieve relaxation: Find a quiet place where you won't be disturbed. Lie on a firm surface, close your eyes, allow your breathing to slow, and begin to be aware of how your body feels.

Consciously try to relax every part of your body in turn. Begin with your face (your eyes, your forehead, your jaw), and work down to your toes. The whole procedure should take at least 10 minutes.

Relaxation tapes, biofeedback training, or attending a yoga class can help teach you to relax if you find it difficult.

✪ VISUALIZATION

Take time each day to do this visualization: In a quiet room, settle as comfortably as possible, close your eyes, and imagine the color and shape of your pain. You may see it as an object or symbol or a more abstract vision. Imagine what color or shape will soothe or relieve your pain. Imagine asking the pain if it has a message for you, how it would like you to treat it. Try to remain with your visualization for at least 10 minutes, and gradually increase the time day by day.

✚ PROFESSIONAL HELP

Acupuncture can be very effective in relieving pain.

Hypnosis can also help.

Transcutaneous electrical nerve stimulation (TENS), available in many hospitals, works like acupuncture without the needles. Ask your doctor for more details, or inquire at your local hospital.

Spiritual healing has helped many people.

••• ORTHODOX

Painkilling drugs, muscle relaxants, nonsteroidal anti-inflammatory drugs, and local anesthetic (sprays, injections, or drops) are all possible treatments. Neurosurgery is occasionally used to sever the nerves causing pain.

PALPITATIONS

A sensation that the heart is beating quickly or irregularly. This usually occurs after hard exercise, a shock, or anger, but it may also be a symptom of heart disease (see **Coronary Heart Disease**), an overactive thyroid gland (see **Hyperthyroidism**), a food allergy (see **Allergies, Food**), or taking too much caffeine. If palpitations continue for several hours or recur over several days, or if they are accompanied by dizziness, shortness of breath, nausea, or chest pain, consult your doctor.

TREATMENT

■ PRACTICAL ADVICE

Stop smoking. Nicotine stimulates the heart.

✕ DIETARY

Avoid caffeine (coffee, tea, chocolate, cola).

If palpitations are related to heart disease, see dietary recommendations under **Coronary Heart Disease.**

Take magnesium supplements: 30 to 60 milligrams *elemental* weight a day, with food. This usually gives relief within two or three days. **Caution:** Do not use magnesium oxide or magnesium carbonate.

❀ AROMATHERAPY

When the cause of palpitations is emotional, use calming essential oils such as lavender, mandarin, and ylang ylang. Add 6 drops of one of these oils to your bath and relax; or put a few drops on a handkerchief and inhale the aroma regularly.

An aromatherapy massage will greatly assist in reducing stress-induced palpitations.

❧ HERBALISM

For palpitations brought by stress or anxiety, infusion of motherwort is effective: Add 1 cup of water to 2 teaspoons of the dried herb, and infuse for 15 minutes; drink 3 times a day.

☐ HOMEOPATHY

Take every 5 minutes for up to 6 doses, during palpitations:

Palpitations after a shock or a fright: *Aconite* 6c

Palpitations after rich food, alcohol, coffee, or stress: *Nux vomica* 6c

Palpitations after sudden excitement or a pleasant surprise: *Coffea* 6c

Palpitations that are worse lying on the left side and improved by lying on the right side: *Phosphorus* 6c

☯ CHINESE MEDICINE

Practitioners of traditional Chinese medicine generally recommend herbs to nourish the heart and the blood, such as lilyturf root, asparagus root, and wild jujube seeds.

☞ MASSAGE

Regular massage is very helpful in promoting relaxation and lowering blood pressure.

✳ ACUPRESSURE

Massage the two points illustrated using deep thumb pressure, for at least 1 minute.

～ RELAXATION TECHNIQUES

Whatever the cause of palpitations, regular relaxation will be generally beneficial.

Carry out the following routine morning and evening: Find a quiet place where you won't be disturbed. Lie on a firm surface, close your eyes, allow your breathing to slow, and begin to be aware of how your body feels. Consciously try to relax every part of your body in turn. Begin with your face (your eyes, your forehead, your jaw), and work down to your toes. The whole procedure should take at least 10 minutes.

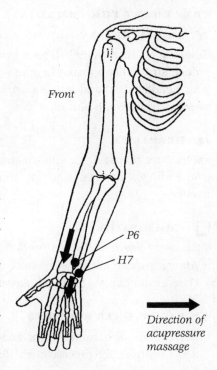

Front

P6

H7

Direction of acupressure massage

Attend a yoga class or learn meditation. Biofeedback is also helpful in learning to relax.

••• ORTHODOX

Your doctor may want to take an electrocardiograph (ECG) to record the electrical impulses of the heart. If the palpitations are intermittent, yet significant, an ambulatory ECG (where the patient wears a portable recording machine for a full twenty-four hours) may be necessary. Simple abnormalities can be treated with medications, but physical disorders may very occasionally require surgical intervention.

PANIC ATTACK

An attack of intense anxiety or fear that usually comes on unexpectedly, but can be triggered by a pattern of situations or events. Symptoms include breathing difficulties, chest pains, palpitations, dizziness, trembling, and faintness.

TREATMENT FOR IMMEDIATE RELIEF

❋ **AROMATHERAPY**

Essential oil of lavender has been shown in studies to relieve anxiety and reduce stress: Keep a small bottle of the oil with you, or sprinkle it on your handkerchief and inhale during stressful moments. Rosewood and sweet marjoram are also effective.

❧ **HERBALISM**

Valerian tea helps reduce tension and anxiety: Pour 1 cup of boiling water over 1 to 2 teaspoons of the root, and infuse for 15 minutes; drink when needed.

▢ **HOMEOPATHY**

Take every few minutes for up to 6 doses:

After a sudden shock with chest pains and fear of dying: *Aconite* 6c

Hysterical changes of mood, gasping for breath: *Ignatia* 6c

✿ **BACH FLOWER REMEDIES**

Rock Rose: for extreme terror and panic nearing hysteria

Red Chestnut: for excessive fear for others, especially loved ones

LONG-TERM TREATMENT

✗ **DIETARY**

Increase your intake of B vitamins:

vitamin B1, found in pork, green peas, oranges, dried beans and peas, wheat germ, and brewer's yeast

vitamin B2, found in milk, green leafy vegetables, mushrooms, asparagus, avocados, and broccoli

vitamin B7 (biotin), found in liver, oatmeal, egg yolk, soybeans, mushrooms, bananas, peanuts, and brewer's yeast

vitamin B-complex supplement: 1 25-milligram tablet a day

〜 **RELAXATION TECHNIQUES**

A yoga or meditation class will help you relax, reducing anxiety and incidence of panic attacks.

Do the following routine at least once every day, and before potentially stressful situations: Find a quiet place where you won't be disturbed. Lie on a firm surface, close your eyes, allow your breathing to slow, and begin to be aware of how your body feels. Consciously try to relax every part of your body in turn. Begin with your face (your eyes, your forehead, your jaw), and work down to your toes. The whole procedure should take at least 10 minutes.

✚ PROFESSIONAL HELP

Hypnotherapy may help you overcome panic attacks.

••• ORTHODOX

Your doctor may recommend psychotherapy or counseling.

PARKINSON'S DISEASE

A degenerative disease that affects a small part of the brain, causing muscle tremor, stiffness, and loss of physical coordination and movement. Typical symptoms are shakiness, rigid posture, and a shuffling, unsteady walk.

TREATMENT

All treatment should be carried out in consultation with your doctor. Natural therapies may complement orthodox treatment, but should not be substituted for medication.

✗ DIETARY

Eat nutritious food: whole-grain cereals, fruits and vegetables, and low-fat protein to provide energy.

Eat plenty of fiber to prevent constipation.

Some Parkinson's sufferers find that spicy food or high-protein meals make their symptoms worse. A vegetarian diet may be beneficial.

Fresh broad beans and fava beans (*Vicia fava*) contain levodopa, the drug used to treat Parkinson's disease. Studies have shown that patients felt relief of symptoms after eating these beans.

☙ CHINESE MEDICINE

Treatment given in the early stages can help, especially for younger people. Acupuncture would be combined with herbal remedies (fleeceflower root, wolfberry root, and umcaria stem).

✤ REFLEXOLOGY

Practitioners recommend massaging the head area, located at the tips of the toes on the right and left soles; the whole of both big toes; the spine area, located along the inner side of both feet; the adrenal glands; and the large intestine. See figure on the next page.

315

✤ EXERCISE

Regular exercise can help increase mobility and improve balance and coordination. Gentle walking, and simple stretching that mobilizes all the major joints, are recommended, but be careful not to overdo it. If you feel tired, stop; if you have a bad day, do not exercise.

✚ PROFESSIONAL HELP

Parkinson's sufferers are often deficient in minerals. Consult a dietitian or a naturopath for advice on mineral status testing.

••• ORTHODOX

Levodopa is the most commonly used drug. It replaces the brain chemicals that are missing and minimizes symptoms. It cannot, however, halt the degeneration of the brain cells. Sometimes brain surgery may be carried out to reduce tremor and rigidity. New advances are being developed, including fetal tissue implants, which have had some success.

Top of head/brain

Waist level

Large intestine

Left sole

The reflex areas

PELVIC INFLAMMATORY DISEASE (PID)

An infection of the female reproductive organs; also known as salpingitis. The infection may not have any obvious cause, though sometimes it results from a sexually transmitted disease such as chlamydia (see **Chlamydia; Sexually Transmitted Diseases**). Pelvic inflammatory disease may also occur after childbirth, abortion, or miscarriage. Symptoms include pelvic pain, fever, and foul-smelling discharge.

PREVENTION

If left untreated, pelvic inflammatory disease can cause infertility. Orthodox treatment with antibiotics is the only way to make sure that you clear up the infection. Complementary treatments, however, can greatly assist in preventing a recurrence.

Get any vaginal discharge or pelvic pain checked out by your doctor immediately.

If you or your partner also have intercourse with other people, protect yourself from sexually transmitted diseases by always using a condom.

When you go to the toilet, always wipe from front to back, to prevent bacteria from the anus entering the vagina.

Avoid anal sex.

Do not use intrauterine devices (IUDs) for birth control.

TREATMENT

Treatment with antibiotics is necessary (see above). Use the following complementary measures in addition to antibiotics.

✗ DIETARY

Strengthen the immune system by making sure you eat plenty of vitamin C, found in citrus fruits and vegetables; vitamin A, found in liver, egg yolk, and dairy products; and vitamin D, found in fortified milk and exposure to sunlight.

Eat whole-grain cereals, lean meats, or fish, and plenty of green leafy vegetables.

Eat live yogurt that contains *Lactobacillus acidophilus* to prevent thrush, which often occurs after taking antibiotics (see **Thrush**). Alternatively, take ½ teaspoon of *Lactobacillus acidophilus,* with 1 teaspoon of *Bifidobacteria* powder, and ½ teaspoon of *Lactobacillus bulgaricus* (available from natural foods stores), in a glass of spring water, 3 times a day.

❧ HERBALISM

Garlic is an effective antimicrobial.

Incorporate raw garlic into your diet as much as possible. If you don't like the taste or smell of raw garlic, take garlic capsules (3 capsules, 3 times a day).

A tried and tested remedy is to peel a clove of garlic and wrap it in sterile gauze, tie the end with a long piece of thread or dental floss, and insert into the vagina like a tampon, with the string outside the body. Change it daily; use for up to 4 days.

≈ HYDROTHERAPY

For pain relief, take hot baths and place a hot water bottle wrapped in a towel on your stomach. This will encourage the circulation of blood through the infected area, helping to fight and flush away the infection.

PROFESSIONAL HELP

Professional homeopathic treatment is recommended to reduce recurrence of infections.

••• ORTHODOX

Your doctor will probably prescribe antibiotic drugs for at least 2 to 6 weeks. Painkillers may also be recommended. If you use an intrauterine device, it should be removed, as it is a foreign body and could perpetuate any infection.

PEPTIC ULCER

A raw area that develops in the mucous membrane of the digestive tract, where it is irritated further by acidic digestive juices. Ulcers may be caused by excessive secretion of acid, resulting from eating the wrong foods, long-term stress, drugs, or alcohol. Symptoms include burning pain in the stomach, loss of appetite, gas, nausea, and vomiting.

TREATMENT

PRACTICAL ADVICE

Stop smoking.

DIETARY

Ulcers are made worse by foods that stimulate acid secretion. Eliminate fatty foods, spices (especially pepper), fruit juices, coffee, tea, cocoa, cola, and alcohol.

Protein also stimulates acid secretion. Avoid meat for the first two weeks of treating an ulcer. Instead of meat, eat 2 ounces of cheese (preferably a low-fat cheese) a day. This will give your system a rest and a chance to start healing.

Make sure that 80 percent of your food is alkaline (fruit and vegetables), and only 20 percent acidic (meat, fish, eggs, cheese, bread, concentrated starches, and sugary foods).

Eat only when you are relaxed, and take your time.

HERBALISM

Licorice has a soothing action on the mucous membranes, and is used in orthodox drugs for ulcers. Herbalists generally recommend licorice decoctions 3 times a day: Put 1 teaspoon of licorice root in 1 cup of water, and simmer for 15 minutes. When using this treatment, eat plenty of fresh fruits and vegetables to ensure adequate intake of potassium.

Marshmallow root decoction is also an effective treatment: Put 1 teaspoon of marshmallow root in 1 cup of water, and simmer for 15 minutes.

☐ HOMEOPATHY

Take 3 times a day for up to 14 days; repeat if necessary:

When the pain is worse immediately after eating, relieved 2 hours later: *Nux vomica* 6c

Pain relieved immediately after eating: *Anacardium* 6c

Pain in a small and precise spot: *Kali bichromicum* 6c

Burning pains and vomiting, better temporarily for cold drinks: *Phosphorus* 6c

Stomach feels like a stone and is very sensitive to touch: *Bryonia* 6c

☯ CHINESE MEDICINE

Practitioners of traditional Chinese medicine advise avoiding "cold" foods, such as salads, bananas, and grapefruit. Burning pain can be relieved by dandelion or dandelion juice. Noto ginseng is recommended to heal the ulcer.

☞ MASSAGE

Regular massage can help with relaxation.

～ RELAXATION TECHNIQUES

Stress increases acid production in the digestive system, and there is a high probability that it greatly contributes to the development of ulcers. Learning how to relax, through yoga, meditation, biofeedback, or relaxation tapes, will help you to make it a regular part of your daily routine.

••• ORTHODOX

Antacids relieve mild symptoms.

H_2-receptor antagonists are more effective in inhibiting stomach acid production and promoting healing.

Surgery is used as a last resort, when the ulcer has perforated the stomach.

PERIODS, PAINFUL
See **Cramps, Menstrual.**

PERIODS, HEAVY

The amount of blood lost during menstruation differs from woman to woman. However, if you experience abnormally heavy periods that last more than seven days, produce large clots, and saturate sanitary protection within minutes, it is advisable to consult your doctor. Heavy periods may result from hormonal imbalances, fibroids (see **Fibroids**), endometriosis (see **Endometriosis**), polyps (see **Polyp**), using an intrauterine device, stress (see **Stress**), and occasionally cancer. If there is no sign of underlying disease, the following treatments can help.

TREATMENT

✗ DIETARY

Increase your intake of the following nutrients:

Iron and zinc: found in red meat, poultry, fish, and green leafy vegetables. Eat or drink citrus fruits and juices with meals to enhance iron absorption.

Vitamin B6, found in lean meats, wheat germ, and brewer's yeast. Take 50 milligrams, 2 times a day, and 25 milligrams of B-complex once a day.

Vitamin A, found in liver, kidney, egg yolk, butter, whole milk, and cod liver oil.

Citrus bioflavonoids, found in the pith of citrus fruits, can help balance hormonal levels and regulate menstruation.

🐾 HERBALISM

Herbalists recommend a decoction of either American cranesbill or periwinkle for excessive blood loss during menstruation: Pour 1 cup of boiling water on 1 teaspoon of either herb, and infuse for 15 minutes; drink 3 times a day.

☐ HOMEOPATHY

Take every 8 hours for 10 doses; start dosage just before period is due:

Spasmodic bleeding, producing dark clots, with cramps, faintness, and pallor: *China* 6c

Bright red blood, abdominal pains, throbbing headache: *Belladonna* 6c

Heavy bleeding, bright red blood, with nausea: *Ipecac* 6c

Pain bearing down, as if internal organs are going to "drop out": *Sepia* 6c

••• ORTHODOX

To treat heavy periods caused by a hormonal imbalance, doctors often prescribe oral contraceptives or doses of progesterone during the later stages of each menstrual cycle. Other treatments will depend on the cause of the bleeding. Iron supplements may be given to prevent anemia.

PERIODS, IRREGULAR OR ABSENT

The most obvious reasons for absent or irregular periods are pregnancy, or the onset of the menopause. Women who have never had a period by the age of eighteen should seek medical advice. For those who have started menstruating but experience irregular periods or a lapse in menstruation, the cause could relate to weight problems (either obesity or low body weight as a result of dieting or an eating disorder; see **Anorexia Nervosa**), hormonal imbalances, stress, or excessive exercising.

TREATMENT

Once a medical examination has ruled out pregnancy, structural abnormalities, or disease, the following therapies may help regulate menstruation.

✗ DIETARY

Research has shown that deficiency of zinc and vitamin B6 can often result in absence of periods. Foods rich in vitamin B6 include lean meat, wheat germ, and brewer's yeast. Alternatively, you could take 1 25-milligram supplement of vitamin B6 daily, with 1 25-milligram vitamin B-complex supplement. Foods rich in zinc include lean meat, poultry, fish, and organ meats.

❧ HERBALISM

For delayed onset of periods in adolescent girls, blue cohosh decoction is prescribed: Put 1 teaspoon of the dried root in 1 cup of water, and simmer for 10 minutes; drink 3 times a day.

Chasteberry infusion helps regulate hormonal function: Pour 1 cup of boiling water on 1 teaspoon of the ripe berries, and infuse for 15 minutes; drink 3 times a day.

☐ HOMEOPATHY

Take every 12 hours for 2 weeks:

Periods stop after an emotional shock: *Aconite* 6c
Periods stop after grief or loss: *Ignatia* 6c

☯ CHINESE MEDICINE

Chinese medicine suggests eating warming foods to encourage regular menstruation: ginger tea, spiced dishes, and soups are recommended.

⚜ EXERCISE

Women who are underweight or who are under rigorous training schedules often experience irregular or absent periods. It is important to maintain a minimum amount of body fat for menstruation to occur.

✚ PROFESSIONAL HELP

Sometimes periods can stop as a result of an emotional shock, grief, sexual trauma, or other psychological problems. Help from a counselor or psychotherapist with experience in such problems may restore ovarian function.

••• ORTHODOX

Once psychological problems have been ruled out, and the problem does not resolve itself spontaneously within a few months, hormonal correction using drugs such as clomiphene may be prescribed.

PHARYNGITIS

Inflammation of the pharynx (the part of the throat that lies between the tonsils and the voice box), resulting in a sore throat. Pharyngitis can result from a virus or a bacterial infection, and is commonly associated with a cold or flu.

TREATMENT

▬ PRACTICAL ADVICE

Avoid alcohol and smoking, as both will irritate the pharynx.
Rest the voice as much as possible.

✕ DIETARY

The following nutrients help fight infection:

- vitamin C, found in fresh vegetables and fruits, particularly citrus fruits and juices
- zinc, found in lean meat, fish, and organ meats

Gargle with cider vinegar and honey 4 times a day.

❉ AROMATHERAPY

A gargle made up of 2 drops of essential oils of both sandalwood and lavender in a glass of water helps soothe the throat.

Steam inhalations using essential oils of sandalwood and lavender are very beneficial: Add 1 to 2 drops to a bowl of steaming hot water. Lean over the bowl, put a towel over your head to trap the steam, close your eyes, and inhale deeply for 2 to 5 minutes. **Caution:** If you suffer from asthma, avoid steam inhalations.

❧ HERBALISM

Decoction of echinacea is an effective remedy for both bacterial and viral infections: Add 2 teaspoons of the root to 1 cup of water, and simmer for 15 minutes; drink 3 times a day.

☐ HOMEOPATHY

Take 1 dose an hour for 4 doses; repeat if necessary:

Barking cough, with burning and irritation, after getting chilled: *Aconite* 6c

Stringy yellow mucus, metallic-sounding cough, and husky voice with raw pain: *Kali bichromicum* 6c

Burning pain, tightness in the chest, and hoarseness eased by eating ice cream: *Phosphorus* 30c

••• ORTHODOX

Doctors recommend gargling with saltwater, along with painkillers. Particularly severe cases may require antibiotics.

PHOBIA

An irrational and disabling fear of a specific object or situation. Phobias may result from past bad experiences, or may be learned from parents or siblings. Common phobias are fear of going outside (agoraphobia) and terror of being enclosed (claustrophobia). Symptoms include extreme anxiety and fear: rapid breathing, sweating, and panic on exposure to the situation or object. This may be accompanied by general depression, and sometimes drug or alcohol abuse. See also **Panic Attack.**

TREATMENT

Phobias are difficult to treat by yourself. The following self-help therapies will ease the way, but should be used in conjunction with the professional help listed below.

✗ DIETARY

Naturopaths would carry out a complete assessment of the diet, and would probably recommend high-potency vitamin B-complex and vitamin C supplements.

Research has shown that people who suffer phobias experience similar symptoms to people with low blood sugar. Making sure blood-sugar levels remain stable may help prevent attacks:

- Eat many small meals over the day.
- Eat complex carbohydrates (potatoes, whole-grain breads and cereals, brown rice, and pasta); avoid simple carbohydrates (sugar, candy, cakes, cookies).
- Keep a nutritious snack, such as nuts or fresh or dried fruit, with you at all times.

❀ AROMATHERAPY

Essential oil of lavender has been shown in studies to provide immediate relief for anxiety and stress: Keep a small bottle of the oil with you, or sprinkle it on your handkerchief to inhale at stressful moments.

Sandalwood and sweet marjoram will help reduce the fear.

୬ HERBALISM

Valerian tea helps reduce tension and anxiety: Pour 1 cup of boiling water over 1 to 2 teaspoons of the root, and infuse for 15 minutes; drink when needed.

✿ BACH FLOWER REMEDIES

Rock Rose: Take for extreme terror and panic nearing hysteria.
Rescue Remedy: Take if Rock Rose is not appropriate.

～ RELAXATION TECHNIQUES

A yoga or meditation class will help you relax, reducing anxiety and incidence of phobic attacks.

Learning biofeedback will greatly assist in relaxation.

✚ PROFESSIONAL HELP

Hypnotherapy may help you overcome your phobia.

Behavioral psychotherapy uses techniques that allow gradual exposure to the feared object or situation, accompanied by reassurance, relaxation techniques, and visualizations of oneself overcoming the phobia.

••• ORTHODOX

Psychotherapy is recommended, along with tranquilizers or antidepressants in severe cases.

PILES

See **Hemorrhoids.**

PIMPLES

Inflamed swellings, either on or under the surface of the skin, which are often red and pus-filled, are common in adolescence, and generally clear up once the hormonal changes of puberty have settled down. Severe and unsightly pimples on the face, neck, and back are likely to be acne (see **Acne**). In adults, pimples occur as a result of the hormonal changes of menstruation or pregnancy or, some believe, as a result of inadequate elimination, which allows toxins to build up in the body. They may also spring up as a result of fatigue or being "run down." Some people respond to food allergies with rashes or pimples (see **Allergies, Food**).

PREVENTION

Make sure to get plenty of rest.

Practice stress-reduction techniques (see **Stress**).

Eat a whole-foods diet, with whole grains, plenty of fresh fruits and vegetables, and low-fat protein. Avoid fats, sugars, and refined and junk foods.

Drink plenty of water, at least 8 glasses a day.

Keep your skin clean by washing morning and night with an oil-free cleanser or mild soap. Rinse well with water.

Get regular exercise to aid circulation and elimination.

Use deodorants rather than antiperspirants, as the latter sometimes inhibit elimination by blocking the sweat glands.

TREATMENT

▬ PRACTICAL ADVICE

The best way to deal with a pimple is to leave it alone. Do not squeeze or pick it, as this may lead to infection and scarring.

✾ AROMATHERAPY

Essential oil of tea tree is useful as an antiseptic: Dab it on the pimple at regular intervals.

🐛 HERBALISM

Echinacea decoction helps detoxify the system: Place 2 teaspoons of the root in 1 cup of water, bring to a boil, and simmer for 10 minutes; drink 3 times a day.

☯ CHINESE MEDICINE

Practitioners of traditional Chinese medicine believe that pimples are generated by excessive heat in the body. Chrysanthemum, honeysuckle, or dandelion tea is recommended to reduce heat. A popular remedy is to cleanse the skin with watermelon or cucumber.

✳ ACUPRESSURE

Massage the points illustrated, using deep thumb pressure, for at least 1 minute several times a week.

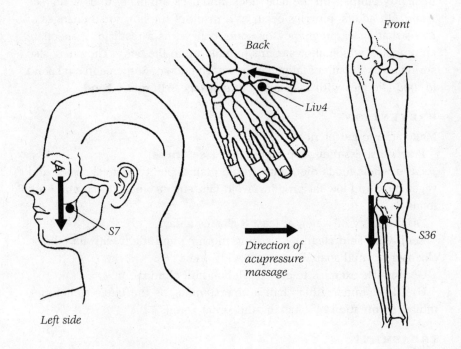

Back

Front

Liv4

S7

Direction of
acupressure
massage

S36

Left side

○ PHOTOTHERAPY

Sunlight and fresh air help clear up pimples.

••• ORTHODOX

Most doctors leave pimples alone to take their own course. For treatment of severe cases, see **Acne.**

PINKEYE
See **Conjunctivitis.**

PLANTAR WARTS
See **Warts.**

PNEUMONIA

Infection of one or both lungs by a virus or bacteria. Symptoms include fever, chills, breathlessness, chest pain, a cough that produces yellow or green phlegm, and sometimes blood. In young, healthy people, pneumonia may be mild; in the elderly, or those with weakened immune systems, it can be life-threatening.

TREATMENT

Use the following treatments in collaboration with your doctor.

✗ DIETARY

Most naturopaths recommend plenty of fluids and small, nutritious whole-foods meals. Eat and drink plenty of fruits and vegetable juices, particularly those containing vitamin C (citrus fruits and tomatoes).

❧ HERBALISM

Coltsfoot infusion has a soothing effect on coughs and helps fight chest infection: Pour 1 cup of boiling water on 2 teaspoons of the dried flowers or leaves, and infuse for 10 minutes; drink 3 times a day.

Incorporate as much raw garlic into your diet as possible to fight infection. If you do not like the taste or smell of fresh garlic, you can take garlic capsules (3 capsules, 3 times a day).

☐ HOMEOPATHY

Take 1 dose every hour, for 4 doses; repeat if necessary:
When the illness has a rapid onset and brings a high fever: *Aconite* 6c
Brings sharp stitching pain, made worse by coughing: *Bryonia* 6c
Pale and weak with bloody phlegm and nosebleeds: *Ferrum phosphoricum* 6c

≈ HYDROTHERAPY

Steam inhalations help relieve a painful chest and facilitate breathing. Add a few drops of essential oil of eucalyptus to a bowl of boiling water. Lean over the bowl, put a towel over your head and the bowl to trap the steam, close your eyes, and inhale for 2 to 5 minutes. **Caution:** If you suffer from asthma, avoid steam inhalations.

☞ MASSAGE

Massage the muscles of the upper back using an oil or lotion carrier with a few drops of essential oil of eucalyptus to ease chest congestion and facilitate the release of phlegm.

Lie face down on a comfortable surface. Use towels and a warm blanket to cover up the areas not being treated. Kneeling at your side, your partner can place the heels of the hands on the muscle running along the opposite side of the spine and push them gently away from him or her.

Cupping the hands, your partner can do a gentle, loose clapping stroke with alternate hands all over the upper back, particularly around the ribcage, and avoiding the spine.

••• ORTHODOX

Antibiotics are given either orally or by injection. Your doctor may also recommend chest physiotherapy to remove mucus and phlegm.

POLYP

A noncancerous growth that projects out of a mucous membrane, often in the nose, the cervical canal, or the intestine. Nasal polyps can develop as a result of allergies, and can cause difficulty breathing, nosebleeds, and diminished sense of smell. Cervical polyps can cause watery bleeding after intercourse, or between periods. Intestinal polyps are usually small and harmless, though larger ones can cause obstructions.

TREATMENT

✚ PROFESSIONAL HELP

Acupuncture or Chinese herbs can be used to treat this condition.

Hypnotherapy or autogenic training may also help.

A number of homeopathic remedies have been found to be helpful; seek professional prescribing.

••• ORTHODOX

Small polyps do not necessarily require treatment. Regular examinations are recommended for cervical polyps; however, they rarely become cancerous. Removal is a relatively easy surgical procedure if the polyp is large or obstructive.

POSTNATAL DEPRESSION

Postnatal depression can range from a few days of mild sadness to serious bouts of depression. Common symptoms include feelings of loneliness and inadequacy; loss of interest in life; tearfulness; bouts of crying; guilt; extreme fatigue; suicidal thoughts; and inability to function or care for the child.

TREATMENT

✗ DIETARY

Research has shown that postnatal depression can result from a deficiency in certain nutrients:

Take 1 25-milligram vitamin B-complex tablet a day.

Increase your intake of zinc, found in lean meat, poultry, fish, organ meats, and whole-grain bread. Take 1 25-milligram zinc supplement each day to ensure adequate intake.

Increase your intake of magnesium, found in nuts, cooked dried beans, whole-grain cereals, soybeans, dark green leafy vegetables, and seafood. Take 1 300-milligram supplement to ensure adequate intake.

Increase your intake of vitamin B2 (riboflavin), found in dairy products, brewer's yeast, meat, and wheat.

Increase your intake of vitamin B6, found in lean meat, fish, brewer's yeast, wheat germ, soybeans, cooked dried beans, and peas.

A number of studies have shown that the amino acid phenylalanine can relieve depression. The dosage is best determined by a naturopath.

Maintain your blood-sugar levels by eating a complex carbohydrate food every 3 hours, such as whole-grain bread or other cereal.

🍃 HERBALISM

Skullcap infusion is prescribed for exhaustion and depression. It helps relax the body, while reviving the nervous system: Pour 1 cup of boiling water on 2 teaspoons of the dried herb, and infuse for 15 minutes; drink 3 times a day.

Take 1 500-milligram capsule of evening primrose oil, 3 times a day.

☐ HOMEOPATHY

Take 4 times a day for 3 days; repeat if needed:

Lack of interest in life and former pleasures, feeling tired, irritable, end of one's tether: *Sepia* 6c

Tearful, needing company, hugs, and reassurance: *Pulsatilla* 6c

Unsociable, reluctant to share one's feelings: *Natrum muriaticum* 6c

✚ PROFESSIONAL HELP

In traditional Chinese medicine, acupuncture and moxibustion have been shown to help balance the body.

••• ORTHODOX

Your doctor may suggest antidepressant drugs, hormonal drugs, and sometimes counseling or psychotherapy. In severe cases, when the child's well-being is at risk, the mother is admitted to the hospital.

PREECLAMPSIA

A life-threatening illness in which high blood pressure, water retention, and protein in the urine develop during the later stages of pregnancy; also known as toxemia. Symptoms include headaches, visual problems, swollen ankles, nausea, and abdominal pain. If left untreated, convulsions and loss of consciousness can occur, threatening the life of the mother and child.

TREATMENT

Preeclampsia requires emergency medical attention. Complementary treatments can be used to help prevent preeclampsia and as an adjunct to orthodox treatment; be sure to tell your doctor about any therapies you are using.

PREVENTION

▬ PRACTICAL ADVICE

Prenatal care is vital. Make sure you have regular checkups so that if you develop preeclampsia, it can be diagnosed early.

Reduce stress as much as possible (see **Stress**).

Get plenty of sleep.

✘ DIETARY

Some studies show that a protein deficiency may contribute to preeclampsia. During pregnancy, eat plenty of lean meat and fish, eggs, dried cooked beans, whole-grain cereals, and low-fat dairy products, along with lightly steamed vegetables and fruit.

If you are a vegetarian or vegan, make sure you get sufficient protein by combining foods that complement each other: legumes with grains, legumes with seeds or nuts, or for nonvegans, grains with milk products.

TREATMENT

✗ DIETARY

Avoid dairy foods, spices, and alcohol.

Eat plenty of fresh vegetables and fruit, especially onions, celery, and garlic, that strengthen the blood vessel walls and improve circulation.

Eat plenty of potassium-rich foods, such as lean meat, potatoes, avocados, bananas, apricots, orange juice, and other fruits.

⅔ HERBALISM

Dandelion leaves can help reduce swelling caused by water retention. Add the fresh leaves to salads, or prepare a decoction: Put 2 teaspoons of the root in 1 cup of water, and simmer gently for 15 minutes; drink 3 times a day.

✚ PROFESSIONAL HELP

Chinese medicine offers herbs to reduce high blood pressure. Acupuncture can also be helpful in treating this condition.

Professional homeopathic treatment is recommended.

••• ORTHODOX

In mild cases your doctor will recommend bed rest and will give drugs to reduce blood pressure and correct salt and water imbalances in the body. If you are nearing the end of the pregnancy, the birth may be induced, as symptoms rapidly improve after delivery.

PREGNANCY PROBLEMS

Common problems experienced in pregnancy include edema, muscle pain, nausea (see **Morning Sickness; Nausea**), constipation (see **Constipation**), and heartburn.

PREVENTION AND TREATMENT: EDEMA

Puffiness of the flesh, especially in the feet, ankles, fingers, and face, caused by an increase in fluid volume, and made worse by heat, standing, and fatigue. The condition may be linked to high blood pressure. Consult your doctor immediately if you begin to notice edema.

Prevention
- Avoid overeating and overexertion.
- Eat a whole-grain diet that includes plenty of fiber (to absorb fluids): cereals, fruits and vegetables, dried fruit, and oat bran.
- Reduce fluid intake to 6 cups a day.

Treatment
- Rest with your feet up as much as possible.
- Dandelion tea is an effective diuretic. Put 2 teaspoons of the root into 1 cup of water, bring to a boil, and simmer for 10 minutes; drink once a day.
- Take the biochemic tissue salt *Nat mur* 6x, 3 times a day for 1 week.
- Massage helps improve circulation and drainage of fluids.
- Gentle exercise, particularly walking, has the same effect as massage.

PREVENTION AND TREATMENT: MUSCLE PAIN

As the baby grows, the body adapts to accommodate it. This can some-times lead to muscular discomfort, particularly neck and back pain, and sometimes headaches resulting from hormonal changes. If you experi-ence severe or persistent pain, consult your doctor.

Prevention
- Pay attention to your posture.
- Avoid lifting heavy objects. If you have to lift, squat down rather than bending forward.
- Do not stand for long periods.
- Get regular exercise: Swimming is particularly good because the buoyancy of the water provides support.

Treatment
- Aromatherapy for headaches: Soak a handkerchief in water with a few drops of lavender and place on the forehead; relax in a quiet, dimmed room.
- Aromatherapy for muscle pain: Ask your partner to rub the area gently with 2 drops of Roman chamomile and 2 drops of sweet marjoram in 2 teaspoons of a carrier oil or lotion.
- Gentle massage from a friend or partner can be very helpful in treat-ing back, shoulder, and neck pain. If it can be done by the person who will accompany you at the birth, this is even better, as he or she will learn how to relieve the pain of contractions. The pregnant woman can sit leaning over the back of a chair with her head on her arms. The massager uses long sweeping strokes from the base of the back, up and outward. Do not massage over the spine itself, but

across all the surrounding muscles. The massager should listen
to what the woman wants him or
her to do.

- Yoga is very effective: There are
  many classes specifically for
  pregnant women.
- Chiropractic treatment relieves
  pain caused by misalignments
  in the spine, which often occur
  during pregnancy.

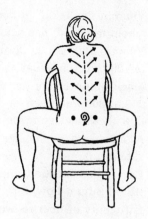

**PREVENTION AND
TREATMENT: HEARTBURN**

Hormonal changes during pregnancy often result in food and gastric acid
backing up in the esophagus, giving pain and a sense of burning in the
chest. As the fetus grows, pressure is put on the stomach, leading to
indigestion.

Eat small meals often.

Do not eat late at night.

Avoid spicy, greasy, sugary, and acidic foods.

Take 1 cup of chamomile, peppermint, or fennel infusion after meals.

Yogurt or milk eases the burning sensation.

Take papaya supplements, which contain digestive enzymes.

Combine foods carefully. Avoid eating carbohydrates and protein
together; instead, eat either carbohydrates and vegetables or protein and
vegetables. Eat fruit only in the morning.

See **Acid Stomach** and **Indigestion** for further advice.

PREMENSTRUAL SYNDROME (PMS)

A collection of symptoms, both physical and emotional, which generally
occur in women during the week or two before their period starts. The
most common signs of PMS are irritability, tension, depression, fatigue,
thirst, fluid retention, breast tenderness, and head, back, and stomach
aches.

TREATMENT

✗ DIETARY

The following nutrients are thought to be helpful in preventing and
relieving PMS:

- Vitamin B6: Taken in doses of 50 milligrams daily throughout the whole month, it has been shown to reduce symptoms.
- Vitamin E: Breast tenderness is often relieved by taking supplements of 100 to 600 iu a day.
- Magnesium: For breast tenderness, tension, and weight gain, take 200 to 300 milligrams a day.

Follow these dietary recommendations:

- Avoid alcohol, coffee, tea, cola, and chocolate, which tend to aggravate symptoms.
- Eat regular nutritious meals to maintain your blood-sugar level (see **Blood Sugar, Low,** for guidelines).
- Eat plenty of fiber to avoid constipation.

Studies have shown evening primrose oil to be an effective treatment for women suffering breast discomfort, irritability, and depression. Take 6 500-milligram capsules a day throughout your cycle. You'll probably begin to notice results after three months of treatment.

☐ HOMEOPATHY

Take morning, noon, and night for up to 3 days, starting 24 hours prior to the expected start of symptoms:

Oversensitive to the slightest criticism, with tearfulness: *Pulsatilla* 6c
Flies off the handle at the stupidity of others: *Nux vomica* 6c
Overtired, underappreciated, worn out, and snappish: *Sepia* 6c

☯ CHINESE MEDICINE

Acupuncture can greatly help. Herbs, such as Chinese angelica, white peony, skullcap, and poria, may be recommended.

⁌ EXERCISE

Moderate exercise relaxes the muscles, improves blood flow, and prevents fluid retention. It also stimulates the production of the body's endorphins, which improve your mood.

Try to exercise regularly throughout the month, but increase your activity in the week or two before your period starts.

∼ RELAXATION TECHNIQUES

Stress is thought to contribute to symptoms of PMS. Attending a yoga or meditation class helps reduce stress.

Try to plan your life in such a way that you can take some time in the week before your period to relax and get more sleep (see **Stress**).

••• ORTHODOX

Many doctors recommend vitamin B6 (100 milligrams, 2 times a day).
Oral contraceptives are sometimes prescribed to suppress ovulation.
Progesterone supplements are sometimes given for several days in the
second half of the menstrual cycle, to correct hormonal imbalances.

PRESBYOPIA
See **Eyesight Problems.**

PRICKLY HEAT

An itchy skin rash that generally occurs when people who are unaccustomed to high temperatures experience extreme heat. It is thought to
be caused by the blockage of sweat glands. Symptoms include red itchy
spots, and inflamed areas of skin, particularly around the waist, upper
trunk, armpits, and insides of the elbows.

TREATMENT/PREVENTION

Some cases of prickly heat are made worse by a hypersensitivity to sunlight. Use a high protection-factor sun cream as a preventive measure,
and cover up when you go outdoors.

▬ PRACTICAL ADVICE

Take frequent cold showers, or sponge down the skin with cool water.
Wear loose clothing to allow sweat to evaporate quickly.

✗ DIETARY

Increase your intake of vitamin C, found in citrus fruits and juices, black
currants, green peppers, parsley, and broccoli. Research has shown that
daily supplements of 500 milligrams of vitamin C clear up itching and the
rash.

✿ AROMATHERAPY

As a soothing lotion or oil: Add essential oils of sandalwood (1 drop) and
lavender (4 drops) to 2 tablespoons of *Calendula* carrier oil or lotion.

❧ HERBALISM

Chickweed ointment helps soothe the rash. Simmer 2 tablespoons of
chickweed in 220 grams of petroleum jelly for 10 minutes, stirring well.

Strain through fine gauze, pour into a container, and allow to cool; apply when needed. You might prefer to keep an old pan specially for herbal preparations.

Chickweed infusion is also a soothing application: Pour 1 cup of boiling water onto 4 teaspoons of dried chickweed, infuse for 15 minutes, and allow to cool; dab on the rash when needed.

☐ HOMEOPATHY

Take every 15 minutes for up to 4 doses, and repeat if necessary:
Stinging itchy rash: *Urtica urens* 6c
Burning and itching rash: *Rhus toxicodendron* 6c
Dusky pink rash with swelling of lips, eyelids, or throat: *Apis* 6c

••• ORTHODOX

Doctors may recommend calamine lotion (available over the counter) to relieve the prickly itching. In severe cases antihistamines are given orally to combat irritation, although these can sometimes cause allergy in their own right and should be avoided if possible.

PROSTATE, ENLARGED

Enlargement of the prostate gland, also known as benign prostatic hypertrophy, generally only afflicts men over the age of fifty. As the gland grows, it presses on the urethra, interfering with the flow of urine. First symptoms are an increased desire to urinate day and night, difficulty starting urination, a weak urine stream, and finally incontinence. Back pain and pain between the legs may also be present. See also **Prostatitis.**

TREATMENT
✗ DIETARY

Studies have shown zinc deficiency to be related to enlarged prostate. Increasing the intake of zinc has also been shown to decrease the size of the prostate and reduce symptoms. Zinc is found in oysters, herrings, clams, wheat bran, whole oatmeal, pumpkin seeds, and sunflower seeds. To ensure sufficient intake, take 1 100-milligram zinc orotate supplement every other day.

Cholesterol in the blood accumulates in the prostate, damaging cells, which can lead to cancer. Lower your cholesterol levels by avoiding saturated fats: Substitute chicken and fish for red meat, and reduce your intake of high-fat dairy products (see **Cholesterol, High,** for further details).

Sufferers are often deficient in essential fatty acids: Supplement your diet with 4 capsules of MaxEPA fish oil daily, and 4 500-milligram capsules of evening primrose oil a day.

Eat plenty of lean protein, fruits, and vegetables, with moderate intake of whole-grain carbohydrates. Fiber is important to prevent constipation and straining.

⁊ HERBALISM

Saw palmetto is an effective remedy for reducing inflammation of the prostate: Take the liposterolic extract of saw palmetto berries, 160 milligrams a day.

Flower pollen is also widely used.

☯ CHINESE MEDICINE

Practitioners of traditional Chinese medicine generally recommend the herbal remedy panax ginseng: Take 2 to 4 grams of the dried root, 3 times a day.

≈ HYDROTHERAPY

Sit in contrast sitz baths, which alternate hot and cold water, to stimulate blood circulation in the pelvic area and tone the muscles: Run a hot bath, around 105°F to 115°F; also prepare a plastic basin of cold water, around 55°F to 85°F. Sit for 10 seconds in the hot, then 5 seconds in the cold, repeat 3 times, finishing with the cold. Do this every other day. Make sure the rest of the body is well covered.

✳ YOGA

The Supine Butterfly exercise improves circulation to the enlarged prostate, and helps reduce inflammation: Lie on your back, bend your knees, bring the soles of the feet together, and bring the feet as close to your buttocks as possible. Relax your legs, letting the knees fall outward, toward the ground. Hold this position for 5 minutes.

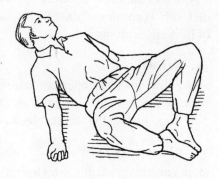

••• ORTHODOX

Your doctor will probably palpate and assess the enlargement clinically, by means of a rectal examination. A blood test can help distinguish between benign and malignant enlargement. In benign enlargement, if pressure on the urethra makes symptoms uncomfortable, part or all of the gland is surgically removed.

PROSTATITIS

Infection and inflammation of the prostate gland, usually as a result of bacterial infection transmitted from the urethra or bladder. The infection may also be sexually transmitted. Symptoms include fever; flu-like aches and pains; aching in the back, rectum, and between the legs; and considerable pain when urinating. Treatment of prostatitis is similar to that of enlarged prostate. See **Prostate, Enlarged.**

TREATMENT

✗ DIETARY

An increased intake of zinc has been shown to clear up symptoms of prostatitis effectively. Zinc is found in oysters, herrings, clams, wheat bran, whole oatmeal, pumpkin seeds, and sunflower seeds. To ensure sufficient intake, you can take a 100-milligram zinc orotate supplement every other day.

Reducing cholesterol levels also helps relieve symptoms of prostatitis, and prevent recurrent attacks: Substitute chicken and fish for red meat, and avoid high-fat dairy products (see **Cholesterol, High**).

Pollen, rich in essential fatty acids and protein, is also a useful treatment. Take 4 Cernilton pollen tablets a day.

Sufferers are often deficient in essential fatty acids: Supplement your diet with 4 capsules of MaxEPA fish oil daily and 4 500-milligram capsules of evening primrose oil a day.

🍂 HERBALISM

Saw palmetto is an effective remedy for reducing inflammation and fighting infections of the prostate: Take the liposterolic extract of saw palmetto berries, 160 milligrams a day.

≈ HYDROTHERAPY

Sit in contrast sitz baths, which alternate hot and cold water, to stimulate blood circulation in the pelvic area and tone the muscles: Run a hot bath, around 105°F to 115°F; also prepare a plastic basin of cold water, around 55°F to 85°F. Sit for 10 seconds in the hot, then 5 seconds in the cold, repeat 3 times, finishing with the cold. Do this every other day. Make sure the rest of the body is well covered.

Doctors generally prescribe drinking plenty of fluids, and long-term antibiotic treatment.

PSORIASIS

A skin disease characterized by thick, red patches covered by a unique silvery scale, particularly around the elbows, knees, scalp, trunk, and back. The skin does not usually itch badly, but is unsightly. The disease tends to run in families. One percent of the population may develop psoriasis at some time in their lives; the condition tends to come and go.

TREATMENT

Reduce your intake of meat, animal fats, sugar, and alcohol.

Increase your intake of fiber: whole-grain cereals, fruit, vegetables, and cooked dried beans and peas.

Increase your intake of oily fish.

Take 1 to 2 tablespoons of linseed oil a day.

Increase your intake of fish, particularly mackerel, herring, and salmon. The following supplements help:

- zinc, 15 to 30 milligrams a day
- vitamin B-complex, 100 milligrams, morning and night
- vitamin A, 10,000 iu, 3 times a day, 6 days a week

Psoriasis is sometimes linked to food allergies, particularly citrus fruits and dairy products (see **Allergies, Food**).

❧ HERBALISM

Burdock is one of the best remedies for dry, scaly skin:
Make a decoction by adding 1 teaspoon of the root to 1 cup of water, and simmer for 15 minutes; drink 3 times a day.

An ointment containing burdock will help relieve irritation and scaliness: Simmer 2 tablespoons of the root in 220 grams of petroleum jelly for 10 minutes, strain through gauze, and allow to cool; apply to the skin when needed. You may like to keep an old pan specifically for herbal preparations.

≈ HYDROTHERAPY

A hot Epsom salts bath stimulates circulation and helps eliminate toxins through the skin: Add 1 pound of Epsom salts to a bath and soak in it for 15 minutes, preferably before going to bed. Not advised if you are weak or frail.

An oatmeal bath helps soothe irritated skin. Put 2 pounds of fine oatmeal in cheesecloth bags and place in a hot bath; soak in the bath for 15 minutes.

⁘ EXERCISE

Aerobic exercise helps improve circulation to the skin. Running, walking, swimming, or vigorous exercises done for 30 minutes, 3 times a week, will help.

✚ PROFESSIONAL HELP

Chinese medicine: Individually prescribed herbs can greatly assist this problem, as has been shown by a number of trials in British hospitals.

Professional homeopathic treatment can help in some cases.

••• ORTHODOX

Psoriasis is sometimes helped by exposure to sunlight or an ultraviolet lamp.

Your doctor may recommend a coal tar or dithranol ointment.

If your case is severe, your doctor may prescribe corticosteroid drugs.

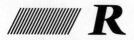 # R

RAYNAUD'S DISEASE

A circulatory disorder where the blood vessels become hypersensitive to the cold and contract, preventing adequate blood flow to the fingers and toes. The affected areas become white, turning blue when warmed, then red. Tingling or numbness is also common.

TREATMENT

■ PRACTICAL ADVICE

Dress in layers to trap the heat.

Wear natural fabrics that absorb perspiration, the body's natural cooling agent.

Mittens keep you warmer than gloves.

Stop smoking. Nicotine constricts the blood vessels.

✗ DIETARY

Make sure you get enough iron. The richest sources are lean red meat, poultry, fish, and leafy green vegetables. Drinking orange juice with meals helps increase iron absorption. Tea inhibits absorption, so do not drink tea immediately before, during, or after meals.

Avoid coffee, which constricts blood vessels.

❊ AROMATHERAPY

Essential oils of black pepper and rosemary help improve circulation.

Ask a friend or partner to give you a regular massage using 3 drops of each oil mixed with 2½ teaspoons of a carrier oil or lotion.

Add 3 drops of each oil to your bathwater.

❧ HERBALISM

Cayenne is useful in stimulating the circulatory system: Pour 1 cup of boiling water on 1 teaspoon of cayenne, and infuse for 10 minutes; mix 1 tablespoon of the infusion with a glass of hot water, and drink when needed.

Add grated fresh root ginger to your diet, or drink an infusion when needed: Add 1 cup of boiling water to 1 teaspoon of grated fresh root, and infuse for 5 minutes.

▢ HOMEOPATHY

Take every 30 minutes for up to 6 doses; repeat if necessary:

Burning sensation in fingers or toes, increased by heat, but the body is cold: *Carbo vegetabilis* 6c

Heat or holding the fingers down increases discomfort: *Pulsatilla* 6c

Swollen, burning, itching fingers and toes, made worse by cold: *Arsenicum album* 6c

☯ CHINESE MEDICINE

Professional treatment can be very effective. Cinnamon twigs and Chinese angelica are often prescribed.

⚜ EXERCISE

Any aerobic exercise (which raises the heart rate and exercises the lungs) is helpful for this condition: walking, running, cycling, swimming, or skipping.

Swing your arms in circular motion, as if throwing a ball over your arm. Do 20 circles on each arm. Then, with your arms outstretched, do 20 more small circles. Repeat morning and evening.

••• ORTHODOX

Vasodilator drugs are effective in relaxing and opening the blood vessel walls. You might want to try battery-heated gloves and socks, or warmer pads containing a substance that heats up when activated (available in stores that sell sporting goods or camping equipment).

REITER'S SYNDROME

A disorder common in men, which produces a combination of arthritis (joint inflammation), urethritis (inflammation of the bladder outlet), and conjunctivitis (an eye infection). Reiter's syndrome is prompted by infection, but only occurs in those who are genetically predisposed. Symptoms include bladder discharge, painful stiff joints, and fever.

TREATMENT

▬ PRACTICAL ADVICE

Place cool, wet tea bags on the eyes to soothe redness and itching.

✗ DIETARY

Drinking cranberry juice helps clear up urethritis. Drink 4 glasses daily.

✽ AROMATHERAPY

Add 2 drops each of essential oil of juniper berry, eucalyptus, and sandalwood to a warm bath, and sit in it for 10 minutes a day to relieve urethritis.

⋛ HERBALISM

Devil's claw decoction is an anti-inflammatory remedy. Add 1 teaspoon of the herb to 1 cup of water, and simmer for 15 minutes; drink 3 times a day. **Caution:** Do not take during pregnancy.

For conjunctivitis, wash the eyes with eyebright tea. Add 1 teaspoon of the herb to 1 cup of boiling water, allow to cool, and strain. With an eye cup, use the solution to rinse the eye.

Parsley and dandelion are useful in helping to flush infection from the bladder. Incorporate both herbs into your diet.

≈ HYDROTHERAPY

For inflamed and stiff joints, prepare a cold compress by soaking a piece of cotton material large enough to cover the joint in cold water. Wring it out well and place over the painful joint. Wrap 2 thicknesses of woolen material around the cold compress and pin it securely. Leave on for 4 to 8 hours, or overnight. The compress should warm up and dry by the time it is taken off. If the compress does not warm up within 15 minutes, remove and try again, making sure the material is well wrung out and insulated.

☛ MASSAGE

Gently stroke the muscles around painful joints in the direction of the heart. Use the fingertips to do gentle, circular strokes in particularly stiff areas. If you cannot use your fingers well, you can roll a clean tennis or squash ball back and forth over the muscles.

••• ORTHODOX

Your doctor may recommend painkillers and nonsteroidal anti-inflammatory drugs to help relieve pain and inflammation.

RESTLESS LEGS

An aching, tickling, burning, or twitching in the muscles of the legs that occurs especially at night or when sitting for long periods. It is particularly common in pregnant and middle-aged women, smokers, and people who drink a lot of caffeine.

TREATMENT

✗ DIETARY

Increase your intake of vitamin E, found in vegetable oils, seeds, wheat germ, and nuts. Take 1 200-iu supplement every day.

Increase your intake of iron, found in lean red meat, poultry, fish, dried fruits, and green leafy vegetables. Avoid drinking tea within 2 hours of eating.

Take 1 multivitamin and mineral supplement daily.

Avoid eating heavy meals late at night.

Cut down your intake of caffeine (coffee, tea, cola, chocolate).

Take 1 60-milligram vitamin B-complex tablet every day.

☐ HOMEOPATHY

Take every 30 minutes for up to 6 doses:

Burning pain in the shins and crawling sensation on the skin, worse after drinking wine: *Zinc metallicum* 6c

Involuntary reaction to music or bright colors: *Tarantula hispanica* 6c

Restlessness worse from lying still and improved by walking around; worse during stormy weather: *Rhus toxicodendron* 6c

≈ HYDROTHERAPY

Bathe the legs alternately in hot and cold water to improve circulation.

☛ MASSAGE

Do this massage on the fleshy parts of the lower leg (avoid pressure on the knees and any varicose veins):

Sit on a firm surface, bend one knee, and place your foot flat on the ground. Place your thumbs on the muscle running along the outside of

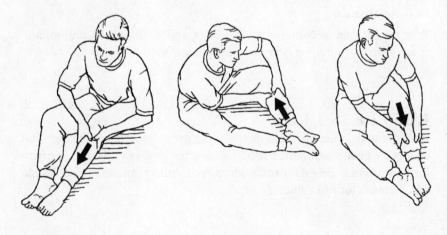

your shin bone, below the knee, and rest your fingers and palms on the sides of your legs for support. Applying pressure with your thumbs, run them slowly down the muscle, as far as the ankle bone. Then move the hands around to the inside of the ankle and massage up the inside of the leg to the knee. Finally, place your hand on either side of the calf and squeeze with the thumbs in front and the fingers behind, kneading either side and the back of the leg. Repeat this procedure several times on both legs.

✛ EXERCISE

Walking is one of the best ways to relieve this condition. An evening stroll can help prevent night discomfort.

∼ RELAXATION TECHNIQUES

Stress often makes this condition worse. Attending a regular yoga class will help you learn to relax, and will provide some good stretching movements to help relieve symptoms. Biofeedback and meditation are also good ways to learn to relax.

••• ORTHODOX

Once more serious problems such as deep vein thrombosis or sciatica have been ruled out, doctors may recommend mild muscle relaxants or calcium supplements.

RHEUMATOID ARTHRITIS

A type of arthritis in which the joints of the body (most commonly the fingers, wrists, knees, and ankles) become painful, swollen, stiff, and sometimes deformed. This is accompanied by mild fever and fatigue. Rheumatoid arthritis is an autoimmune disorder (where, for some unknown reason, the immune system attacks the body's own tissues).

TREATMENT
 DIETARY

Rheumatoid arthritis is rare in countries where an unrefined, low-fat diet is consumed. Studies have indicated that adopting a diet high in whole-grain cereals, vegetables, and fiber, and low in sugar, animal products, and refined carbohydrates, helps prevent and treat this condition.

A vegetarian diet has been shown to reduce inflammation.

Cook with vegetable oils and margarine instead of animal fats, such as butter and lard.

Eat oily fish: mackerel, herring, sardines, and salmon daily. These contain eicosapentaenoic acid (EPA), which helps to produce substances that reduce inflammation. An alternative to eating fish is a daily supplement of cod liver oil.

Increase your intake of vitamin E, found in wheat germ, nuts, seeds, and seed oils, and take a daily supplement of 400 to 1000 iu.

Sometimes rheumatoid arthritis can be triggered by food allergies (see **Allergies, Food**).

Take a daily supplement of 50 to 100 milligrams of selenium.

Bromelain, an extract of pineapple, has significant anti-inflammatory effects: Take 600 milligrams a day, in 3 doses, between meals.

Take 1 multivitamin and mineral supplement each day.

ξ♣ HERBALISM

Devil's claw decoction or tablets have been shown to help: Add 1 teaspoon of the herb to 1 cup of water, and simmer for 15 minutes; drink 3 times a day.

☐ HOMEOPATHY

Take 2 times a day for up to 14 days; repeat if needed:

Worse from warm weather, inflamed joints, intolerant of touch, and ill-humored: *Colchicum* 6c

Worse during stormy weather: *Rhododendron* 6c

When symptoms include pain and stiffness, made worse after rest and in cold, damp weather, symptoms improve with continued motion: *Rhus toxicodendron* 6c

Stitching pain, made worse by any motion, eased by rest: *Bryonia* 6c

☯ CHINESE MEDICINE

Bupleuri root, licorice, and Chinese skullcap are recommended for their powerful anti-inflammatory effects.

≈ HYDROTHERAPY

Place a cold compress on the affected joint: Wet a piece of cotton material in cold tap water, wring it out, and wrap it around the joint. Cover this with two layers of flannel or wool pinned in place. Leave in position for 4 to 8 hours. The compress should warm through. If it does not warm up within 15 minutes, remove it and try again.

☛ MASSAGE

Gentle self-massage aids circulation and reduces inflammation: Using a light cream or oil, lightly stroke the muscles and tissues around the area involved, in the direction of the heart. You can also roll a clean tennis or squash ball over the area, exerting pressure.

⁂ EXERCISE
Swimming in a heated pool helps keep joints mobile.

✚ PROFESSIONAL HELP
Chiropractic, homeopathy, and acupuncture may all help relieve symptoms.

••• ORTHODOX
Doctors generally recommend aspirin and nonsteroidal anti-inflammatory drugs.

RHINITIS
See **Allergies, Hay Fever, and Rhinitis.**

RICKETS
See **Osteomalacia.**

RINGWORM
See **Fungal Infection.**

ROSACEA
A skin disorder where the forehead, nose, and cheeks become abnormally red, due to minute blood vessels opening up near the surface of the skin. Sometimes redness is accompanied by pus-filled spots resembling acne. In elderly men the condition can develop into rhinophyma, a bulbous swelling of the nose.

TREATMENT
✗ DIETARY
Some studies have shown people with rosacea to be deficient in hydrochloric acid, a gastric secretion that digests the food in the stomach. Some

naturopaths recommend taking hydrochloric acid capsules (10 grains) with every large meal. Start with 1 capsule, and increase the dose by 1 at every large meal, until you are taking 7 capsules, or you feel a warmth in your stomach. Once you have felt the warmth, decrease the dose by 1 capsule, and keep taking that number at all meals of similar size (take a smaller dose at smaller meals). As your stomach begins to adapt, you will feel the warmth earlier and can gradually cut down the dosage.

People with rosacea are often deficient in vitamin B: Take 100 milligrams of vitamin B-complex without niacin.

The pancreatic enzyme lipase is also often deficient: Take 1 to 2 tablets daily of pancreatin.

Avoid caffeine (coffee, tea, cola, chocolate), alcohol, hot drinks, spicy foods, and any other food or drink that causes flushing.

☐ HOMEOPATHY

Hot, burning, and itching skin: *Sulphur* 6c, 3 times a day.

With a swollen, glazed appearance and stinging skin: *Apis* 6c, 3 times a day.

∼ RELAXATION TECHNIQUES

A reduction in hydrochloric acid production is often caused by stress, depression, and anxiety. The following techniques may alleviate these symptoms:

Try to anticipate stressful situations and prepare for them, if possible.

Reduce your commitments. Learn to say no.

If you have a problem or concern, talk about it.

Take time out to do "nothing."

Develop a hobby, sport, or interest that distracts you from your concerns and absorbs your attention while you are doing it.

Join a yoga class, or learn meditation or biofeedback.

••• ORTHODOX

Doctors generally recommend antibiotics. Men with rhinophyma can have surgery to cut away the thickened skin.

ROSEOLA INFANTUM

A viral infection common in children aged six months to two years. Symptoms include a high fever, swollen neck glands, and a pink rash on the chest, back, and stomach, which lasts about a week.

TREATMENT

✗ DIETARY

Drink plenty of fluids, particularly fruit juices. Eat light, nutritious meals of vegetable soups, broths, and lightly cooked vegetables.

⅍ HERBALISM

Catmint infusion helps reduce fever: Add 1 cup of boiling water to 1 teaspoon of the dried herb, and infuse for 10 minutes; drink 3 times a day.

☐ HOMEOPATHY

Take every hour for up to 4 doses; repeat if needed:

High fever, eyes bright and staring, child delirious, neck glands sore: *Belladonna* 6c

Child clingy and tearful, craving fresh air: *Pulsatilla* 6c

Earache on swallowing, swollen glands, craving cold drinks: *Phytolacca* 6c

✿ BACH FLOWER REMEDIES

Keep a glass of water containing 1 or 2 drops of Rescue Remedy near the bed.

••• ORTHODOX

Report a fever to your doctor. Tepid sponging is often recommended along with temperature-lowering drugs.

RUBELLA

This infectious illness manifests as a slight fever, a mild rash, and tender glands, which usually last about three to five days; also known as German measles. Rubella is very dangerous if contracted during pregnancy, as it can cause defects or death to the unborn baby. Women who have not had the illness are advised to seek immunization before becoming pregnant.

TREATMENT

✗ DIETARY

Make sure to get an adequate intake of fresh fruit juices and vegetable soups, followed by a whole-foods diet once the fever has gone.

◊♣ HERBALISM

Infusion of yarrow: Pour 1 cup of boiling water on 1 teaspoon of the dried herb, and infuse for 10 minutes; drink hot 3 times a day.

For children with a high fever, infusion of catmint: Pour boiling water over 1 heaped teaspoon of the dried herb, and infuse for 5 minutes; drink 3 times a day.

☐ HOMEOPATHY

Take every hour for up to 6 doses; repeat if necessary:
Child has a rash, red eyes, yellow mucus, and is tearful: *Pulsatilla* 6c
Bright red rash, hot red face, craving for lemons: *Belladonna* 6c
Swollen glands and painful ears, alleviated by cold drinks: *Phytolacca* 6c

≈ HYDROTHERAPY

Cool sponging will help reduce fever and relieve discomfort caused by the rash.

••• ORTHODOX

Doctors recommend that children should be kept at home while they have a rash, and for 3 days after the spots have disappeared. If they have a temperature of over 99°F, they should stay in bed. German measles is a mild illness and does not usually warrant treatment; however, fever should be monitored and treated accordingly (see **Fever**).

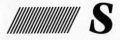 # *S*

SALPINGITIS
See **Pelvic Inflammatory Disease.**

SAND FLY BITES
See **Insect Bites and Stings.**

SCABIES

An infectious skin condition brought on by mites burrowing into the skin and laying eggs. Symptoms include an intensely itchy rash with red lumps, particularly around the trunk, between the fingers, on the wrists, and in the genital area. The area above the neck is usually spared. Once scratched, the lumps develop into sores and scabs. See **Sexually Transmitted Diseases** for scabies in the pubic area.

TREATMENT

■ **PRACTICAL ADVICE**

Thoroughly wash all clothes and bedding in the house in very hot water. If they cannot be washed, air them for several days; mites cannot survive for long without human contact.

❀ **AROMATHERAPY**

Dab essential oil of lavender on the sores.

🐾 **HERBALISM**

Soak a handful of ivy leaves in 1 quart of wine vinegar overnight, and strain. Dab all over the body 2 times a day.

▢ **HOMEOPATHY**

Everyone living with the infected person should take *Sulphur* 6c, every 8 hours, for up to 3 days.

••• **ORTHODOX**

Most doctors recommend applying an insecticide lotion to the entire body, which should be left on for 24 hours before being washed off. A second application is advised. Skin irritation will continue for a few days as a result of residual foreign body material in the skin tissue.

SCAR

A mark left on the skin after the tissue has healed following an injury. Excess scar tissue, known as hypertrophic scars or keloids, sometimes develop when the injury is infected, or in people who have a genetic tendency to produce excess scar tissue.

TREATMENT

▬ PRACTICAL ADVICE

Make sure wounds heal properly. Clean all cuts and scrapes well, and keep the wound slightly moist with vitamin E oil while it is healing.

Do not pick the scabs.

✗ DIETARY

A well-balanced diet is essential in encouraging healthy scar tissue to grow. Eat plenty of protein (lean meat, fish, low-fat dairy products, dried cooked beans, soybeans), and incorporate plenty of zinc into your meals (lean meat, fish, and organ meats, whole-grain breads and cereals, pumpkin seeds and sunflower seeds, Brazil nuts, and peanuts).

Take vitamin E supplements: 100 to 400 iu a day.

☐ HOMEOPATHY

Apply *Calendula* cream as soon as the wound starts to heal; use a fresh tube to ensure sterility.

Take *Thiosinaminum* 6x, 4 times a day.

☛ MASSAGE

Massaging the scar area with vitamin E oil can help in the healing process.

✚ PROFESSIONAL HELP

Massage can soften the tissues and break down old scars.

••• ORTHODOX

Your doctor may suggest injecting steroids into thickened scar tissue to reduce the size and thickness.

SCARLET FEVER

A bacterial infection most often found in small children. Symptoms include fever, a sore throat, swollen glands, and a rash. The tongue is usually coated white with red spots that peel off to reveal a bright red ("strawberry") surface. Later, the skin on the body also peels.

TREATMENT

✗ DIETARY

Drink plenty of fluids, particularly citrus fruit juices (oranges, lemons, grapefruit).

🐾 HERBALISM

Catmint is effective in treating the fever. Take 2 to 3 drops of catmint tincture in a glass of water 3 times a day.

Echinacea decoction will combat the virus, ease out the rash, and help clear chest congestion. Use it once the fever has started to come down: Put 2 teaspoons of the powdered root in 1 cup of water, and simmer for 15 minutes; drink 3 times a day.

☐ HOMEOPATHY

If a child has been in contact with others with scarlet fever: *Belladonna* 6c, 2 times a day, for up to 10 days.

✳ BIOCHEMIC TISSUE SALTS

Take 4 tablets, 4 times a day:
In early stages, with sore throat and shivering: *Ferr Phos* 6x
When there is a skin rash and white tongue: *Kali Mur* 6x

≈ HYDROTHERAPY

To soothe the rash, take lukewarm baths to which you have added 3 tablespoons of baking soda.

••• ORTHODOX

Scarlet fever itself is a relatively mild infection, but the bacteria that cause it can affect many other parts of the body in more serious ways if not treated. Many doctors prescribe painkillers and antibiotics to protect against heart, kidney, and other complications that may arise.

SCHIZOPHRENIA

A psychiatric illness that causes changes in personality and behavior and a loss of touch with reality. The patient's thoughts are dissociated from the physical reality of his or her own body and surroundings. Sufferers often experience delusions, illusions, hallucinations, and paranoia.

TREATMENT

▬ PRACTICAL ADVICE

Recent research has shown that a caring, nonjudgmental environment can help reduce the severity of this illness.

✗ DIETARY

A number of nutritional deficiencies, particularly minerals, are thought to be linked to schizophrenia. Professional help from a naturopath or dietitian with a particular interest in this condition is recommended. The following guidelines indicate the type of treatment that may be proposed:

- Avoid gluten. Research studies have shown that eliminating gluten and milk from the diet sometimes helps schizophrenia. Gluten is found in all wheat and rye products, and in smaller quantities in oats and barley. Replace these cereals with corn, millet, rice, and potato products.
- Increase intake of niacin, found in protein-rich foods such as lean meat, chicken, fish, beans, peas, brewer's yeast, peanut butter, low-fat milk and cheese, soybeans, and nuts. Eat protein-rich foods 3 times a day.
- Take 1 25-milligram vitamin B-complex supplement a day to complement the niacin.
- Avoid caffeine (coffee, tea, cola drinks, and chocolate).
- Avoid alcohol.
- Megadoses of vitamins B3, B6, C, and E may be recommended.
- Supplements of amino acids may also be advised.

Food allergies can play a role in schizophrenia. For further information see **Allergies, Food.**

••• ORTHODOX

Drugs are used in oral or long-acting injection form to control excitable or violent states, as well as to reduce delusions and hallucinations. Electroconvulsive therapy is still sometimes used, especially where disorders of muscular control, known as catatonia, are present. Environmental stimulation, occupational therapy, rehabilitation, and psychotherapy (individual and group) are all used as forms of supportive therapy.

SCIATICA

Nerve pain that radiates through the buttock and often the back of the thigh, calf, and sometimes down to the foot. Sciatica is usually a symptom of a structural problem in the lower back, where the nerve is pinched as it emerges from the spinal column and runs down the back of the leg. The pain can be accompanied by numbness or tingling.

TREATMENT

■ PRACTICAL ADVICE

When sleeping or resting, lie on your side, with a pillow between the knees to minimize pelvic strain.

≈ HYDROTHERAPY

To relieve pain and discomfort and reduce inflammation, try hot and cold treatments: Prepare an ice pack by wrapping a bag of ice cubes or frozen peas in a kitchen towel; also prepare a hot water bottle wrapped in a towel. Place each alternately on the site of pain for 10 minutes; repeat. Do this at least 2 times a day.

☛ MASSAGE

Place two tennis balls in a sock. Lie down on your back on the floor, with your knees bent and the sock under your lower back; one tennis ball should be on either side of the spine. Relax for several minutes, letting your body sink down into the floor and over the tennis balls.

Remove the balls and relax on the floor for a further 2 minutes. Then place a tennis ball under each buttock, and repeat the procedure.

✳ ACUPRESSURE

The following exercises help stimulate the pressure points related to sciatica:

Lie on your back on the floor with your knees bent. Inhale, and pull your knees up to your chest, keeping your lower back as flat as possible on the floor. Hold your knees, hug them close to the chest, and exhale; inhale, and release your knees; exhale, and hug them close to your chest again. Repeat this action for several minutes.

Lie on your back on the floor with your knees bent. Place your hands, palms down, under your lower back. Taking deep breaths, rock your knees from side to side for several minutes. Bring your hands to the side, then raise your knees, steady them with your hands, and continue rocking for several minutes.

You can also massage the points illustrated, using deep thumb pressure, for at least 1 minute each.

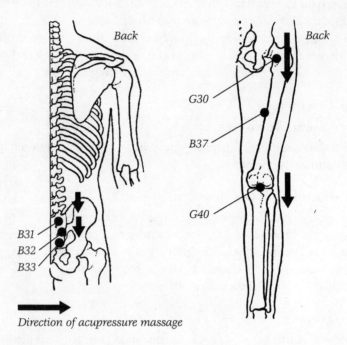

Direction of acupressure massage

✚ **PROFESSIONAL HELP**

Chiropractors specialize in dealing with sciatic pain.
Acupuncture can also be very helpful.

••• **ORTHODOX**

Doctors generally prescribe anti-inflammatory drugs and muscle relaxants.
Surgery may be suggested if the pain results from a prolapsed disc (see **Slipped Disc**).

SEASICKNESS
See **Motion Sickness.**

SEASONAL AFFECTIVE DISORDER (SAD)
A syndrome that strikes during the winter months and is characterized by depression, fatigue, and listlessness, along with the desire to eat more,

and subsequent weight gain. Symptoms generally begin in September or October, and are relieved in the spring.

TREATMENT

✘ DIETARY

SAD sufferers have a tendency to binge on sweet, fattening foods, leading to considerable weight gain during the winter months. The following guidelines help minimize food cravings:

Eat small, nutritious meals regularly: whole-grain cereals, lean meat, fish, and low-fat dairy products, and plenty of fruits and vegetables.

Eat complex carbohydrates regularly (cereals, pasta, bread, and potatoes). Avoid simple carbohydrates, such as sugar and foods containing sugar, as these are fattening and provide little nutritional value.

Avoid alcohol.

Keep nutritious snacks at hand for when you feel a slump in energy coming on: a sugar-free granola bar, a slice of whole-grain bread with honey, fruit, and nuts.

If you feel a craving, eat the food you want, but do it slowly and in small quantities. Put a small amount of the food on a plate, and go out of the kitchen to eat it. Eat slowly, have a drink, and allow yourself to digest the food. Then try to distract yourself from the craving by doing a calming activity: read, have a shower, call a friend.

～ RELAXATION TECHNIQUES

Accept that you can do less in the winter.

Reserve stressful undertakings for the summer months, when you have more energy.

Try to distract yourself when you become obsessed with a stressful thought.

Talk to others.

Try to rationalize your concerns by examining the possible outcomes of the problem realistically.

○ PHOTOTHERAPY

Extensive research has shown light therapy to be an effective treatment for SAD. A high-intensity light box (at least 2,500 lux) is required for treatment; it is available from some hospitals and specialist lighting manufacturers. Four to six hours of light therapy a day is generally recommended, though this can vary from person to person, depending on the type of light box used and the severity of the illness. A psychiatrist can help with initial treatment.

Introducing more natural daylight into your daily life will also help relieve symptoms. Try taking a 30-minute walk at midday, when the sun is at its highest and brightest.

••• ORTHODOX

Light therapy is the accepted medical treatment. Antidepressant drugs are sometimes offered, particularly fluoxetine. Psychotherapy or counseling can also be helpful.

SEPTICEMIA

A potentially life-threatening condition in which large numbers of disease-causing bacteria invade the bloodstream; more commonly known as blood poisoning. It generally occurs in people whose immune system is weakened, and results from bacteria escaping from an infected site, such as an abscess or pneumonia, into the blood. Symptoms include high fever, rapid breathing, headaches, nausea, low blood pressure, and sometimes loss of consciousness. Immediate medical attention is necessary.

TREATMENT

Orthodox treatment with antibiotics, sometimes given by injection, is vital to prevent the multiplication of harmful bacteria in the body. The following treatments can complement the orthodox approach.

❀ AROMATHERAPY

Oils that strengthen the immune system include bergamot, Roman chamomile, and rosemary. Put 3 drops of two of these into a bath, or 1 drop of each in a vaporizer.

❧ HERBALISM

Echinacea decoction is recommended to help the body rid itself of microbial infections: Add 2 teaspoons of the powdered root to 1 cup of water, bring to a boil, and simmer for 15 minutes; drink 3 times a day.

Garlic also helps purify the blood: Incorporate the raw herb into your diet as much as possible. If you do not like the taste or smell of garlic, take 3 garlic capsules, 3 times a day.

☐ HOMEOPATHY

Loquacious and delirious, aching and sore, disproportionately fast pulse: Take *Pyrogen* 30c, 2 times a day, for 3 days.

••• ORTHODOX

Septicemia must be treated with antibiotics. Consult your doctor immediately if you suspect blood poisoning.

SEX DRIVE PROBLEMS

Lack of interest in sex, which can result from a number of factors: painful intercourse, vaginal dryness, erection difficulties, and premature ejaculation are dealt with elsewhere in this book (see **Ejaculation Problems; Intercourse, Painful; Menopausal Problems; Vaginal Irritation**). Your sex life or your libido may also be affected by the medication you are taking, so it is worth mentioning it to your doctor. More often, however, sexual problems are related to fatigue and decreased opportunity for sex (common in couples with children), or psychological factors: stress, anxiety, negative past experiences, insecurity, and lack of communication and trust between partners can all contribute.

TREATMENT

If your desire for sex is frequently overwhelmed by your desire for sleep, or kept on hold by career or family worries, it is time to do something about it. The following therapies may help:

■ PRACTICAL ADVICE

Give yourself time to relax in the evening by doing the following:

Avoid eating a heavy meal late at night.

Avoid excessive alcohol.

Start to wind down several hours before bedtime. Stop working and do an enjoyable activity: reading, yoga, or meditation.

Avoid heavy discussions or arguments.

Avoid talking about work.

Have a warm bath, using essential oils of clary sage, rose, or ylang ylang.

Give or receive a massage with your partner. You don't have to massage the whole body, but start with the neck and shoulders or the feet.

❀ AROMATHERAPY

Essential oil of ylang ylang and clary sage are reputed to encourage relaxation and sensuality: Place 4 drops of each in the bath or in a vaporizer in the bedroom; or use in 4 teaspoons of a carrier oil or lotion in massage.

✳ ACUPRESSURE

Pelvic and abdominal tension is thought to contribute to lack of sex drive. When the pelvic area is relaxed, pleasurable sensations and orgasm can be fully experienced. The following treatments help relax the pelvic area and stimulate sexual energy:

Press lightly for 3 seconds on either side of each vertebra, from the tailbone up to the waist.

Place the fingertips of one hand just above the center of your pubic bone, and the fingers of the other hand between your navel and your pubic bone. Breathe deeply and apply deep pressure.

Also try the points illustrated, especially the ear point. (Massage this with the fingernail to get the exact point.)

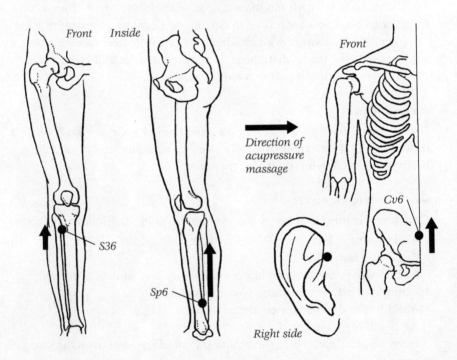

Front   Inside

Direction of
acupressure
massage

S36

Sp6

Cv6

Right side

❖ EXERCISE

Moderate exercise generally increases energy and relieves stress and fatigue. It also increases physical awareness and stimulates sexuality.

Adopt a regular exercise program: running, walking, swimming, racquet or ball games, and aerobics are all good. Pick something you enjoy and do it at least twice a week for 30 minutes.

✚ **PROFESSIONAL HELP**

If lack of sexual desire results from inability to enjoy sex, lack of communication between partners, or anxiety about performance, you may consider seeking help from a sex therapist or skilled counselor.

••• **ORTHODOX**

The sensate focus technique is a common method taught to couples experiencing sexual difficulties. The aim is to make each partner more aware of his or her pleasurable sensations, and those of the partner. First the couple give each other as much pleasure as possible without touching breasts or genitals. Then the breasts and genitals can be touched, stopping short of intercourse or orgasm. Finally, intercourse occurs, but with an emphasis on enjoyment, not orgasm. By slowing down the procedure and increasing stimulation and enjoyment, this technique can be very successful.

SEXUALLY TRANSMITTED DISEASES (STDs)

Infections or infestations that are typically, though not always exclusively, transmitted by sexual intercourse. For details of specific infections, see **AIDS; Chlamydia; Herpes, Genital; Thrush; Trichomoniasis.**

PREVENTION

Limit your number of sexual partners: STDs are more commonly diagnosed in people who have multiple partners.

Practice "safe sex" (for details, see **AIDS**).

Use a condom.

If you discover symptoms such as a discharge from the vagina, urethra, or penis, contact your doctor or a hospital STD clinic immediately for a checkup, and abstain from sexual intercourse.

If you develop an STD, it is advisable that your sexual partners be traced and treated to prevent spreading the infection further.

PREVENTION AND TREATMENT: GENITAL WARTS

Warts that appear anywhere around or inside the vagina, cervix, or anus. In men they may appear on the penis or under the foreskin. Genital warts are sexually transmitted and require immediate treatment, as there is some evidence of their link with cervical cancer in women.

For women who have had warts, or whose partner has them, frequent Pap smear tests are recommended.

The warts can be removed surgically, or by painting them with podophyllin; however, they do tend to recur.

PREVENTION AND TREATMENT: GONORRHEA

More commonly known as "the clap," this bacterial infection can be transmitted during vaginal, oral, or anal sex. It can also be passed from a mother to a child at birth. Symptoms in men and women include a green, creamy discharge from the urethra, pain on urinating, and sometimes abdominal pain and a fever. Men may experience swelling and pain in the testicles. If left untreated, gonorrhea can lead to infertility and ultimately death.

Antibiotic treatment is essential, followed by medical checkups to make sure that the infection has not recurred.

Sexual partners should be traced and treated.

PREVENTION AND TREATMENT: NONSPECIFIC URETHRITIS (NSU)

This is an extremely common sexually transmitted disease. The infection brings inflammation of the urethra, with a urethral discharge, and often pain during urination. It is more common in men, but may cause infertility in women. If you or your partner suspects NSU, consult a doctor immediately.

Prevention

- Barrier methods of contraception help prevent transmission of NSU. Use a condom along with a spermicide; a diaphragm also provides some protection.
- Both partners should wash the genital area before intercourse.
- Both partners should urinate and wash the genital area after intercourse.

Treatment

- Doctors generally test to find the organism responsible for the infection, and prescribe the appropriate antibiotic.
- Sexual partners should be traced and treated. Abstain from sexual intercourse until the infection has cleared up. See also **Urinary Tract Infection.**

PREVENTION AND TREATMENT: PUBIC LICE

Itching in the pubic area, particularly when warm in bed, may be caused by pubic lice (commonly called "crabs") infestation. Lice are transmitted through close contact, though it does not have to be sexual (sharing clothes, towels, and bedding can pass on the parasites). Your doctor can prescribe an insecticide lotion to apply to the pubic area. All family members and sexual contacts should be treated.

SCABIES

Itching in the pubic area may be caused by scabies. This may be transmitted by close contact, not necessarily sexual. See **Scabies** for details of treatment. Sexual contacts and other members of the family should also be treated.

SYPHILIS

Syphilis brings an extremely infectious ulcer on the shaft of the penis in men, or near the vagina in women. Syphilis may also cause swollen glands, and infection in other parts of the body. Antibiotics are effective, but must be taken in the early stages to prevent the infection spreading to other parts of the body. It is very important to treat syphilis as soon as possible; left untreated it can eventually cause insanity and death. Sexual partners should be traced and treated.

SHINGLES

Extreme sensitivity over an area of skin, usually the ribs, neck, or upper half of the face, followed by a rash that blisters and then turns to crusty scabs. Medically known as *Herpes zoster,* shingles is caused by the chicken pox virus, which lies dormant in a nerve root and reemerges when the immune system is weak. Shingles can cause long-term nerve damage, so it is advisable to consult your doctor, particularly if the head or eyes are affected. The following complementary treatments will also help.

TREATMENT

✗ DIETARY

The following measures will help raise immunity and fight the virus:

Increase your intake of vitamin C, found in fruits and vegetables, particularly citrus fruits, Brussels sprouts, parsley, and strawberries. Take 1 1,000-milligram supplement, 4 times a day.

Take 1 25-milligram vitamin B-complex supplement a day to help build healthy nerve cells.

Eat a well-balanced diet of lean meat, fish, or vegetable protein, low-fat dairy products, and fruits and vegetables.

Studies have shown that supplementation with vitamin E can relieve the long-term symptoms associated with shingles. The recommended dosage is 1,400 to 1,600 iu of vitamin E a day, spread over 3 doses.

Vitamin E oil applied directly to the sores can also help.

�֍ AROMATHERAPY

Dab the sores with a solution of 2 drops each of essential oil of lemon and geranium in 1 cup of water.

☐ HOMEOPATHY

Take every hour for up to 4 doses; repeat if necessary:

- When symptoms improve with warm bathing and with movement: *Rhus toxicodendron* 6c
- Sharp pain worse at night, patient chilly, skin better for warmth: *Arsenicum album* 6c
- Skin burns and itches and is aggravated by warm bathing, thick crusts and suppuration: *Mezereum* 6c
- Bluish tinge to the blisters; pain between the ribs: *Ranunculus bulbosus* 6c

Prevention: If you have been in contact with someone suffering chicken pox or shingles: *1Variolinum* 30c, once every 12 hours, for 3 doses.

☯ CHINESE MEDICINE

Practitioners of traditional Chinese medicine often recommend oriental wormwood and Chinese gentian. Acupuncture helps long-term pain.

••• ORTHODOX

Doctors may prescribe antiviral drugs, in liquid form to apply to the skin or in tablet form to swallow, to reduce both the severity and the duration of the attack. Antibiotics are only used if secondary bacterial infection is present.

SINUSITIS

Inflammation of the mucous membranes of the sinuses (the air-filled cavities in the bones surrounding the nose), caused by injury to the nose; bacterial or viral infections, such as a cold (see **Colds**); allergies (see **Allergies, Food,** and **Allergies, Hay Fever,** and **Rhinitis**); or swimming. Symptoms include a stuffed nose, pain in the nose and face area (including toothache and in the upper jaw), sometimes a fever, and the production of thick nasal discharge.

TREATMENT

✗ DIETARY

Recurrent attacks of sinusitis may indicate a food allergy. See **Allergies, Food,** to identify and treat potential allergies.

Naturopaths recommend a diet free of dairy products, with limited carbohydrates and plenty of raw green vegetables and fruits.

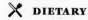 HERBALISM

Golden seal infusion is an effective remedy: Pour 1 cup of boiling water on 1 teaspoon of the powdered herb, and infuse for 15 minutes; add 250 milligrams of bromelain (the proteolytic enzyme from pineapple, available in natural foods stores). Take every 2 hours during an acute attack.

Garlic is also useful: Include as much raw garlic as possible in your cooking. If you do not like the taste or smell of garlic, take 3 garlic capsules, 3 times a day.

☐ HOMEOPATHY

For recent symptoms, take once an hour for up to 4 doses; for long-term symptoms, take 3 times a day for up to 4 days:

Stinging pain in the cheekbone area or pressure on the bridge of the nose, with thick stringy mucus: *Kali bichromicum* 30c

Tearing facial pain, worse in the cold, teeth feel too long: *Mercurius solubilis* 6c

Chronic sinusitis with no discharge, persistent stuffiness, feels as if floating when walking: *Sticta pulmonaria* 6c

≈ HYDROTHERAPY

Inhaling steam helps drain the sinuses:

Take long, hot showers.

Prepare a basin of boiling hot water. Lean over it, with a towel over the head, and inhale deeply for 10 minutes. **Caution:** If you suffer from asthma, avoid steam inhalations.

Use a humidifier in your bedroom.

☯ CHINESE MEDICINE

The condition is seen as a deficiency of *qi* in the lungs. Peppermint, honeysuckle, fritillary bulb, tangerine peel, and zanthium fruit are all helpful.

✳ ACUPRESSURE

Place the thumb and index finger of your left hand on the indentation of the inner eyes, where the bridge of the nose meets the eyebrows; place your right hand behind the neck, grasping the muscles on either side of the spine with your fingers and the heel of your hand. Put pressure on all 4 points simultaneously for 1 minute, while breathing deeply.

••• ORTHODOX

Doctors generally recommend antibiotics to fight the infection.

Decongestant drops or sprays may be given for long-term problems.

Surgery is sometimes carried out in extreme cases, to sterilize and dry out the sinus cavities.

SKIN, CHAPPED

Rough, sore, or cracked skin on areas that have been left wet and exposed to the wind or cold. Chapping usually occurs on the hands, face, or lips, when the natural oils that keep the skin soft are depleted.

TREATMENT

▬ PRACTICAL ADVICE

To prevent chapped hands, wear gloves when doing household chores, and avoid immersing hands in water as much as possible.

Always dry hands thoroughly and apply a rich, lanolin-based hand cream.

If the skin on the face is chapped, always apply moisturizer before going outside.

In winter, use a humidifier or place bowls of water around the house to counteract the dry air caused by central heating, which draws moisture out of your skin.

For chapped lips, always apply a lip balm before going outside during the winter; apply sunscreen in summer.

✗ DIETARY

Continuously chapped skin may indicate a dietary deficiency. Make sure to incorporate plenty of fatty acids in your diet by eating sufficient vegetable oil (olive, sunflower, or safflower).

Increase your intake of vitamin D, obtained by exposure to sunlight, and vitamin A, found in cod liver oil, egg yolk, mackerel, liver, and carrots.

Rub vitamin E oil or cream into the skin.

❋ AROMATHERAPY

Once a week, steam the face over a basin of hot water to which 2 drops of geranium have been added. Then add 2 drops of either chamomile, patchouli, or lavender (or 1 drop each of the last two) to 2 teaspoons of a carrier oil or lotion, and massage into the skin.

☐ HOMEOPATHY

Take 3 times a day for up to 4 days; repeat if necessary:

Deep cracks with a watery discharge: *Petroleum* 6c

Cracks and chapping with the formation of a yellow crust: *Graphites* 6c

Cracks in the middle of the lips from exposure to sea air: *Natrum muriaticum* 6c

••• ORTHODOX

Doctors generally recommend the practical advice given above.

SKIN, DRY

Dry skin usually occurs when the sebaceous (oil) glands are inactive as a result of a hormonal imbalance or a nutritional deficiency. It can also be caused by exposure to harsh sun, wind, or cold, indoor heat, or air-conditioning. Crash dieting sometimes results in changes to skin condition.

TREATMENT

▬ PRACTICAL ADVICE

Use a moisturizer day and night to protect against water loss.

Avoid using detergents on the skin. Use a lotion, not soap.

Add 2 cups of oatmeal to a lukewarm bath, and soak in it to soften the skin. Pat yourself almost dry, and apply moisturizer to seal in the dampness.

Distribute bowls of water around your home and workplace during the winter, or use a humidifier.

Keep the temperature in your home as low as possible.

✗ DIETARY

Increase your intake of essential fatty acids, found in olive, sunflower, or safflower oils.

Increase your intake of vitamins A and D, found in fish liver oils; egg yolk; salmon, herring, and mackerel; and carrots.

Increase your intake of vitamin E, found in sunflower seeds, soybean oil, and olive oil. Rubbing vitamin E oil on the skin will also help.

�֍ AROMATHERAPY

Essential oil of geranium added to the bath, or used in a steam bath, helps balance the skin and regulate sebum secretion.

••• ORTHODOX

In severe cases, doctors may recommend a low-dose cortisone cream for itchy, very dry, or eczematous skin (see **Eczema**).

SKIN, OILY

Overactivity of the oil-producing glands in the face often occurs as a result of hormonal imbalances. It commonly develops during pregnancy or when taking oral contraceptives. Stress, poor diet, and using the wrong cosmetics can also contribute.

TREATMENT

▬ PRACTICAL ADVICE

Oily skin requires gentle treatment, so avoid using soap. Instead, wash with a mild lotion cleanser that does not contain drying agents. Rub it onto the skin with your fingers, wipe it off with tissues, then rinse the face with cold water.

Use a light moisturizer and water-based cosmetics.

Once a week, make up a face mask with 1 teaspoon of brewer's yeast and enough water or plain, natural yogurt to make a paste. Apply the mask after cleansing the face, allow it to dry completely, then rinse with warm water.

✗ DIETARY

Avoid fatty food; eat plenty of fruits and raw and cooked vegetables.

Vitamin B-complex is important for healthy skin. It is found in whole-grain cereals and liver. Brewer's yeast is also an excellent source: Take 1 tablespoon mixed in a drink 3 times a day.

Zinc helps regulate the oil-producing glands of the skin: it is found in lean meat, poultry, fish, organ meats, and whole-grain cereals.

✖ AROMATHERAPY

After cleansing, morning and night, dab the face with a solution made of the following: 4 drops of essential oil of lavender with 4 drops of essential oil of bergamot or lemon, well mixed with ⅓ cup of spring water.

ଝ HERBALISM

Calendula is one of the best remedies for skin problems: Pour 1 cup of boiling water on 2 teaspoons of the petals, and infuse for 15 minutes; drink 3 times a day.

••• ORTHODOX

Most doctors recommend benzoyl peroxide creams or lotions. Antibiotic lotions are prescribed when the glands become infected. Hormonally acting agents can be effective in severe cases.

SLIPPED DISC

A rupture of the disc (discs do not actually slip), which allows part of its soft core to bulge out and put pressure on surrounding nerves and tissue; this term is often used incorrectly to refer to general backache. Rupture may be due to wear and tear of the discs, or a sudden strain or fall. The result is excruciating pain in the back, which sometimes radiates down the legs. A more correct term for slipped disc is prolapsed or herniated disc.

TREATMENT

A prolapsed disc brings severe and incapacitating pain. Only 15 percent of severe backaches are due to a prolapsed disc. For general advice on back pain, see **Backache.** If you suspect you have a prolapse, seek professional help. An X-ray will confirm the diagnosis.

▬ PRACTICAL ADVICE

If you suspect you have a prolapsed disc, lie down to take pressure off the disc. Sometimes lying on your side with the knees bent is more comfortable than flat on your back. Placing a pillow between your knees can also help. If you experience weakness, tingling in the limbs, or loss of bladder or bowel control, get immediate emergency help.

◻ HOMEOPATHY

Take *Arnica* 6c every 30 minutes for up to 6 doses, then every 4 hours for up to 5 days.

✿ BACH FLOWER REMEDIES

Rescue Remedy will help with the shock of severe pain.

≈ HYDROTHERAPY

Ask a friend or family member to help you use hot and cold treatment for pain relief: Prepare an ice pack by wrapping a bag of frozen peas in a kitchen towel, and place on the area of the most pain for 10 minutes; then place a hot water bottle wrapped in a towel on the area. Continue alternating hot and cold for 40 minutes.

✳ ACUPRESSURE

Massage the points illustrated, using deep thumb pressure, for at least 1 minute.

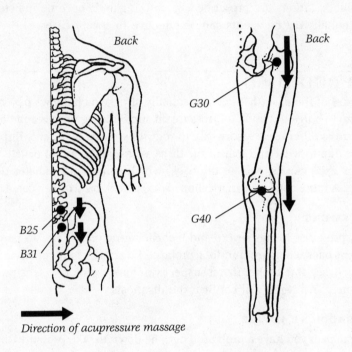

Direction of acupressure massage

✚ PROFESSIONAL HELP

Chiropractic can be successful in treating moderate prolapses through manipulation.

Acupuncture may be helpful in relieving acute pain.

••• ORTHODOX

Doctors generally recommend painkillers, anti-inflammatory drugs, and muscle relaxants, along with physiotherapy, including traction, to pull the vertebrae apart and allow the prolapsed part of the disc to move back into place.

Surgery is used in severe cases, to open up the vertebrae and relieve pressure on the nerve.

SNAKE BITE

Symptoms of snake bite include an immediate burning pain at the site of the bite, which may be followed by dizziness, nausea, and pallor. The bite can also affect the blood pressure, the heart rate, and the nervous system, bringing symptoms of thirst, headache, slurred speech, and double vision. Always try and remember the color and markings of a snake that bites you, in case specific antivenom is needed.

PREVENTION

Wear boots, and protective clothing covering the legs and ankles, when you walk in overgrown areas.

Keep to cleared pathways.

Use a stick to clear stones, logs, or brush from your path.

Never sleep unprotected on the ground in snake-infested areas; always use a tent.

Put food in bags tied up in trees, and burn rubbish—it attracts rodents, which in turn attract snakes.

If you see a snake, do not disturb it, but move quietly away.

TREATMENT

① FIRST AID

Keep the victim still; do not raise the injured area.

Place a sterile dressing on the bite.

Bandage the area firmly.

Start CPR if the victim has stopped breathing.

Get medical help.

☐ HOMEOPATHY

Take *Golondrina* 30c, every 30 minutes for up to 4 doses, until professional help can be obtained.

••• ORTHODOX

Antibiotics and tetanus antitoxin injections are given for all snake bites. For a severely poisonous bite, a serum injection containing antibodies against the venom will be given. Such treatment generally provides complete recovery if administered in time.

SORE THROAT

A rough or raw sensation at the back of the throat, which often is the first sign of a cold (see **Cold**s), influenza (see **Flu**), tonsillitis, laryngitis, or pharyngitis (see **Laryngitis; Pharyngitis; Tonsillitis**). Sore throats are generally caused by viruses, but they can sometimes result from the *Streptococcus* bacteria, which produce a sore throat along with high fever and a more generalized feeling of illness, known as strep throat. Strep throat can sometimes lead to more serious problems, such as rheumatic fever and rheumatic heart disease, so it is advisable to consult your doctor for treatment.

TREATMENT

✗ DIETARY

Drink plenty of fluids, particularly fruit juices.

Avoid milky drinks.

Increase your intake of vitamin C, found in citrus fruits and vegetables.

Increase your intake of zinc, found in lean meat and fish: Freshly made chicken and vegetable soup is an excellent food for anyone with a sore throat.

❀ AROMATHERAPY

Make up a gargle: Stir 2 drops each of essential oil of lemon and sandalwood into a glass of water; gargle with the mixture 3 times a day.

Add 2 drops each of eucalyptus and peppermint to 2 teaspoons of a carrier oil or lotion, and apply to the chest and throat area.

❧ HERBALISM

Garlic is effective in attacking viral and bacterial infections. Incorporate as much raw garlic into your diet as possible; if you do not like the taste or smell of raw garlic, take 3 garlic capsules, 3 times a day.

Red sage, used as a gargle, helps soothe an inflamed and sore throat: Pour 1 cup of boiling water on 2 teaspoons of the leaves, and infuse for 10 minutes; use hot as a gargle for 10 minutes, 2 times a day.

Golden seal is particularly good for strep throat: Add 1 cup of boiling water to 1 teaspoon of the powdered herb, and infuse for 10 minutes; drink 3 times a day. **Caution:** Do not take during pregnancy.

☐ HOMEOPATHY

Take every 30 minutes for up to 4 doses; repeat as necessary:

Strawberry red appearance with flushed face and fever: *Belladonna* 6c

Pain in neck and ears, swallowing painful, feeling exhausted and weak: *Gelsemium* 6c

Sudden sore throat made worse by cold wind, tonsils swollen, throat burning, everything tastes bitter: *Aconite* 6c

Worse right side with purplish appearance and a swollen uvula, better from cold drinks: *Apis* 6c

Worse left side, intolerant of any constriction, pain worse from swallowing saliva and better from swallowing food: *Lachesis* 6c

••• ORTHODOX

Doctors generally advise gargling with saltwater. Painkillers may also be recommended, and antibiotics may be prescribed for severe cases of strep throat.

SPRAINS

Overstretching the ligaments that attach the bones of a joint to each other. Sprains bring painful swelling and muscle spasm around the joint, along with pain on movement. Ligaments, which are rope-like and fibrous, have a poor blood supply and generally take a long time to heal.

TREATMENT

❋ AROMATHERAPY

Sweet marjoram and rosemary help dull the pain: Add 4 drops of both essential oils to a bowl containing enough cold water to cover the joint. Soak the joint for at least 10 minutes.

At night, make up a cold compress with the above mixture: Soak a clean cotton cloth in the solution, wring out, and wrap around the sprain. Wrap with a piece of dry cotton and plastic wrap. Leave on for at least 1 hour before bedtime.

☐ HOMEOPATHY

Take *Arnica* 6c, every 30 minutes for up to 4 doses.

Apply cold compresses with *Arnica* solution 2 times a day to help reduce swelling.

Take *Ruta graveolens* 6c, 3 times a day for 1 week.

≈ HYDROTHERAPY

Apply an ice pack to the area as soon as possible: Make an ice pack by wrapping a plastic bag full of ice cubes or a bag of frozen peas in a kitchen towel. Place it on the joint or muscles for 10 minutes, take it off for 10 minutes, then reapply for 10 minutes. If no ice is available, apply a cold compress (a clean cloth soaked in cold water and wrung out) for 30 minutes. If you have a sprained ankle or wrist, use a light bandage to support the joint. Rest with the joint elevated.

☞ MASSAGE

Massage can help once the swelling has subsided. Do not work directly on the joint, but on the muscles around it. For example, if it is a knee strain, work on the muscles from the knee up the thigh, and the muscles from the ankle to the knee. Use long, upward sweeping strokes. As the injury heals, you can begin to work with careful kneading and friction strokes around the joint.

✚ PROFESSIONAL HELP

Chiropractic can be helpful.
Acupuncture can help relieve pain.

••• ORTHODOX

Doctors may recommend:
physiotherapy
heat treatment, infrared, and laser treatment to improve the blood supply
wrapping the joint with an elastic bandage to provide support
surgery for entirely ruptured ligaments

STIFFNESS

Rigid and painful muscles may be caused by physical overexertion, osteoarthritis, or rheumatoid arthritis (see **Osteoarthritis; Rheumatoid Arthritis**). The following treatments are for stiffness following overuse of muscles.

PREVENTION

▬ PRACTICAL ADVICE

Make sure you warm up properly and stretch before you begin any sport or exercise. After exercising, don't just stop. Take at least 5 minutes of slow exercise (such as walking if you have been running, slow pedaling if you have been bicycling) to cool down thoroughly and stretch the muscles. This prevents the buildup of lactic acid, which is the main cause of stiffness. Consult a sport or exercise trainer if you are unsure of how to do this correctly.

TREATMENT

☐ HOMEOPATHY

Arnica 6c, taken hourly for 4 doses, may help prevent stiffness after unaccustomed exertion.

≈ HYDROTHERAPY

Soaking in a hot bath, or taking a hot shower or a sauna immediately after exercising, helps relax the muscles and prevent stiffness.

☛ MASSAGE

Massage is one of the best ways to relieve stiffness. It helps increase circulation to the muscles, which in turn flushes out the waste products produced during exercise that cause stiffness. Add a soothing essential oil, such as eucalyptus or lavender, to the massage oil or lotion.

✦ EXERCISE

Exercise gently while the stiffness lasts. Try walking or swimming.

✳ YOGA

The yoga postures collectively called the Salutation to the Sun are an excellent way to loosen up stiff muscles on awakening. (See figure on following page.) Repeat several times a day:

Stand erect, with feet next to each other and palms together (position 1).

Inhale, stretch your arms above your head, and bend back, arching your head, shoulders, and back (position 2).

Exhale, and bend forward, letting your arms and head hang down to your legs and feet (as far as is comfortable) (position 3).

Inhale, bend your knees, and put your palms flat on the ground beside your feet. Take your right leg back as far as you can, with the knee resting on the floor. Keep the arms straight, look up, and push your hips forward (position 4).

Leave the right leg where it is, and take the left back to meet it. Raise the abdomen, making an arch, and keep the feet flat on the floor. Exhale (position 5).

Lower the body slowly to the floor (position 6).

Inhale, and lift the chest and shoulders off the floor, looking up (position 7).

Exhale, and bring the chest and shoulders down; bring the right foot forward, leaving the left knee on the ground; look up (reverse of position 4).

Inhale, bring the left knee up, and stand (position 2).

Exhale, and return to position 1.

••• ORTHODOX

Your doctor will probably recommend heat treatment, exercise, and massage to relieve stiffness.

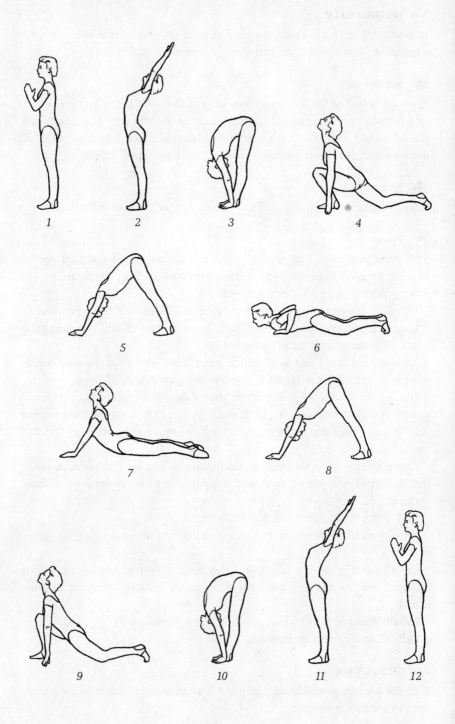

STINGS
See **Insect Bites and Stings; Jellyfish Stings.**

STOMACH ACHE
Stomach pain can result from a number of different causes that are dealt with elsewhere in this book. These are the most common:

indigestion caused by overeating, drinking too much alcohol, or eating the wrong food (see **Acid Stomach; Indigestion**)

in women, menstrual pain (see **Cramps, Menstrual**), ovulation pain (see **Ovulation Pain**), or gynecological disorders (see **Endometriosis**)

urinary infections and cystitis (see **Cystitis; Urinary Tract Infection**)

stress or anxiety (common in children; see **Stress**)

colic (in infants only; see **Colic**)

ulcers (see **Peptic Ulcer**)

tumors

appendicitis (see **Appendicitis**)

TREATMENT
If pain lasts for more than six hours, or is accompanied by feelings of dizziness, sweating, and pallor, or vomiting blood, consult your doctor immediately. For specific advice on the conditions listed above, refer to the appropriate entry. The following treatments are for nonspecific stomach pain.

▬ PRACTICAL ADVICE
Lie down and put a hot water bottle or heating pad on the stomach.

✗ DIETARY
Eat a whole-foods diet high in whole grains, fiber, and fruits and vegetables, and low in fat, caffeine, and alcohol.

⚘ HERBALISM
Chamomile or peppermint tea helps soothe indigestion and relax muscular spasm.

Slippery elm soothes the mucous membrane of the digestive tract: Use 1 part of the powdered bark to 8 parts water, and simmer for 10 minutes; drink ½ cup 3 times a day.

☐ HOMEOPATHY

Take 1 tablet every 15 minutes for up to 4 doses; repeat if needed:

After rich foods, with gas and rancid belching: *Carbo vegetabilis* 6c

After spicy food, stimulants, alcohol: *Nux vomica* 6c

Burning pain, worse in the small hours of the morning: *Arsenicum album* 6c

Burning pains and vomiting, better temporarily for cold drinks: *Phosphorus* 6c

Stomach feels like a stone and is very sensitive to touch: *Bryonia* 6c

Pain is better from eating, but starts again 2 hours later: *Anacardium* 6c

✳ ACUPRESSURE

Massage the points illustrated, using deep thumb pressure, for at least 1 minute.

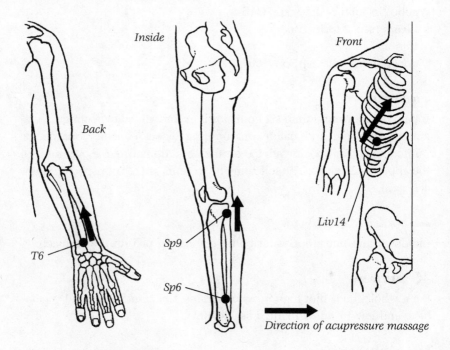

Direction of acupressure massage

～ RELAXATION TECHNIQUES

Practicing yoga, or learning to meditate, helps relieve stress-related stomach ache in adults. Relaxation tapes and biofeedback can also help.

Psychotherapy or counseling may help you learn how to cope with stress.

✿ **BACH FLOWER REMEDIES**

Children can take Aspen to help them relax.

••• **ORTHODOX**

Treatment depends on the cause of stomach ache. Antacids are commonly prescribed for digestive problems.

STRABISMUS

A condition where there is abnormal deviation of one eye in relation to the other; colloquially called lazy eye, squint, cross-eye, or wall-eye. The deviance may be convergent (cross-eye), where one eye is directed too far inward; or divergent (wall-eye), where the eye is directed outward. Sometimes an eye can be directed up or down (vertical strabismus). Strabismus can cause permanent visual problems in children and should be treated by an ophthalmologist.

TREATMENT

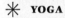 **YOGA**

Yoga may help to relax the eye muscles.

Sit comfortably at a table, place your elbows on the table, and rub the palms of your hands together. Cup your hands over your closed eyes, sealing out all light. Relax in this position for 20 seconds. Repeat as often as you like, but at least twice a day.

Sit comfortably at a table. Place a lighted candle at eye height, about 3 feet away, and gaze at the flame (without blinking, if possible) for 10 seconds. Then do the above palming exercise for 30 seconds. Next, gaze at the candle with one eye for 10 seconds, then with both eyes for 10 seconds, then with the other eye for 10 seconds; repeat the palming. Repeat this procedure 3 times.

✚ **PROFESSIONAL HELP**

The Bates Method can be helpful. Minor deviations often disappear within a short time of starting this training; more established or severe problems may take longer.

••• **ORTHODOX**

Depending on the severity of the problem, your ophthalmologist may recommend any of the following treatments:

Refraction: correction of a weak or lazy eye using glasses or contact lenses.

Occlusion: blocking off the good eye to force the lazy one to work harder.

Orthoptic training: a form of ocular physiotherapy to activate the lazy eye.

Surgery: to lengthen or shorten the muscles that control the movements of the eyes. Surgery must be performed at a young age if useful vision in the deviating eye is to be preserved.

STREP THROAT
See **Sore Throat.**

STRESS

Being under a constant state of tension as a result of daily pressures. The stress reaction is a fundamentally natural response to fear. It prepares the body for "fight or flight" by tensing the muscles and constricting the blood vessels. Today, however, most of the stressful experiences we encounter do not require us to fight or flee, and the body is left in a state of physical tension that can result in a lowering of immunity that renders us more susceptible to disease.

Common signs of stress include recurrent headaches; dizziness; rashes; colds and infections; panic attacks or anxiety; palpitations; sexual problems; indigestion; aches and pains in neck, shoulder, or back; loss of appetite; compulsive eating; irritability; fatigue; tearfulness; sleep problems; lack of concentration. To treat these symptoms, see **Acid Stomach; Allergic Dermatitis; Anorexia Nervosa; Backache; Bulimia; Colds; Colitis; Depression; Dizziness; Headache; Indigestion; Infection; Inflammatory Bowel Disease; Insomnia; Lower Back Pain; Neck Pain and Stiffness; Obesity; Palpitations; Panic Attack.**

TREATMENT

There are many ways to tackle stress, and most complementary therapies will help. It is a question of finding out which is best for you. The methods listed below are most commonly used.

✗ DIETARY

How well you handle stress can be related to how well you are nourished. People who eat a diet high in whole-grain breads and cereals, fruits, and vegetables, and low in refined carbohydrates, sugar, and caffeine, show greater ability to cope with stress.

�֎ AROMATHERAPY

Essential oil of lavender has been shown in studies to reduce stress. Add 5 or 6 drops to a bath; or put 2 or 3 drops on a handkerchief or tissue and inhale periodically.

☯ CHINESE MEDICINE

Acupuncture brings deep relaxation. Practitioners of traditional Chinese medicine may prescribe herbs such as thorowax root, peony root, and schizandra fruit.

☛ MASSAGE

Massage relieves many of the physical symptoms of stress: tense muscles, aching neck, shoulders, and back, and headaches. By relaxing the muscles and improving blood circulation, it also relaxes the mind.

⊹ EXERCISE

Exercise is what the body instinctively wants to do under stress, and it is extremely beneficial in relaxing the mind and body. Regular running, walking, cycling, swimming, or any other aerobic exercise, ideally carried out for at least 30 minutes, 3 times a week, is helpful. Even a walk around the block can help let off steam or reduce anxiety.

∼ RELAXATION TECHNIQUES

Yoga—attending a yoga class and practicing by yourself at home—will divert your mind from stress, relax muscle tension through stretching, and teach you to breathe more completely.

Meditation takes you into a deep state of relaxation. It helps to learn meditation with a teacher, but you can easily practice at home.

Biofeedback teaches you how to relax mentally and physically. Once you have learned how to do this, you can apply it to situations in everyday life.

◯ AFFIRMATIONS

Keep a list of affirmations to say to yourself when under stress: Chanting simple phrases, such as "I can handle this," "I know what I'm doing," "I'm the best," and so on, can divert the stress response.

••• ORTHODOX

Your doctor will probably try to identify the cause of stress and help you find ways to avoid it or deal with it. Counseling may be a good idea, but avoid tranquilizers and alcohol at all costs.

STRETCH MARKS

Silvery streaks commonly found on the stomach, thighs, and breasts of pregnant or overweight women, as a result of the loss of elasticity in the skin when it is extended over a long period of time; also known as striae. The marks first appear as red raised lines, which become purple, and then flatten into silvery streaks.

TREATMENT

✗ DIETARY

Increase your intake of vitamin E, found in vegetable oils, seeds, wheat germ, nuts, avocados, peaches, whole-grain cereals, spinach, broccoli, asparagus, and dried prunes. Massage vitamin E oil into the skin during the pregnancy.

Make sure you get adequate zinc, found in lean meat, poultry, and fish.

Increase your intake of vitamin B6 by taking 1 25-milligram vitamin B-complex supplement a day.

❀ AROMATHERAPY

Essential oils of lavender and myrrh can be used both to prevent and treat stretch marks: Aromatherapist Shirley Price recommends an anti–stretch mark concoction of 3 drops of both frankincense and myrrh, 6 drops of lavender, 4 drops of geranium, and 2 fluid ounces of *Calendula* carrier oil. Apply this mixture to the breasts, stomach, buttocks, and thighs regularly, every morning and night, starting in the fourth month of pregnancy.

✳ BIOCHEMIC TISSUE SALTS

Calc Fluor: Take 3 tablets, 3 times a day, 5 days a week, for up to 3 months.

••• ORTHODOX

Doctors recommend avoiding being overweight during pregnancy. Cosmetic surgery can cut out the widest stretch marks, though some scar will be visible and no absolute guarantee of reducing stretch marks is given.

STROKE

The interruption of blood supply and oxygen to the brain due to a blood clot or hemorrhage, which causes permanent damage to the cells of the affected area. Symptoms include differing degrees of paralysis, speech impairment, and loss of function, depending on the area of the brain affected.

PREVENTION

A poor diet, excessive alcohol or drug use, obesity, and lack of exercise can all contribute to a weakening of the arteries of the brain, leading to blood clots and strokes:

Reduce your intake of saturated fats (found in red meat and dairy products).

Eat plenty of whole-grain cereals, fresh fruits and vegetables, dried cooked beans, and lean protein (fish and poultry).

Stop smoking.

Limit your alcohol intake.

Do aerobic exercise (such as walking, cycling, or swimming) 3 times a week, for at least 30 minutes, if possible.

TREATMENT

✗ **DIETARY**

Reduce your intake of fatty meats and high-fat dairy foods.

Increase your intake of fresh fruits and vegetables, fish, poultry, and whole-grain cereals and breads.

The following daily supplements are recommended as a preventive measure and a treatment:

- vitamin E: 400 iu
- vitamin C: 500 milligrams
- evening primrose oil: 6 500-milligram capsules
- lecithin: 5 to 10 grams
- fish oils: 3 grams

HERBALISM

As part of a general health program, yarrow infusion is recommended to improve circulation and tone the blood vessels: Pour 1 cup of boiling water on 2 teaspoons of the dried herb, and infuse for 15 minutes; drink hot 3 times a day.

▢ **HOMEOPATHY**

Take *Arnica* 200c, as soon as possible after the stroke.

Arnica 6c, and the biochemic tissue salt *Kali mur* 6x, taken 2 times a day for 1 month, will help to dissolve blood clots.

≋ HYDROTHERAPY

Swimming in a heated pool under the supervision of a physiotherapist can help restore physical strength and movement.

❖ EXERCISE

Gentle exercise is recommended as soon as possible after a stroke, to prevent the muscles contracting and becoming stiff. This is best carried out with the help of a physiotherapist.

✚ PROFESSIONAL HELP

Practitioners of traditional Chinese medicine often prescribe lovage tuber to dissolve or prevent blood clots. Acupuncture can be very helpful after a stroke in treating paralysis. The earlier it is given, the better.

Chiropractic and massage can help maintain muscle function and prevent stiffness.

••• ORTHODOX

Doctors generally direct treatment toward improving quality of life, with occupational therapy, physiotherapy, home adjustments, and walking aids.

Psychotherapy or counseling is invaluable.

Drugs to prevent blood clotting and to regulate the heart are often prescribed.

STY

A small abscess near the eyelash caused by infection of the hair follicle.

TREATMENT

✘ DIETARY

Recurrent sties indicate that immunity is low. The following recommendations will help improve your resistance to infection:

Increase your intake of zinc, found in lean meat, poultry, and fish. Take 1 30-milligram supplement, 2 times a day.

Increase your intake of vitamin C, found in fresh fruits and vegetables.

Eat a well-balanced diet of lean proteins, whole-grain cereals, and plenty of raw and lightly cooked vegetables and fruits.

☐ HOMEOPATHY

Take every 4 hours for up to 4 doses; repeat if needed:

Itching and weeping in the eye, with a sensation as if the eyeball were covered by a film: *Pulsatilla* 6c

Smarting and cutting pains, eyes feel dry: *Staphysagria* 6c

≈ HYDROTHERAPY

Make up a warm solution of water with a few drops of *Calendula* tincture. Soak a compress in the solution and hold over the eye for a few minutes, to help discharge any pus. Do not squeeze the sty, as this may further infect the area.

★ FOLK REMEDIES

Cold tea makes a soothing eye wash. Soak cotton wool in cold tea and hold over the eye. Alternatively, place a cold, used tea bag over the eye.

••• ORTHODOX

Plucking the offending eyelash sometimes does the trick, but in long-standing chronic or recurrent sties, treatment with an antibiotic ointment is recommended.

SUNBURN

Redness, heat, and sometimes blistering can easily occur with prolonged exposure to the sun. The long-term effects of sunburn are premature aging of the skin and skin cancer. Fair skin and young skin are most susceptible; however, even dark skin loses its elasticity with repeated and prolonged exposure to the sun.

PREVENTION

Limit your exposure to the sun: Avoid going out in the sun during the hottest time of the day (10 A.M. to 4 P.M.).

Always wear a sunscreen.

If you are exposed to the sun, wear protective clothing and a hat that shades the face.

If you want to acquire a tan, do so gradually: Use a high protection-factor sunscreen, and limit yourself to 15 minutes of sunbathing per day until a tan is built up.

TREATMENT

▬ PRACTICAL ADVICE

Stay out of the sun for at least a week after sunburn, as your skin will be very sensitive.

❧ HERBALISM

Use aloe vera gel on the burned areas to soothe and heal. You can buy this in natural foods stores, or you can cut open a fresh leaf and smear the gel onto the skin.

≈ HYDROTHERAPY

A cool shower or bath is probably one of the best ways to relieve sunburn. You can add baking soda, fine oatmeal, or vinegar to the water to soothe stinging skin.

To soothe sore eyes, place a piece of cucumber on each eye and lie back and relax for 15 minutes.

Drink plenty of water or soft drinks, as you will probably be a little dehydrated. Avoid alcohol.

••• ORTHODOX

Calamine lotion or after-sun cream soothes the stinging.

Painkillers may also be recommended, along with antihistamine preparations in severe cases.

Blistering requires the application of sterile dressing and medical supervision to prevent and treat infection (see **Burns**).

SUNSTROKE
See **Heatstroke.**

SYPHILIS
See **Sexually Transmitted Diseases.**

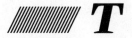 *T*

TACHYCARDIA

An increase in the rate of heartbeat. Most people's hearts beat at around sixty-five to seventy-five beats per minute at rest. Those with tachycardia have one hundred or more beats per minute when resting. Rapid heartbeat is sometimes accompanied by breathlessness, nausea and sweating, or dizziness. See also **Fibrillation; Palpitations.**

PREVENTION

Stress reduction and relaxation help prevent this ailment. Practicing yoga, meditation, or biofeedback is the best way to reduce stress. (See **Stress** for more details.)

Some foods may trigger tachycardia; see the dietary recommendations below.

TREATMENT

✗ DIETARY

Avoid coffee, tea, chocolate, cola, alcohol, tobacco, and other stimulants that activate the heart excessively.

Low blood sugar can trigger tachycardia: To stabilize blood sugar, eat regular meals of complex carbohydrates (pasta, potatoes, rice, bread), fruits and vegetables, and moderate amounts of protein; avoid simple carbohydrates (foods containing sugar).

Increase your intake of magnesium, found in nuts, cooked dried beans and peas, whole-grain breads and cereals, soybeans, dark green leafy vegetables, milk, and seafood.

❀ AROMATHERAPY

Essential oil of lavender has been shown to reduce stress and lower blood pressure: Use in a massage or in the bath, or place a few drops on a handkerchief and sniff when needed.

☐ HOMEOPATHY

Take every 5 minutes for up to 6 doses; repeat if necessary:

Heart rate speeds up after a shock or a fright: *Aconite* 6c

Heart rate speeds up after rich food, alcohol, coffee, or stress: *Nux vomica* 6c

Heart rate speeds up after sudden excitement or a pleasant surprise: *Coffea* 6c

Worse lying on the left side and improved by lying on the right side: *Phosphorus* 6c

≋ HYDROTHERAPY

Plunging your face into a basin of cool water for 10 to 20 seconds sometimes helps stop an attack. Alternatively, try slowly drinking water or holding your breath.

☛ MASSAGE

Regular massage helps reduce stress and slow the heartbeat.

∿ RELAXATION TECHNIQUES

The best way to stop an attack of tachycardia is to slow down and rest for a while. Do this exercise if you feel an attack coming on: Find a quiet place where you won't be disturbed. Lie on a firm surface, close your eyes, allow your breathing to slow, and begin to be aware of how your body feels. Consciously try to relax every part of your body in turn. Begin with your face (your eyes, your forehead, your jaw), and work down to your toes. The whole procedure should take at least 10 minutes.

••• ORTHODOX

Electrocardiograph (ECG) tracings are used to determine exactly the type of tachycardia responsible for the symptoms. For simple tachycardia, stimulation of the vagus nerve, which slows the heartbeat, can be achieved by pressing on the eyeball or massaging the carotid sinus at the back of the neck. If this fails, drug therapy or mild electric shock treatment under sedation is effective.

TANTRUM

A somewhat violent episode in which a child may scream, yell, cry, kick, bite, bang feet and fists, hold his or her breath, or turn red or blue. Temper tantrums are common in small children between the ages of one and five. They occur particularly around the age of two, when children feel frustrated at being unable to communicate their feelings and desires adequately through speech. Tantrums may also start when a sibling is born and the older child feels neglected.

TREATMENT

▬ PRACTICAL ADVICE

Try to understand the cause of the tantrum and explain it quietly and calmly to the child. Do not lose your temper. Allow the child to have the tantrum and don't pay too much attention, as long as he or she does not come to harm. Do not punish the child, but try to divert the child's attention away from the problem to a game or object. Most children grow out of tantrums as they learn to communicate more competently.

✗ DIETARY

Naturopaths and practitioners of traditional Chinese medicine believe that dietary habits can affect children's behavior and mood. They make the following recommendations:

Do not allow the child to overeat.

Give small, regular meals.

Avoid rough whole-grain foods.

Reduce the child's intake of cow's milk.

Avoid toxins, such as artificial additives and preservatives, often found in processed and fast foods.

Sometimes food allergies can cause behavioral problems: see **Allergies, Food,** for common allergies and how to deal with them.

Reduce the child's intake of sugar.

✿ BACH FLOWER REMEDIES

Holly, Vine, and Walnut are all suitable remedies for this condition.

✚ PROFESSIONAL HELP

Professional homeopathic treatment may be helpful.

••• ORTHODOX

When the child is particularly manipulative and behaves in a way that makes parental control difficult, family psychotherapy with a child psychologist may help parents with exercises designed to correct the problems.

TEETHING PROBLEMS

Most babies have problems when the teeth start to come through, starting at around six months and sometimes continuing until three years. The child will probably be irritable and clingy, have difficulty sleeping, and cry more. A tendency to drool more is also common.

TREATMENT
✗ DIETARY

Digestive problems sometimes enhance teething problems:

Do not overfeed the baby.

When weaning, give easily digested foods, such as baby rice or millet; raw vegetables and whole-grain cereals are too hard to digest.

When allowed to eat on demand, some children eat too much, which may contribute to teething discomfort; establish regular feeding times once the child is on solid foods, and feed the child slowly.

For toddlers, avoid rich foods, especially red meats and fats, and whole-grain bread and raw vegetables.

Do not give the child too much to drink—give just enough to moisten the food being eaten.

Burp your baby after feeding.

ॐ HERBALISM

Marshmallow root syrup helps soothe inflamed or sore gums: Add 3 level teaspoons to the child's food or drink every day.

☐ HOMEOPATHY

Chamomilla Teething Granules (3x) dissolve easily, and will help where there is one red cheek and the child is colicky and irritable. Give every 30 minutes until quiet.

✷ BIOCHEMIC TISSUE SALTS

Calc Phos: Take 1 tablet every 30 minutes for up to 6 doses.

✷ ACUPRESSURE

Spread the child's left thumb and index finger apart and gently massage between them. Do the same on the other hand.

••• ORTHODOX

Teething gels rubbed onto the gums can be helpful: they contain antiseptic and painkilling ingredients.

Teething rings (especially when they have been chilled in the refrigerator first) for the baby to chew on can also resolve the problem.

Doctors may prescribe paracetamol (120 to 240 milligrams every 6 hours, for children aged one to six), or antihistamines for severe cases.

TEMPOROMANDIBULAR JOINT SYNDROME (TMJ)

Pain that affects the head, jaw, and face when the temporomandibular joint (connecting the jaw bone to the skull just below and beside the ear) and its surrounding muscles and ligaments do not function correctly.

It is often caused by clenching or grinding the teeth. Symptoms include frequent headaches, pain around the ear, and clicking noises when the mouth is opened or closed.

TREATMENT

 CHINESE MEDICINE

Practitioners of traditional Chinese medicine treat teeth grinding with herbal teas of Chinese yam or skullcap.

≈ **HYDROTHERAPY**

The first course of treatment is to relax tight muscles in the jaw area by increasing the blood flow. This can be done with cold or hot treatment. Prepare an ice pack, using a bag of ice cubes or a bag of frozen peas wrapped in a kitchen towel, and place it on the painful side of the jaw. Alternatively, use a heating pad or a hot water bottle wrapped in a towel. Keep the ice pack or the hot water bottle in place for 10 minutes, then take it off for 10 minutes. Repeat several times.

☛ **MASSAGE**

Lay the tips of your fingers on the jaw muscles. You can locate these by clenching and unclenching the teeth, which activates the jaw muscles. Unclench the teeth and massage the area with small, firm circular movements, gradually easing away tension.

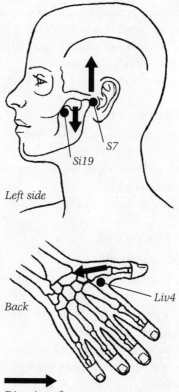

Left side

Back

Direction of acupressure massage

✳ **ACUPRESSURE**

Place the heels of your hands between the upper and lower jaws, in front of the earlobes, and gradually press inward. Clench your back teeth—you will feel a muscle pushing out into your hands. Press again on this muscle with the teeth apart for 1 minute. Take your hands away and move the jaw from left to right for a few seconds. Then place your fingertips on the same muscle and press firmly for another minute.

Try pressing on the other points shown in the illustration.

✚ **PROFESSIONAL HELP**

Chiropractic treatment can be most helpful in this condition.
Acupuncture can help relieve spasm and pain.
Hypnosis can also be effective.

●●● **ORTHODOX**

Muscle-relaxant drugs may be recommended to relieve spasm.

Orthodontists can prescribe a bite splint, a device that prevents teeth clenching at night. Sometimes braces can readjust the bite and solve the problem.

Cortisone injected directly into the joint can dramatically reduce inflammation and reduce symptoms.

TENDINITIS

Inflammation of a tendon, the tissue that attaches muscle to bone. Usually this occurs as a result of an injury, when the muscle is subjected to overuse, or is overstretched. It is a common occurrence in those who exercise sporadically and vigorously without properly warming up. Symptoms include pain, tenderness, and restricted movement. Often a feeling of "creakiness" is also experienced on movement. The most commonly affected areas are the Achilles tendon at the back of the ankle, the front of the shoulder, the thumb, the knee, and the inside of the foot.

PREVENTION

Do at least 15 minutes of warm-up exercises and stretches before exercising.

If you are jogging or doing impact sports (such as aerobics, tennis, basketball), replace your training shoes regularly—don't keep the same ones for years.

Try to run on soft ground.

TREATMENT

✗ **DIETARY**

The following nutrients are thought to help aid the healing of injured tissue:

vitamin C, found in high concentrations in citrus fruits, broccoli, parsley, and green pepper

beta-carotene, found in green leafy vegetables and yellow vegetables

zinc, found in liver, meat, Cheddar cheese, lentils, haricot beans, and whole-grain cereals selenium, found in whole-grain flour, mackerel, pork, and eggs

vitamin E, found in wheat germ, sunflower seeds and oil, olive oil, and margarine

🏵 HERBALISM

Turmeric is traditionally used as an anti-inflammatory in India and China. The extract of the turmeric root known as curcumin is the most effective: Take 250 milligrams 3 times a day, between meals.

Bromelain, an enzyme extracted from pineapples, is also an effective anti-inflammatory: Take 250 milligrams 3 times a day, between meals.

≈ HYDROTHERAPY

Immediately after exercise, rest the joint and apply an ice pack: Wrap a bag of frozen peas in a kitchen towel and apply to the joint for at least 10 minutes. Elevate the joint if possible. Remove the ice pack for 10 minutes, then reapply for 10 minutes.

An elastic bandage placed on the joint can sometimes help reduce swelling and internal bleeding.

Keep the injured part elevated as much as possible.

✚ PROFESSIONAL HELP

Chiropractors would probably treat this using massage, or with an ultrasound machine, which emits high-frequency vibration that heats the area, increasing circulation and drainage.

Acupuncture helps relieve pain and may assist in healing.

Transcutaneous nerve stimulation (TENS), available in some physiotherapy units, helps control pain. It works in much the same way as acupuncture, without the needles.

••• ORTHODOX

Most doctors prescribe nonsteroidal anti-inflammatory drugs for this condition. Your doctor may prescribe cortisone injections; they should never be injected directly into the tendon, but rather into the sheath surrounding the injured tendon.

TENNIS ELBOW

Inflammation of the muscles around the elbow joint, often caused by straining the muscles and tendons around the elbow and lower arm. Racquet sports, gardening, and home decorating jobs such as painting walls and ceilings are common activities that cause this ailment. Pain is felt on the outer edge of the elbow and the back of the lower part of the arm, and is often made worse by bending the arm or lifting a heavy object.

TREATMENT

■ PRACTICAL ADVICE

Rest the arm. This means no gripping, lifting, or carrying heavy objects for several days. Try to keep the arm elevated when resting.

☯ CHINESE MEDICINE

Practitioners of traditional Chinese medicine may recommend herbal teas of cinnamon twigs, mulberry twigs, and ginger.

≈ HYDROTHERAPY

Make an ice pack by wrapping a plastic bag full of ice cubes or a bag of frozen peas in a kitchen towel. Place it on the elbow, and lower the arm for 5 minutes every hour for several hours during the first few days. If the elbow is very painful, alternate ice treatment with 10 minutes of warm treatment, using a heating pad or a hot water bottle wrapped in a towel.

☞ MASSAGE

After two or three days of hydro-therapy and rest, a partner can massage the arm and elbow: The patient should lie on his or her back, and the person doing massage should be at the injured side. Start by kneading the upper arm, then the lower arm, by firmly squeezing all muscles. Then support the elbow on your knee. Using small, circular motions, massage around the elbow joint with the thumbs. Finally, using deep thumb pressure, massage across the muscles of the lower arm, working upward from the wrist to the elbow.

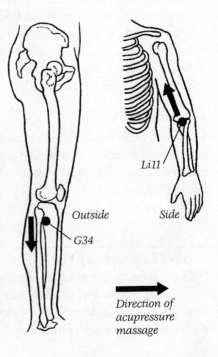

Li11

Outside

G34

Side

✳ ACUPRESSURE

Massage the points illustrated, using deep thumb pressure, for at least 1 minute.

Direction of acupressure massage

✚ **PROFESSIONAL HELP**

Chiropractic and professional massage would both be helpful. Acupucture and moxibustion are very effective.

••• **ORTHODOX**

Doctors generally recommend painkillers or a corticosteroid injection.

THROMBOPHLEBITIS

Inflammation of a vein, resulting from injury, infection, and irritation of the vein walls, and sometimes the formation of blood clots. The condition is most common in the superficial veins of the legs and in people with varicose veins. Symptoms include swelling and redness along the affected vein, sometimes accompanied by fever. It is important to distinguish between this condition and the deep vein thrombosis (see **Thrombosis**) that produces different symptoms and is potentially much more serious. Consult your doctor before carrying out self-help treatment.

TREATMENT

▬ **PRACTICAL ADVICE**

If you are taking oral contraceptives, consider an alternative method of contraception.

Do not smoke.

Do not sit for long periods without taking breaks, particularly when traveling; in a plane, get up and walk around every 30 minutes.

Put your feet up when resting.

Wear support hosiery or support socks.

🐾 **HERBALISM**

Hawthorn is a good tonic for the circulatory system and the treatment of blood vessels: Pour 1 cup of boiling water over 2 teaspoons of the berries, and infuse for 20 minutes; drink 3 times a day. It may take some time for effects to be seen.

To help clear and prevent infection: Take 3 garlic capsules, 3 times a day.

▢ **HOMEOPATHY**

Take 4 times a day, for up to 7 days:

If the condition follows an injury: *Arnica* 6c

If bruising persists: *Hamamelis* 6c

If the veins are worse in heat and when the limb is not elevated: *Pulsatilla* 6c

≋ HYDROTHERAPY

Contrasting temperatures help stimulate sluggish circulation, which contributes to this condition. Spray the legs first with cold water for 5 minutes, then with hot water for 5 minutes. Repeat several times.

⋰⋱ EXERCISE

Exercise helps pump blood around the body and stops it stagnating in the veins. Daily walking or swimming is particularly good for this condition.

••• ORTHODOX

Your doctor will prescribe antibiotics if the vein is infected, along with anti-inflammatory drugs and support bandages.

THROMBOSIS

A blood clot (thrombus) forms on the roughened walls of an injured blood vessel, gradually blocking the flow of blood. The clot may be caused by sluggish blood flow or an accumulation of fats in the blood. The blockage prevents blood and oxygen reaching part of the body, and a heart attack or stroke results. Generally, there are no symptoms of thrombosis until the clot blocks the blood vessel.

TREATMENT/PREVENTION

✗ DIETARY

The same dietary guidelines apply to thrombosis as for high cholesterol (see **Cholesterol, High**).

Fatty fish is known to reduce the stickiness of the blood platelets, making it more difficult for clots to form. Oily fish such as herring, kipper, mackerel, salmon, sardines, and tuna are better than white fish; eat these fish at least twice a week.

Linoleic acid, a fatty acid found in nuts, wheat germ, and vegetable oils, is thought to also help reduce stickiness of blood platelets. A handful of nuts daily is a good preventive measure.

Eat plenty of fresh garlic and onions, as these too help prevent the formation of a thrombus.

Vitamin E is thought to both prevent the formation of clots and dissolve any existing ones. If your blood pressure is no higher than 160 systolic (ask your doctor), take 300 milligrams of vitamin E a day; if your blood pressure is higher than 160 systolic, take 200 milligrams a day.

ૐ HERBALISM

Hawthorn is a good tonic for the circulatory system and the treatment of blood vessels: Pour 1 cup of boiling water over 2 teaspoons of the berries, and infuse for 20 minutes; drink 3 times a day. It may take some time for effects to be seen.

••• ORTHODOX

A thrombus can be detected by X-rays of the blood vessels after a radio-opaque substance is introduced into the body. Treatment is with anti-coagulant drugs to prevent further clotting, along with anti-inflammatory drugs to relieve the inflammation of the blood vessels.

THROMBOSIS, DEEP VEIN

Clotting of blood in the deep-lying veins of the legs that inhibits the return of blood to the heart. (The same condition can occur in the super-ficial veins of the legs; see **Thrombophlebitis.**) It is generally caused by sluggish circulation due to sitting or lying for long periods. Pregnant women and women taking oral contraceptives are more susceptible. Symptoms include pain, tenderness, swelling, and discoloration of the leg, sometimes with ulceration of the skin. This is a serious complaint. Consult with your doctor before you begin treatment.

PREVENTION

Getting out of bed as soon as possible after childbirth or surgery greatly reduces the likelihood of developing this condition.

If you are immobilized for long periods, try to keep the blood circulating by wiggling your toes and flexing your ankles and knees.

Massage is very helpful in stimulating circulation of the veins of the legs. However, avoid massaging directly on varicose veins.

Do not smoke.

Avoid taking oral contraceptives.

Do not sit for long periods without getting up to move your legs. When traveling by bus, plane, or train, get up and walk about every 30 minutes.

Put your feet up when resting.

Wear support hosiery.

TREATMENT

ૐ HERBALISM

Hawthorn infusion stimulates the blood circulation: Pour 1 cup of boiling water over 2 teaspoons of the berries, and infuse for 20 minutes; drink 3 times a day.

Incorporate plenty of raw garlic into your diet. You can take garlic capsules (3 capsules, 3 times a day) if you do not like the taste or smell of fresh garlic.

Ginger is also helpful in stimulating circulation. Add fresh or powdered to your meals, or make an infusion by adding 1 cup of boiling water to 1 teaspoon of the peeled, grated root, and infuse for 15 minutes; drink 3 times a day.

☐ HOMEOPATHY

Take every hour for up to 3 doses; repeat if necessary:

If accompanied by varicose veins, bruised and sore: *Hamamelis* 6c
After injury, feels and looks bruised, cannot bear touch: *Arnica* 6c
Unbearable bursting pain, must keep leg raised: *Vipera* 6c

≈ HYDROTHERAPY

Contrasting temperatures help stimulate sluggish circulation. Spray the legs first with cold water for 5 minutes, then with hot water for 5 minutes. Repeat several times, morning and evening.

⊹ EXERCISE

Exercise keeps the blood moving around the body, preventing stagnation and the formation of clots. Daily walking or swimming is helpful in preventing and treating this condition.

••• ORTHODOX

Small clots are generally left alone to break up spontaneously.
Thrombolytic drugs are prescribed to dissolve larger clots.
In severe cases the clot is surgically removed.

THRUSH

A yeast infection that usually affects the mouth or vagina. The yeast organism (*Candida albicans*) grows naturally in the body; but when the system is upset, its growth gets out of hand, causing a white coating or an itchy, cottage cheese–like discharge. Thrush occurs in the vagina when the immune system is compromised, or when the acid/alkali balance of the vagina is upset by using douches, spermicides, or bath products. Excessive use of antibiotics can also trigger an attack, as can the use of oral contraceptives. See also **Fungal Infection; Thrush, Oral.**

TREATMENT

✗ DIETARY

Reduce your intake of sugar, including fruit and alcohol, which encourages yeast growth.

Reduce your intake of foods containing yeast: bread, mushrooms, blue cheese, alcohol, soy sauce, foods containing monosodium glutamate, smoked fish and sausages, and vinegar.

Thrush tends to occur when immunity is low. To increase immunity, make sure you are eating plenty of raw and lightly cooked vegetables, brown rice, and lean meat or fish.

Incorporate plenty of olive oil and garlic into your meals.

Avoid coffee and tea; instead drink mineral water, rooibos tea, and other herbal teas.

Eat plenty of live yogurt with *Lactobacillus acidophilus* (at least one large carton a day).

Take supplements of *Lactobacillus acidophilus*. Take ½ teaspoon of *Lactobacillus acidophilus*, 1 teaspoon of *Bifidobacteria* powder, and ½ teaspoon of *Lactobacillus bulgaricus* (available from natural foods stores) in a glass of spring water, 3 times a day.

✿ AROMATHERAPY

Add 4 drops of essential oil of tea tree and 2 drops of myrrh to your bathwater.

Use 4 drops of essential oil of tea tree in 1 quart of warm spring water in a douche; or put 1 drop of tea tree oil on a tampon and insert overnight.

○ DOUCHES

Special douches help restore the acid/alkali balance of the vagina for vaginal thrush. (**Caution:** Do not douche during pregnancy.)

Buy a commercial douche, empty it out, and rinse it thoroughly with bottled or boiled water. Then make up a solution with 1 tablespoon of live yogurt or *Lactobacillus acidophilus* powder and 1 quart of warm boiled or bottled water. Place the solution in the douche and insert into the vagina twice a day, allowing it to flush out completely.

You can also douche with a solution of 2 tablespoons of apple cider vinegar added to 1 quart of warm bottled or boiled water.

••• ORTHODOX

Your doctor can prescribe antifungal agents in cream, tablet, vaginal pessary, oral solution, or tampon-impregnated form. Although treatment is effective within a matter of days, thrush tends to recur, so it is worth resolving the cause. In vaginal thrush it is advisable for sexual partners to be treated simultaneously, as the infection can be passed back and forth.

THRUSH, ORAL

A fungal infection of the mouth and throat that generally affects the very young, the elderly, or those whose immunity is compromised. The infection, known as *Candida albicans,* thrives in warm moist areas where the natural healthy bacteria have been disrupted by illness, or by taking antibiotics or oral corticosteroids. Symptoms include white patches in the mouth that peel off to reveal sore, reddened areas beneath.

TREATMENT

✗ DIETARY

Candida albicans thrives on sugar, so avoid all sugar-containing foods, including fruit, fruit juices, honey, and maple syrup.

Avoid coffee, tea, chocolate, vinegar, mushrooms, and cheese.

Avoid fermented foods, including alcohol and soy sauce.

Eat at least 3 cartons a day of live yogurt with *Lactobacillus acidophilus.*

Olive oil acts to prevent the conversion of yeast into fungus; incorporate it into your diet as much as possible.

Take ½ teaspoon of *Lactobacillus acidophilus*, 1 teaspoon of *Bifidobacteria* powder, and ½ teaspoon of *Lactobacillus bulgaricus* (available from natural foods stores) in a glass of spring water, 3 times a day. This restores healthy bacteria to the body and helps fight *Candida.*

❧ HERBALISM

Garlic is an effective antifungal agent. Incorporate plenty of the raw herb into your diet. If you do not like the smell or taste of fresh garlic, take garlic supplements (3 capsules, 3 times a day).

Aloe vera mouthwash, available from herbalists and pharmacies, has an antifungal effect.

Studies have shown barberry to prevent the growth of *Candida,* while stimulating the immune system. Take 1 teaspoon of the tincture in water 3 times a day. **Caution:** Do not take during pregnancy.

Caprylic acid, an extract of coconuts, is a powerful antifungal agent. Take 3 capsules with each meal.

☐ HOMEOPATHY

Take 4 times a day for up to 5 days:
  When the first signs start: *Borax* 6c
  Hot, sore patches in the mouth, made worse by cold water: *Capsicum* 6c
  Oral thrush with mouth ulcers: *Arsenicum album* 6c

••• ORTHODOX

Treatment consists of antifungal agents, such as nystatin, in lozenges or
mouthwash form.

TINNITUS

A ringing, buzzing, hissing, or whistling sound in the ears, often worse
when background noise is low. It is sometimes accompanied by hearing
loss. Tinnitus may be caused by long-term exposure to loud noise, excessive wax in the ears, catarrh, sinusitis, or damage to the nerves of the ear.
Some drugs, particularly aspirin, may also contribute to the condition.

TREATMENT

▬ PRACTICAL ADVICE

Removal of excess ear wax can sometimes bring relief.
  Your doctor can syringe the ears to remove wax.
  Some complementary practitioners use Hopi wax candles, a safe and
natural method of drawing wax out of the ear.
  Another method is to place 2 drops of slightly warmed almond oil in
the ear, keep the head on one side to prevent the oil running out, and
insert a twist of soft cotton material gently into the ear to soak up the oil
and remove the softened wax. **Caution:** Never put matchsticks, cotton
swabs, long fingernails, or sharp instruments in the ear to remove wax.

✗ DIETARY

Naturopaths recommend a cleansing regime, which includes a three-day
vegetable juice fast every six weeks and a diet high in raw and cooked
vegetables, grains, nuts, legumes (peas, beans, lentils), and low-fat yogurt
and fish. Avoid coffee, alcohol, salt, and fried food.
  Increasing your intake of the following nutrients can sometimes help:

- magnesium, found in Brazil nuts, soy flour, whole-grain flour, lentils,
  and parsley
- potassium, found in dried brewer's yeast, dried dates, mushrooms,
  cabbage, lean meats, and bananas

- manganese, found in tea, whole-grain cereals, dried cooked beans, and leafy vegetables

✳ ACUPRESSURE

Massage the points illustrated, using deep thumb pressure for at least 1 minute.

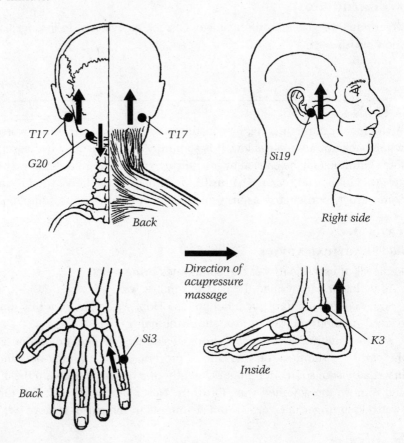

✛ EXERCISE

Increasing the blood circulation to the head may help. Most vigorous exercise increases circulation; for example, running, fast walking, swimming, or aerobics.

✳ YOGA

The following postures, which loosen the neck, are particularly good for increasing circulation to the head:

Keeping your chin tucked in, turn your head slowly to the left as far as it will comfortably go, hold for a few seconds; then turn to the right, hold again, and come back to center. Repeat 3 times.

Tilt your head forward, bringing your chin toward your chest, and hold for a few seconds; then tilt your head backward, keeping the chin tucked in, and return to the starting position. Repeat 3 times.

✚ PROFESSIONAL HELP

Chiropractic and acupuncture have been known to help.
Professional homeopathic treatment may also be helpful.

••• ORTHODOX

Treatment is disappointing, though maskers have had some success. These are battery-operated devices, somewhat like hearing aids, which emit a constant noise of a different frequency to the one heard in the tinnitus. This provides a soothing effect, but is not a cure.

TONSILLITIS

Inflammation and swelling of the tonsils, which are situated at the back of the throat. This condition usually occurs in children, who have enlarged, red tonsils, a sore throat, difficulty swallowing, a fever, and sometimes a congested chest and nose.

TREATMENT

✗ DIETARY

Naturopaths make the following recommendations:

During the illness:

- Drink plenty of water and fresh fruit and vegetable juices.
- Eat lightly steamed vegetables or vegetable broths.

To avoid recurrent attacks:

- Reduce your intake of dairy products: Replace milk with soy milk or goat's milk.
- Reduce your intake of carbohydrates, particularly sweets, pastries, and white bread. Instead, eat whole-grain cereals in moderation, and plenty of fresh fruits and vegetables and low-fat protein.

❈ AROMATHERAPY

Add 2 drops of essential oil of eucalyptus and 1 drop of peppermint to 1 teaspoon of a carrier lotion or oil and massage the chest, back, and throat. Gently rub the oil or lotion into the throat too.

🐌 HERBALISM

Red sage infusion soothes the inflammation: Put 2 teaspoons of the leaves in 2 cups of water, bring to a boil, and let stand for 15 minutes. Gargle with the warm tea for 5 minutes several times a day.

☐ HOMEOPATHY

Take every 30 minutes for up to 4 doses; repeat as necessary:

Pain in neck and ears, swallowing painful, feeling exhausted and weak: *Gelsemium* 6c

Sudden sore throat made worse by cold wind, tonsils swollen, throat burning, everything tastes bitter: *Aconite* 6c

Worse right side with purplish appearance and a swollen uvula, better from cold drinks: *Apis* 6c

Worse left side, intolerant of any constriction, pain worse from swallowing saliva and better from swallowing food: *Lachesis* 6c

Stitching pain like a fish bone, which extends to the ears when swallowing; cheesy exudate on the tonsils: *Hepar sulphuris* 6c

Moist, flabby tongue and foul breath; swollen neck glands: *Mercurius solubilis* 6c

Tonsils are as large as plums: *Baryta muriatica* 6c

☯ CHINESE MEDICINE

Practitioners of traditional Chinese medicine recommend honeysuckle flower tea; a salt gargle is helpful to soothe and sterilize the throat. Avoid spicy foods if you are prone to tonsillitis. Recurrent bouts may be helped by ear acupuncture.

••• ORTHODOX

Your doctor will prescribe a painkiller to provide relief. In severe cases doctors will prescribe antibiotics or suggest surgery.

TOOTHACHE

Pain in or around one tooth or several teeth and gums most commonly results from decay, and is a sign that dental treatment is needed. An abscess around the root of the tooth may also be a cause of pain (see **Abscess, Dental**).

TREATMENT

The following remedies will help relieve discomfort while you await dental treatment.

❀ AROMATHERAPY

Wet one finger with essential oil of clove and rub on the gum of the painful tooth. Dilute 2 drops in 1 teaspoon of carrier oil if the skin is sensitive.

❧ HERBALISM

Wet one finger with tincture of myrrh and rub on the gum of the painful tooth to relieve pain.

☐ HOMEOPATHY

Take every 5 minutes for up to 4 doses; repeat if necessary:
Pain made worse by hot food and drinks and soothed by cold drinks: *Coffea* 6c
Pain made worse by cold air, along with the tendency to produce a lot of saliva: *Plantago* 6c
Pain made worse by cold air, food and drinks: *Calcarea carbonica* 6c
Pain after dental treatment: *Arnica* 6c

☯ CHINESE MEDICINE

If there is no apparent dental problem, practitioners of traditional Chinese medicine may suggest that a toothache is linked with a stomach or liver problem. They may recommend herbs such as gypsum with rhubarb for the stomach, and Chinese ginseng for the liver.

✳ ACUPRESSURE

Apply deep pressure to the area between the thumb and the index finger to relieve pain. Stimulating this point can also reduce pain during dental treatment.
Another point that may be helpful is on the top of the foot, about ½ inch toward the ankle from the point where the second and third toes join.

••• ORTHODOX

Doctors recommend painkillers for temporary relief until you are able to see your dentist. If you suspect an abscess (severe continuous pain, swelling around the gum, and tenderness of the tooth), make an emergency appointment.

TORTICOLLIS

A twisting of the neck, causing the head to be rotated and tilted to one side, bringing pain and stiffness; also known as wry neck. Torticollis can result from an injury, sleeping in an awkward position, or stress. It can also occur at birth.

TREATMENT

≈ HYDROTHERAPY

Use hot and cold treatment for torticollis that follows an injury, awkward sleeping position, or stress: Make an ice pack by wrapping a plastic bag full of ice cubes or a bag of frozen peas in a kitchen towel. Place on the tense muscle for 10 minutes. Then place a hot water bottle wrapped in a towel on the muscle for a further 10 minutes. Alternate hot and cold several times, morning and night.

☞ MASSAGE

If you are able, turn your head to the left side and place the ends of the fingers of your right hand at the top of the large muscle that runs from the back of the right side of your head to the collar bone (sternocleido-mastoid muscle). Massage deeply the length of the muscle with your thumb. Do the same on the other side.

Hook the fingers of both hands over your shoulders and squeeze the muscles lying between the neck and the shoulder joints.

♣ REFLEXOLOGY

If the neck is too sensitive to move or touch, reflexology may help:

Massage the point where the big toe joins the foot on the sole of the left foot.

Massage the cervical spine area: along the inner side of both feet, and along the joint of the big toe.

Rotate the big toes.

～ RELAXATION TECHNIQUES

To relieve stress and relax tense muscles, make a head rest by putting two tennis balls in a sock and tying the end. Lie down on the floor on your back, using the balls as a rest under the neck. Each ball should be on either side of the spine. Relax in this position for 10 minutes a day.

✚ PROFESSIONAL HELP

Chiropractors specialize in dealing with this problem.

Acupuncture helps if the neck is very painful.

The Alexander Technique corrects postural problems that may lead to torticollis.

••• ORTHODOX

Most doctors will recommend heat treatment and physiotherapy. Sometimes an orthopedic collar is used to immobilize the neck. Surgery is occasionally performed for this condition.

TOXEMIA
See **Preeclampsia.**

TOXOPLASMOSIS

An infection found in animals, birds, and reptiles, which is passed on to humans through eating infected meat or touching animals or their litter. Usually the body's immune system protects us against the infection. However, in pregnant women toxoplasmosis can be transmitted to the fetus, causing miscarriage or stillbirth. Pregnant women should get a blood test to be sure they do not have toxoplasmosis. Toxoplasmosis is also a concern for people with AIDS (see **AIDS**).

PREVENTION

Avoid handling cat litter.
Wash your hands thoroughly after touching pets.
Do not allow pets to lick you.
Use separate utensils for animals' food, and wash them separately from your own.
Always wash your hands before eating or preparing food.
Avoid raw meat or fish during pregnancy.
Wash all raw vegetables thoroughly; avoid eating raw vegetables in restaurants.

TREATMENT

••• ORTHODOX

If you suspect toxoplasmosis, your doctor can give you a blood test to make a diagnosis. Most patients have a mild form of the disease, and no treatment is required.

Antibiotics, such as pyrimethamine and sulphadiazine, are given to immune-compromised patients and patients with severe cases.

In pregnancy, spiramycin is used instead of pyrimethamine, and steroids can be useful if the eyes are affected by the disease.

TRAVEL SICKNESS
See **Motion Sickness.**

TRICHOMONIASIS

A parasitic infection of the vagina that is often sexually transmitted, or contracted from a towel, clothing, or washcloth carrying the infection. Symptoms include inflammation and itching of the vaginal area; frothy, yellowish discharge; and sometimes a burning sensation when urinating and pain during intercourse.

PREVENTION

Do not share towels, swimsuits, or clothing.

Avoid using washcloths or sponges to wash the genital area; these may harbor germs.

Always wipe from front to back when going to the toilet, to prevent bacteria from the anus entering the vagina.

Remove your swimsuit immediately after swimming.

In those prone to infection, it is advisable for both partners to wash before and after intercourse.

TREATMENT

✗ DIETARY

Drink plenty of unsweetened cranberry juice every day, to acidify the system.

Eat live yogurt daily, and take a *Lactobacillus acidophilus* supplement: 1 teaspoon in a glass of water 3 times a day, with ½ teaspoon of *Bifidobacteria.*

The following supplements help promote healing and boost immunity:

- vitamin A: 10,000 iu a day
- vitamin C: found in fresh fruit and vegetables; also take 1 1,000-milligram supplement, 3 times a day
- vitamin E: 800 iu a day
- zinc: 50 milligrams a day

○ DOUCHES

The parasite thrives in an alkaline environment, so use one of the following douches to acidify the vagina once a day during the infection. **Caution:** Do not use during pregnancy.

Vinegar douche: Add 1 teaspoon of vinegar to 1 quart of warm water, place in a douche bag or in an infant syringe (available from most pharmacies). Use the douche while lying in a warm bath: Insert into the vagina and remain horizontal for a while to allow the solution to remain inside. When you stand up, it will flush out of the vagina.

Live yogurt or a solution of *Lactobacillus acidophilus* (½ teaspoon of powder to 1 cup of water) helps reintroduce healthy bacteria into the vagina. Mix either ingredient with the strained juice of 1 lemon to introduce acidity. Using an infant syringe, place in the vagina, remain horizontal for a few moments, and rinse off, using a sanitary pad to catch any drips over the next few hours.

••• ORTHODOX

Antibiotics, such as metronidazole, are generally prescribed for this condition. However, the drug should be used with caution, as it has been shown to cause birth defects and cancer in animal studies.

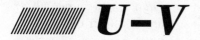 # *U–V*

ULCER

See **Leg Ulcer; Mouth Ulcers; Peptic Ulcer.**

URINARY TRACT INFECTION

The symptoms of a urinary tract infection include burning when urinating, a frequent urge to urinate, abdominal pain, and sometimes a mild fever. The infection can occur anywhere along the urinary tract. The most common types are:

urethritis, inflammation of the urethra, the tube that excretes urine from the bladder

cystitis, inflammation of the bladder (see **Cystitis**)

pyelonephritis, inflammation of the kidneys

Urethritis may result from structural problems or from an infection that is often a sexually transmitted disease, such as gonorrhea or nonspecific urethritis (see **Sexually Transmitted Diseases**). Most other urinary tract infections result from bacterial infections spreading from the rectum. Women are more susceptible due to the shortness of the urethra. In men urinary infections may be a sign of an enlarged prostate (see **Prostate, Enlarged**). It is important to consult your doctor if you experience symptoms of a urinary tract infection to identify the source, and receive treatment, particularly if the infection is sexually transmitted.

PREVENTION

Make sure to urinate regularly; do not put off going to the toilet.

Always urinate after intercourse.

Women should always wipe the genital area from front to back to avoid introducing bacteria from the anus into the vagina.

TREATMENT

✗ DIETARY

Naturopaths advise building up immunity to fight infection. Eat plenty of raw and lightly cooked vegetables, whole-grain cereals, and low-fat protein.

Drink plenty of water, at least 8 glasses a day, to help flush the infection out of the system.

Vitamin A helps build healthy mucous membranes. It is found in liver, egg yolk, butter, fortified margarine, cheese, and cod liver oil.

You will probably be given antibiotics for the infection. To restore healthy bacteria destroyed by the drugs, eat plenty of live, unsweetened yogurt with *Lactobacillus acidophilus,* at least one small carton a day, for at least 1 month.

❀ AROMATHERAPY

Add 2 drops of essential oil each of juniper berry, eucalyptus, and sandal-wood to a warm bath, and sit in it for 10 minutes to relieve symptoms.

ૠ HERBALISM

Parsley is a diuretic that helps to excrete water and clear infection: Eat liberally in salads and cooked foods.

Dandelion leaves have a similar diuretic effect: Eat them raw in salad.

☐ HOMEOPATHY

Take every 30 minutes for up to 5 doses; repeat if necessary:

- Urine feels like scalding water; violently painful: *Cantharis* 6c
- Burning pain at the end of urination and afterward: *Sarsaparilla* 6c
- Stinging pains, better from cold bathing: *Apis* 6c
- Violently painful with blood in the urine: *Mercurius corrosivus* 6c
- *Berberis* mother tincture: Take 3 drops in a little water 2 times a day for a general support and tonic during treatment.

••• ORTHODOX

Doctors can test your urine to identify the microorganism responsible for the infection. Antibiotics are generally recommended. If the infection is sexually transmitted, inform your sexual partners so they can get treatment.

URTICARIA
See **Hives.**

UTERINE PROLAPSE
A condition in which the uterus drops down into the vagina, usually as a result of weakening of the ligaments during childbirth. Symptoms are

few, though there may be a dragging sensation in the pelvis, backache, and difficulty urinating or defecating.

TREATMENT

 DIETARY

Carrying extra pounds can contribute to uterine prolapse. If you are heavier than your recommended weight, try to lose weight (see **Obesity**).

⁜ EXERCISE

Strengthening the pelvic floor muscles through exercise helps hold the uterus in place. To locate these muscles, try stopping and starting the flow of urine when you urinate. Practice tightening and relaxing these muscles throughout the day: Start with 5 contractions 10 times a day; then build this up to 10 contractions, 10 times a day.

Your doctor can provide small weights that are designed to be held inside the vagina, making the pelvic floor muscles work.

✚ PROFESSIONAL HELP

Professional homeopathic treatment can be helpful.

••• ORTHODOX

Your doctor will probably recommend the pelvic floor exercises, above, or passive exercises for the muscles using an electric current.

A pessary that fits around the cervix and holds the uterus up and back provides relief for a mild prolapse, but the pessary has to be enlarged every three to six months to reduce the possibility of infection.

As a last resort, surgery is used to tighten the ligaments.

VAGINAL IRRITATION

An inflammation of the vagina that can be caused by infection (see **Thrush**), drugs, allergy, hormonal problems, or a foreign body, such as a forgotten tampon; also known as vaginitis. Postmenopausal women are particularly susceptible. Symptoms include irritation, redness, and intense itching, and sometimes odor, discharge, and pain during intercourse.

PREVENTION

Wash the genital area regularly and pat dry with a clean towel. Avoid talc, vaginal deodorants, and scented soaps.

Wear cotton underpants and avoid tight clothes.

Always wipe from front to back when going to the toilet, to avoid introducing bacteria from the anus into the vagina.

Always wash the genital area (both partners) before intercourse.

Use a lubricant, such as KY jelly, during intercourse.

TREATMENT

✗ DIETARY

Reduce your intake of coffee and sugar. These can upset the acid/alkali balance of the vagina and increase the likelihood of infection.

If symptoms are caused by a fungal infection (see **Thrush**), avoid all sugars for at least one month. Eat plenty of fresh vegetables, whole-grain cereals, and lean meat and fish. Eat at least one carton of live yogurt with *Lactobacillus acidophilus* a day, and take 1 teaspoon of *Lactobacillus acidophilus* in a glass of water 3 times a day, with 1 teaspoon *Bifidobacteria*.

❋ AROMATHERAPY

Essential oil of tea tree and myrrh are both effective when added to a warm bath.

Apply 2 drops of tea tree oil to the top of a damp tampon and insert into the vagina for 3 hours. **Caution:** Do not use during pregnancy.

ঽ HERBALISM

Golden seal–myrrh douche: Simmer 1 tablespoon of each herb in 3 cups of water for 5 minutes; use as a douche once a week. **Caution:** Do not use during pregnancy.

To relieve itching, bathe the vagina in chickweed infusion: Pour 1 cup of boiling water on 2 teaspoons of the herb, leave to infuse for 5 minutes, and allow to cool.

Garlic is an effective antifungal: Incorporate plenty of fresh garlic into your diet; if you don't like the taste or smell of fresh garlic, take 3 garlic capsules, 3 times a day.

••• ORTHODOX

Your doctor will take vaginal swabs to diagnose the microorganism that is responsible, and will probably prescribe antibiotic treatment to eradicate the infection.

VAGINISMUS

Painful spasm of the muscles surrounding the vaginal entrance that makes sexual intercourse and the use of tampons painful and sometimes impossible. Sometimes the legs also straighten and come together involuntarily during sex or a vaginal examination. The condition may result from infection, fear of pain, past trauma, or psychological causes relating to negative sexual experiences or guilt.

TREATMENT

Professional help is recommended (see below). Use the following suggestions as an adjunct to talking therapy.

~ RELAXATION TECHNIQUES

Practicing yoga or meditation provides mental and physical relaxation, which facilitates talking therapy and relieves the stress brought by this condition.

Aromatherapy and massage are also extremely helpful in providing deep relaxation, especially if carried out by your partner.

✚ PROFESSIONAL HELP

Vaginismus is very difficult to treat alone. The vaginismus support group, Resolve, recommends talking therapy as the most beneficial treatment for this syndrome. Psychotherapy, counseling, or simply talking with an understanding health professional, friend, or family member can be very helpful. If you have a partner, it is a good idea to do talking therapy together. The following are some of the techniques used.

Behavioral therapy includes relaxation, visualization of the lovemaking situation, and the use of dilators or a cervical cap to insert into the vagina. Presenting the fearful situation in a safe and supportive environment allows the patient gradually to overcome it.

Sex therapy is usually carried out with both partners. It includes counseling, examination of the vagina, vaginal exercises (contracting and releasing the muscles that control urination) that demonstrate control of the vagina, and visualization. Relaxation is also encouraged, and sometimes hypnosis. Dilators are sometimes used to accustom the woman to inserting something into the vagina. Sensate focusing, where the focus of lovemaking is giving each other pleasure rather than penetration, is encouraged.

Professional homeopathic treatment can be a successful adjunct to these treatments.

••• ORTHODOX

Your doctor will probably recommend talking therapy, as discussed above.

VAGINITIS
See **Vaginal Irritation.**

VARICOSE ULCER
See **Leg Ulcer.**

VARICOSE VEINS

Blue, prominent, and sometimes kinked veins just below the surface of the skin, most commonly in the legs, but also in the anus (see **Hemorrhoids**) and the testes, where they are commonly known as varicocele. Varicose veins occur when the valves that prevent blood draining backward are weakened, and blood tends to pool and stagnate in the lower veins. The condition is often made worse by pregnancy, menopause, obesity, and long periods of standing.

■ PRACTICAL ADVICE

The development of varicose veins is closely linked with constipation. Follow the advice given in **Constipation,** and try to avoid straining at all times.

If you are overweight, try to lose some weight (see **Obesity** for suggestions).

Avoid wearing tight clothing.

Wear support hose if you have to stand for long periods.

Put your feet up whenever possible.

✘ DIETARY

Research has shown that varicose veins improve on taking 400 iu of vitamin E every day.

Increase your intake of citrus fruits, apricots, blackberries, cherries, rosehips, and buckwheat, all of which contain rutin, a valuable natural remedy for improving elasticity of the veins.

Take 500 milligrams of vitamin C with 100 milligrams of bioflavonoids every day.

Increase your intake of raw beetroot.

≈ HYDROTHERAPY

For swollen veins, apply alternate hot and cold compresses: Prepare two basins, one with hot (but not boiling) water, and one with cold water, with ice cubes in it. Soak 1 towel in each basin and wring out. First place the hot towel on the vein for 1 minute, then the cold for 30 seconds. Repeat the process 3 times, finishing with the cold.

✛ EXERCISE

In his book *Varicose Veins,* naturopath Leon Chaitow suggests the following daily stretches for the prevention and treatment of early varicose veins:

Stand with feet apart and hands clasped behind your back. Bend forward from the hips as far as you can go, hold for 30 seconds, breathing slowly and deeply.

Stand with feet 12 to 15 inches apart, and slowly go into a squat position. If this is easy, hold out your arms in front of you; if you are losing your balance, hold onto a table or chair to stabilize you. Repeat 3 to 10 times.

Lie on the floor on your back, stretch your arms above your head, and press the lower back to the floor. Keep the leg straight, lift one leg 15 inches off the floor, circle the foot 4 times each way, then do the same with the other leg.

Skipping, dancing, or brisk walking are all good activities for varicose veins; do one of these at least every other day.

✳ YOGA

Do the Inverted Corpse pose: Lie near a wall, and place the legs at an angle of 45 degrees against the wall. Remain in this position for 3 minutes a day.

A regular yoga class will help improve your breathing, an important factor in the treatment of this condition.

••• ORTHODOX

Veins below the knees can be injected with a sclerosing agent, which fuses the walls of the vein together.

Your doctor may want to perform surgery to strip out the vein from groin to ankle, which brings longer-lasting results.

VERRUCA
See **Warts.**

VOMITING
Regurgitation of the contents of the stomach. Vomiting can be due to a number of causes, of which the most common are:

general illness, which can be trivial (flu) or serious (hepatitis, cancer, kidney disease, meningitis)

drugs and medications, especially chemotherapy for cancer, but also nonsteroidal anti-inflammatory drugs for arthritis

food poisoning: bacterial, viral, or chemical, or toxins produced by bacteria that have entered the body; this is the most common cause (see **Food Poisoning** for treatment)

upset caused by traveling (see **Motion Sickness**)

ear infections (see **Earache and Ear Infections**)

emotional upset

smoking, recreational drugs, alcohol

migraine headaches (see **Migraine**)

stomach ulcer (see **Peptic Ulcer**)

gallbladder disorders (see **Gallstones**)

The following treatments provide relief after an attack of vomiting. However, they do not address the cause. An episode of vomiting that lasts more than an hour or two is unusual. Bring it to your doctor's attention for diagnosis and treatment.

TREATMENT

✗ DIETARY

To avoid dehydration from vomiting, drink plenty of fluids. Bottled or boiled cool water to which a little sugar and salt are added is the best (add ½ teaspoon of each to 1 quart of water).

Avoid eating solids until nausea subsides, then introduce bland, nonfat foods, such as yogurt, bananas, and toast.

🌿 HERBALISM

Ginger is an effective remedy for nausea: Place 1 teaspoon of the fresh grated root in 1 cup of boiling water, and infuse for 5 minutes; strain and drink when needed.

Meadowsweet infusion soothes and protects the mucous membranes of the digestive system: Pour 1 cup of boiling water on 1 to 2 teaspoons of the dried herb, and infuse for 10 to 15 minutes; drink 3 times a day.

☐ HOMEOPATHY

Take every 15 minutes for up to 4 doses; repeat if needed:

Vomiting with persistent nausea and an unusually clear tongue: *Ipecac* 6c

Vomiting with pain and burning sensation in stomach, frightened of being sick: *Arsenicum album* 6c

Nausea made better by vomiting: *Nux vomica* 6c

Nausea and vomiting relieved by keeping the abdomen uncovered: *Tabacum* 6c

Burning pains and vomiting, better temporarily for cold drinks: *Phosphorus* 6c

✳ ACUPRESSURE

Place your right thumb on the inside of your left wrist, two thumb-breadths from the center of the wrist joint toward the elbow. Massage with the thumb, using a deep, circular motion, for 1 minute, taking deep breaths. Do the same on the other wrist.

••• ORTHODOX

Treatment will depend on the cause of vomiting.

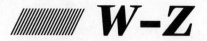 # W-Z

WALL-EYE
See **Strabismus.**

WARTS

Harmless yet contagious growths that are spread by a virus and are commonly found on the hands, face, knees, scalp, or feet (where they are known as verrucas or plantar warts). Usually warts are symptomless, though they may sometimes itch or be painful, particularly if on the soles of the feet. Genital warts, found around the vagina, anus, penis, or scrotum, can lead to cervical cancer in women and should be reported to your doctor immediately. Use a condom to prevent transmission of genital warts. See also **Sexually Transmitted Diseases.**

TREATMENT

Warts often disappear after about a year without treatment. The following treatments may help stubborn cases.

☙ HERBALISM

Rubbing a crushed garlic clove on the wart is said to help remove it. Eating plenty of raw garlic may also help. If you do not like the taste or smell of fresh garlic, you can take garlic capsules (3 capsules, 3 times a day).

☐ HOMEOPATHY

Professional homeopathic treatment is strongly recommended, though you may try the following remedies initially:
Take every 12 hours for up to 3 weeks:

- Large jagged warts on the face, eyelids, fingertips, which bleed easily: *Causticum* 6c
- Cauliflower-like warts, itchy, which bleed when washed: *Nitric acid* 6c
- Flat, horny warts on the hands and soles of the feet: *Antimonium crudum* 6c
- Warts on the palms, when the hands tend to be sweaty: *Natrum muriaticum* 6c
- *Thuja* mother tincture is a common remedy: Apply 2 times a day, then keep the wart covered.

✪ **VISUALIZATION**

Spend 5 minutes each day relaxing with your eyes closed, and visualizing your warts shrinking and gradually disappearing.

◯ **OTHER APPLICATIONS**

Castor oil and baking powder mixed into a paste: Apply at night and cover with an adhesive bandage. Leave exposed to the air during the day.

Vitamin E oil: Apply 3 times a day and cover.

Vitamin A oil: Apply 3 times a day and cover.

✚ **PROFESSIONAL HELP**

Hypnotherapy can be effective. The power of suggestion is often very successful in getting rid of warts.

••• **ORTHODOX**

Doctors generally recommend freezing or burning the warts off, or using surgery to remove them.

WASP STINGS
See **Insect Bites and Stings.**

WHIPLASH INJURY

An injury to the joints and ligaments of the neck caused when the neck is suddenly thrown forward and then backward, or vice versa. This condition is common after a car accident, and leads to symptoms of neck pain and stiffness that may be short-lived or long-term and are often accompanied by headaches, nausea, insomnia, numbness in the arms and fingers, and ringing in the ears.

TREATMENT

✗ **DIETARY**

Stiffness can be relieved by taking a high-dose supplement of calcium pantothenate: 2,000 milligrams a day. Reduce the dose as the stiffness wears off.

✿ **AROMATHERAPY**

Essential oils of sweet marjoram and rosemary are effective in relieving pain.

Add 2 drops of each oil to your bath.

Add 2 drops of each oil to 2 teaspoons of a carrier oil or lotion, and rub in night and morning.

☐ HOMEOPATHY

Take *Arnica* 6c, every 5 minutes for up to 6 doses; then *Hypericum* 6c, every 4 hours for up to 3 days.

≋ HYDROTHERAPY

Immediately after the injury, apply an ice pack to the painful area. Make an ice pack by wrapping a plastic bag full or ice cubes or a bag of frozen peas in a kitchen towel. Hold it on the painful area for 10 minutes. Then apply a hot water bottle wrapped in a towel for 10 minutes. Continue to alternate several times. Do this morning and evening.

✳ ACUPRESSURE

Place the fingers of both hands on the tops of your shoulders and apply firm pressure to the muscles near the base of the neck. Hold for 1 minute, while taking slow deep breaths.

Shrug your shoulders up toward your ears, hold for a few seconds, and relax. Repeat several times.

Place the fingers of both hands on the muscles of your neck on either side of the spine. Apply firm pressure, while nodding your head slowly and breathing deeply for 1 minute. Repeat several times.

✚ PROFESSIONAL HELP

A whiplash injury will almost certainly require professional treatment.

Chiropractors specialize in diagnosing and resolving structural problems connected with bones, ligaments, and nerves.

Massage therapists will help restore movement.

Acupuncturists can help combat pain.

Long-term problems concerned with posture can be treated successfully by the Alexander Technique.

••• ORTHODOX

Depending on the severity of the condition, doctors generally prescribe:

painkilling drugs

muscle relaxants

a collar to immobilize the neck

physiotherapy

WHOOPING COUGH

An infectious disease that mainly affects young children and results in fits of violent coughing with the characteristic "whoop" as the child catches breath, often followed by vomiting. The illness brings extreme exhaustion and sometimes permanent lung damage. It can be life-threatening, particularly in babies.

PREVENTION

Many children are vaccinated against whooping cough. Although this does not guarantee immunity, it is recommended by doctors due to the severity of this illness.

TREATMENT

▬ PRACTICAL ADVICE

The child may become frightened by the violence of the coughing attacks. Reassure your child by remaining calm. Consider having the child sleep in your room during the illness for comfort at night.

Babies should be laid chest down with their head to one side to prevent choking.

✘ DIETARY

Avoid dairy products, excessive sugar, and raw vegetables.

Give warm vegetable broth or soup every day.

Eat the main meal in the middle of the day; eat lightly in the evening to reduce night vomiting.

✽ AROMATHERAPY

Put 2 drops of essential oil of lavender or rosemary on a tissue and have the child inhale it.

Eucalyptus oil is also good, but it is stronger, so use it in an electronic vaporizer.

⁊ HERBALISM

Wild lettuce infusion is effective in calming the throat and chest and reducing the cough: Pour 1 cup of boiling water on 1 teaspoon of the leaves, and infuse for 15 minutes; drink 3 times a day.

Syrup of wild cherry is also effective, and is a favorite with children.

☐ HOMEOPATHY

Consult a professional homeopath for treatment. The treatments listed under **Cough** may help during the first few days.

••• ORTHODOX

If the illness is recognized early, antibiotics may be given. Once the coughing has started, however, they are not particularly helpful. If a child becomes blue or keeps vomiting after coughing, call for emergency help.

WIND
See **Flatulence.**

WORMS

The most common types of worms to infest humans are the digestive parasites, threadworms (also called pinworms), and roundworms, all of which can be acquired by eating undercooked infected meat or ingesting the eggs by eating dirt. Worms are particularly common in small children aged two to five, who tend to play on the ground and put things in their mouths. The dirt they ingest can harbor eggs, which hatch in the intestine. The principal symptom of threadworms is itching around the anus at night. Roundworms produce few symptoms until they have multiplied, when they cause stomach pain, diarrhea, and vomiting.

PREVENTION

Improve hygiene: Make sure children always wash their hands after going to the toilet and before eating. Keep nails short and clean, and discourage children from putting their fingers in their mouth.

Worm pets regularly.

Vacuum carpets regularly, particularly around and under beds.

TREATMENT

❧ HERBALISM

Wormwood is an effective remedy that can be taken as pills, or in an infusion: Pour 1 cup of boiling water on 2 teaspoons of the dried herb, and infuse for 15 minutes; drink 3 times a day.

Take the equivalent of 1 clove of garlic a day, fresh or as garlic capsules.

☐ HOMEOPATHY

For threadworms, take 3 times a day for 2 weeks (consult a professional if there is no improvement):

Itchy anus, child irritable, hungry, rings under eyes: *Cina* 6c

Itchy anus and nose, worse in evening after going to bed: *Teucrium* 6c

••• ORTHODOX

Doctors generally prescribe anthelmintic drugs, which kill or paralyze the worms and allow them to be passed out in the feces. These drugs may produce side effects of nausea, vomiting, and abdominal pain.

WRY NECK
See **Torticollis.**

XANTHOMATOSIS

A condition in which fatty, yellow deposits accumulate in different parts of the body, particularly the skin, internal organs, blood vessels, eyes, and brain. When the deposits occur only in the eyelids, the condition is known as xanthelasma.

PREVENTION AND TREATMENT

Prevention and treatment are aimed at reducing levels of fat and cholesterol in the body.

✕ DIETARY

Avoid saturated fat, found in animal products (meat and dairy products). Replace red meat with poultry, fish, and vegetable protein, and use nonfat milk.

Eat moderate amounts of polyunsaturated fats, which lower blood cholesterol. They are found in most fats of plant origin (except coconut and palm oils); use olive oil for cooking and low-fat vegetable spreads to replace butter.

Avoid ice cream (have sorbet instead), confectionery made with fat, high-fat snacks (such as potato chips), and fried food.

Increase your intake of whole-grain cereals, complex carbohydrates (potatoes, pasta, rice), cooked dried beans and peas, and fresh fruits and vegetables.

Increase your intake of oat bran and rice bran, which lower cholesterol.

Eat reasonable quantities of nuts and avocados. These contain monounsaturated fat, which is thought to help lower cholesterol.

Eat plenty of fish, particularly salmon, tuna, trout, mackerel, and sardines. Fish oil reduces cholesterol.

૨ુ. HERBALISM

Eat plenty of raw garlic, shown to reduce harmful blood fats. If you do not like the taste or smell of fresh garlic, you can take garlic capsules (3 capsules, 3 times a day).

⁘ EXERCISE

Aerobic exercise helps lower cholesterol. Any activity that raises the pulse and respiration rate significantly for more than 20 minutes is the most effective. Jogging, swimming, skipping, and brisk walking are all good.

~ RELAXATION TECHNIQUES

Studies have shown that relaxation also helps lower cholesterol levels. Learning to meditate, or attending a yoga class, will teach you deep relaxation. Relaxation tapes and biofeedback can also help. See **Stress.**

••• ORTHODOX

Your doctor will probably advise eating a diet that is low in cholesterol and high in polyunsaturated fats (see above), and may prescribe drugs to reduce fats in the blood.

YEAST INFECTION
See **Dandruff; Fungal Infection; Thrush.**

SUGGESTED READING

THE BOOKS LISTED HERE are intended as suggestions: You will find many more books on these subjects than we can possibly list. Some of these books have different publishers in the United States and the United Kingdom. If you are unable to find any of them in your local library or bookstore, ask the librarian or clerk to order them for you.

HEALING TECHNIQUES

✳ ACUPRESSURE

Cerney, J. V., *Acupuncture Without Needles,* New York: Prentice Hall, 1986.

Gach, Michael Reed, D. C., *Acupressure's Potent Points,* New York: Bantam Books, 1990.

Houston, F. M., *The Healing Benefits of Acupressure,* New Canaan, CT: Keats, 1974.

➤ ACUPUNCTURE

Connelly, Diane, *All Sickness Is Homesickness,* Columbia, MD, 1987.

Firebrace, Peter, B.Ac., *Acupuncture—The Illustrated Guide,* Harmony Books.

Nightingale, Michael, *The Healing Power of Acupuncture,* Javelin Books.

▲ ALEXANDER TECHNIQUE

Barker, Sarah, *Alexander Technique: Learning to Use Your Body for Total Energy,* New York: Bantam, 1991.

Connington, Bill and Judith Leibowitz, *Alexander Technique,* New York: HarperCollins, 1990.

◆ APPLIED KINESIOLOGY

Jensen, Clayne R. and Gordon M. Schulz, *Applied Kinesiology,* New York: McGraw-Hill, 1983.

Valentine, Tom, and Carol Valentine, *Applied Kinesiology,* Rochester, VT: Inner Traditions, 1989.

❀ AROMATHERAPY

Davis, Patricia, *Aromatherapy: An A to Z,* C. W. Daniel.

Price, Shirley, *Aromatherapy for Common Ailments,* New York: Fireside, 1991.

——, *Practical Aromatherapy,* Thorsons.

Stead, Christine, *The Power of Holistic Aromatherapy,* New York: Sterling, 1987.

Tisserand, Robert, *Aromatherapy: To Heal and Tend the Body,* Wilmot, WI: Lotus Light, 1989.

✿ BACH FLOWER REMEDIES

Hynne-Jones, T. W., *Dictionary of the Bach Flower Remedies,* C. W. Daniel.

Scheffer, Mechthild, *The Bach Flower Therapy,* Rochester, VT: Inner Traditions, 1987.

Vlamis, Gregory, *Flower Remedies to the Rescue,* Thorsons.

✳ BIOCHEMIC TISSUE SALTS

Goodwin, J. S., *The Biochemic Tissue Salts Handbook,* Thorsons.

Lessell, Colin B., *Biochemic Handbook,* Thorsons.

☯ CHINESE MEDICINE

Li Shih Chen, *Chinese Medicinal Herbs,* Georgetown Press.

Lucas, Richard, *Secrets of the Chinese Herbalists,* New York: Prentice Hall, 1977.

Palos, Stephen, *The Chinese Art of Healing,* Bantam Books.

Reid, Daniel P., *Chinese Herbal Medicine,* Shambhala.

☆ CHIROPRACTIC

Howitt-Wilson, M. B., *Thorsons Introductory Guide to Chiropractic,* Thorsons.

⚘ HERBALISM

Campion, Kitty, *A Woman's Herbal,* Century.

Hoffman, David, *Thorsons Guide to Medical Herbalism,* Thorsons.

Mills, Simon Y., *The Dictionary of Modern Herbalism,* Rochester, VT: Inner Traditions, 1985.

▢ HOMEOPATHY

Castro, Miranda, *The Complete Homeopathy Handbook,* New York: St. Martin, 1991.

Clover, Dr. Anne, *Thorsons Introductory Guide to Homeopathy,* London: Thorsons, 1991.

Cummings, Stephen, M.D., and Dana Ullman, *Everybody's Guide to Homeopathic Medicine,* Los Angeles: Tarcher/Perigee, 1991.

Gemmell, David, *Everyday Homeopathy,* Beaconsfield.

Grossinger, Richard, *Homeopathy: An Introduction for Beginners and Skeptics,* Berkeley: North Atlantic, 1994.

Kruzel, Tom, M.D., *The Homeopathic Emergency Handbook,* Berkeley: North Atlantic, 1992.

Lockie, Dr. Andrew, *The Family Guide to Homeopathy*, New York: Fireside, 1989.

Moskowitz, Richard, M.D., *Homeopathic Medicines for Pregnancy and Childbirth*, Berkeley: North Atlantic, 1992.

Rose, Barry, M.D., *Family Guide to Homeopathy*, Berkeley: Ten Speed, 1993.

Ullman, Dana, *Discovering Homeopathy: Medicine for the 21st Century*, Berkeley: North Atlantic, 1991.

———, *Homeopathic Medicine for Children and Infants*, Los Angeles: Tarcher/ Perigee, 1992.

❋ HYPNOTHERAPY

Gibson, H. B., and M. Heap, *Hypnosis in Therapy*, Hillsdale, NJ: L. Erlbaum Assocs., 1991.

Sleet, Roger, *Hypnotherapy: Is It for You?* New York: Element, 1990.

☛ MASSAGE

Dawes, Nigel, *Massage Cures*, Tulsa, OK: Thorsons, 1990.

King, Robert K., *Performance Massage*, Simi Valley, CA: Leisure Pr., 1992.

Thomas, Sara, *Massage for Common Ailments*, New York: Fireside, 1989.

Young, Jacqueline, *Self Massage*, San Francisco: Thorsons, 1992.

◯ NATUROPATHY AND DIET

Chaitow, Leon, D.O., N.D., *Amino Acids in Therapy*, Healing Arts Press.

——— and Natasha Trenev, *Probiotics*, San Francisco: Thorsons, 1990.

Grant, Doris and Jean Joice, *Food Combining for Health*, Rochester, VT: Inner Traditions, 1987.

Mayes, Adrienne, Ph.D., *The A—Z of Nutritional Therapy*, Thorsons.

Somer, Elizabeth, *The Essential Guide to Vitamins and Minerals*, New York: HarperPerennial, 1992.

Turner, Roger Newman, *Naturopathic Medicine*, San Francisco: Thorsons, 1991.

❖ REFLEXOLOGY

Grinberg, Avig, *Holistic Reflexology*, Thorsons.

Hall, Nicola M., *Thorsons Introductory Guide to Reflexology*, San Francisco: Thorsons, 1988.

Kunz, Kevin and Barbara, *Hand and Foot Reflexology*, New York: Prentice Hall, 1984.

✳ YOGA

Balaskas, Arthur, *Bodylife*, Sidgwick and Jackson.

Friedeberger, Julie, *Office Yoga*, San Francisco: Thorsons, 1992.

Monro, Dr. Robin, *Yoga for Common Ailments,* Dr. Nagarathna, Dr. Nagendra, Fireside.

Tobias, Maxine and Mary Stewart, *The Yoga Books,* Pan Books.

von Lysebeth, Andre, *Yoga Self-Taught,* New York: HarperCollins, 1973.

✿ VISUALIZATION

Gawain, Shakti, *Creative Visualization,* New York: Bantam, 1983.

——, *Creative Visualization Workbook,* San Rafael, CA: New World Library, 1982.

◖ WOMEN'S HEALTH

The Boston Women's Health Book Collective, *The New Our Bodies Ourselves,* New York: Simon & Schuster, 1985.

Hayman, Suzie, *The Well Woman Handbook: A Guide for Women throughout Their Lives,* Penguin.

Reuben, Carolyn and Dr. Joan Priestley, *Essential Supplements for Women,* Thorsons.

Spodnik, Jean Perry and David P. Cogan, M.D., *The Thirty-Five Plus Good Health Guide for Women,* New York: HarperCollins, 1991.

Westcott, Patsy, and Leyardia Black, *Alternative Health Care for Women,* Rochester: VT: Inner Traditions, 1987.

GENERAL

Bricklin, Mark, *The Practical Encyclopedia of Natural Healing,* New York: Penguin, 1990.

Murray, Michael, N.D. and Joseph Pizzorno, N.D., *Encyclopedia of Natural Healing,* New York: Prima, 1991.

Scott, Julian, M.A., Ph.D., *Natural Medicine for Children,* New York: Avon, 1990.

Shreeve, Caroline, *The Alternative Dictionary of Symptoms and Cures,* Century Paperbacks.

Trattler, Ross, N.D., D.O., *Better Health through Natural Healing,* New York: McGraw-Hill, 1988.

SPECIFIC AILMENTS

AIDS

Bamforth, Nick, *AIDS and the Healer Within,* Washington: Amethyst, 1989.

Callen, Michael, *Surviving AIDS,* New York: HarperCollins, 1990.

Charles, Rachel, *Mind, Body and Immunity—How to Enhance Your Body's Natural Defenses,* Methuen.

Froman, Paul Kent, *Pathways to Wellness,* New York: Dutton, 1990.

Kushi, Michio, and Martha Cottrell, *AIDS, Macrobiotics, and Natural Immunity,* New York: Japan Publications, 1989.

Meek, Jennifer, *Immune Power—Health and the Immune System,* Macdonald Optima.

Tavanyar, Judy, *The Terrence Higgins Trust HIV/AIDS Book,* Thorsons.

ALLERGIES

Brown, Dr. H. Morrow, *All About Asthma and Allergy.*

Chaitow, Leon, N.D., D.O., *Asthma and Hayfever,* San Francisco: Thorsons, 1990.

Mumby, Dr. Keith, *The Allergy Handbook,* Thorsons.

Paterson, Barbara, *The Allergy Connection.*

Prevention Magazine, *Allergy Self-Help Book,* Emmaus, PA: Rodale, 1983.

ALZHEIMER'S DISEASE

Markin, R. E., *The Alzheimer's Cope Book,* Secaucus, NJ: Citadel, 1992.

Powel, Lenore S., Ed.D., with Katie Courtice, *Alzheimer's Disease, A Guide for Families,* Reading, MA: Addison-Wesley, 1983.

Woods, Bob, *Alzheimer's Disease—Coping with a Living Death,* Souvenir Press.

AMNESIA

Erdmann, Robert, Ph.D. and Meirion Jones, *Overcoming Memory Problems,* San Francisco: Thorsons, 1991.

ANOREXIA NERVOSA AND BULIMIA

Chernin, Kim, *The Hungry Self,* New York: HarperCollins, 1986.

French, Barbara, *Coping with Bulimia,* San Francisco: Thorsons, 1984.

Lawrence, Marilyn, *The Anorexic Experience,* Women's Press.

Orbach, Susie, *Fat Is a Feminist Issue,* New York: Berkeley, 1982.

Palmer, R. L. *Anorexia Nervosa,* New York: Viking, 1981.

Roth, Geneen, *Feeding the Hungry Heart,* New York: Dutton, 1983.

Siegel, Brisman and Weinshel, *Surviving an Eating Disorder: Strategies for Family and Friends,* New York: HarperCollins, 1989.

ARTHRITIS

Chaitow, Leon, N.D., D.O., *Arthritis (New Self-Help Series),* Thorsons.

BACK PAIN

Fisk, J. W., *Your Painful Neck and Back,* North Pomfret, VT: Trafalgar, 1988.

Turner, Roger Newman, *Back Pain,* Thorsons.

BLOOD PRESSURE, HIGH

Chaitow, Leon, N.D., D.O., *High Blood Pressure,* San Francisco: Thorsons, 1988.

BREAST-FEEDING

La Leche League, *The Womanly Art of Breastfeeding,* New York: Dutton: 1991.

Pryor, Karen and Gale Pryor, *Nursing Your Baby,* Pocket Books.

Renfrew, Mary, Chloe Fisher, and Suzanne Arms, *Getting Breast Feeding Right for You.*

BREAST PROBLEMS

Cirket, Cath, *Breast Awareness,* Thorsons.

Love, Dr. Susan, *Dr. Susan Love's Breast Book,* Reading, MA: Addison-Wesley, 1990.

CANCER

Brohn, Penny, *The Bristol Programme: An Introduction to the Holistic Therapies Practised by the Bristol Cancer Help Centre,* Century.

Clyne, Rachael, *Cancer: Your Life, Your Choice,* Thorsons.

Faulder, Carolyn, *Always a Woman: A Practical Guide to Living with Breast Cancer,* Thorsons.

CATARRH

White, Arthur, N.D., D.O., *Catarrh (New Self-Help Series),* Thorsons.

COLITIS

White, Arthur, N.D., D.O., *Colitis (New Self-Help Series),* Thorsons.

CYSTITIS

Kilmartin, Angela, *Cystitis: a Complete Self-Help Guide,* Warner Books.

Shreeve, Caroline, *Cystitis,* Rochester, VT: Inner Traditions, 1987.

DEPRESSION

Rowe, Dorothy, *Depression, The Way Out of Your Prison,* New York: Routledge, 1984.

DIVERTICULITIS

White, Arthur, N.D., D.O., *Diverticulitis (New Self-Help Series),* San Francisco: Thorsons, 1988.

ECZEMA

Orton, Christine, *Eczema Relief,* San Francisco: Thorsons, 1991.

ENDOMETRIOSIS

Breitkopf, Dr. Lyle and Marion Gordon Bakoulis, *Endometriosis,* Thorsons.

EYE PROBLEMS

Barnes, Jonathan, *Improve Your Eyesight,* Angus and Robertson.

Benjamin, Harry, *Better Sight without Glasses,* San Francisco: Thorsons, 1986.

FATIGUE

Chaitow, Leon, N.D., D.O., *The Beat Fatigue Workbook (New Self-Help Series),* San Francisco: Thorsons, 1989.

HEADACHES

Chaitow, Leon, *Headaches and Migraine (New Self-Help Series),* Thorsons.

HEART PROBLEMS

Mervyn, Leonard, Ph.D., *Heart Disease (New Self-Help Series),* San Francisco: Thorsons, 1990.

HIATUS HERNIA

Lay, Joan, N.D., *Hiatus Hernia (New Self-Help Series),* Thorsons.

HYPERACTIVITY

Barnes, Belinda and Irene Colquhoun, *The Hyperactive Child—Handbook for Parents,* London: Thorsons.

Feingold, B. F., *Why Your Child Is Hyperactive,* New York: Random House, 1985.

INCONTINENCE

Millard, Dr. Richard J., *Overcoming Urinary Incontinence,* Thorsons.

INFERTILITY

Stangel, John J., M.D, *The New Fertility and Conception,* New York: Dutton, 1988.

Winston, Robert, *Getting Pregnant,* Anaya Publishers.

LABOR PAIN/CHILDBIRTH

Balaskas, Janet, *New Active Birth,* Thorsons.

ME

Macintyre, Dr. Anne, *M.E. Post-Viral Fatigue Syndrome: How to Live with It,* Thorsons.

Shepherd, Dr. Charles, *Living with M.E.: A Self-Help Guide,* Heinemann Cedar.

Wilkinson, Steve, *M.E. and You, A Survivor's Guide to Post-Viral Fatigue Syndrome,* Thorsons.

MENOPAUSE

Reitz, Rosetta, *Menopause—A Positive Approach,* New York: Viking, 1979.

Shreeve, Dr. Caroline, *Overcoming the Menopause Naturally.*

MENSTRUAL CRAMPS

Weller, Stella, *Pain-Free Periods—Natural Ways of Overcoming Menstrual Problems,* Rochester, VT: Inner Traditions, 1986.

MULTIPLE SCLEROSIS

Graham, Judy, *Multiple Sclerosis: A Self-Help Guide to Its Management,* Rochester, VT: Inner Traditions, 1990.

OSTEOPOROSIS

Cooper, Wendy, *Understanding Osteoporosis,* Arrow Books.

Dixon, Dr. Allan and Dr. Anthony Woolf, *Avoiding Osteoporosis,* MacDonald Optima.

PAIN

Chaitow, Leon, *The Book of Pain Relief,* Thorsons.

POSTNATAL DEPRESSION

Dalton, Katharina, *Depression After Childbirth: How to Recognize and Treat Post-Natal Depression,* New York: Oxford University Press, New York: 1989.

PREGNANCY

Pickard, Dr. Barbara, *Eating Well for a Healthy Pregnancy,* Sheldon.

PREMENSTRUAL SYNDROME

Dalton, Katharina, *Once a Month,* Claremont, CA: Hunter House, 1990.

Lark, Susan M., *PMS Self-Help Book: A Women's Guide,* Berkeley, CA: Celestial Arts, 1989.

Shreeve, Dr. Caroline, *Premenstrual Syndrome,* San Bernardino, CA: Borgo, 1986.

PROSTATE PROBLEMS

Chaitow, Leon, N.D., D.O., *Prostate Troubles (New Self-Help Series)*, Thorsons.

Hamand, Jeremy, *Prostate Problems*, San Francisco: Thorsons, 1991.

Rous, Stephen, M.D., *The Prostate Book: Sound Advice on Symptoms and Treatment*, New York: Norton, 1988.

Swanson, Janice M. and Katherine A. Forrest, eds., *Men's Reproductive Health*, New York: Springer, 1984.

PSORIASIS

Gibbons, Sandra, *Psoriasis*, Thorsons.

SEASONAL AFFECTIVE DISORDER

Smyth, Angela, *Seasonal Affective Disorder, Who Gets It, What Causes It, How to Cure It*, San Francisco: Thorsons, 1992.

STRESS

Kirsta, Alix, *The Book of Stress Survival*, New York: Simon & Schuster, 1987.

Wikin-Lanoil, Georgia, *Coping with Stress: A Practical Self-Help Guide for Women*, Sheldon.

TINNITUS

White, Arthur, N.D., D.O., *Tinnitus (New Self-Help Series)*, Thorsons.

ULCERS

Mervyn, Leonard, Ph.D., *Stomach Ulcers and Acidity (New Self-Help Series)*, San Francisco: Thorsons, 1990.

VAGINISMUS

Valins, Linda, *When a Woman's Body Says No to Sex: Understanding and Overcoming Vaginismus*, New York: Penguin, 1992.

VARICOSE VEINS

Chaitow, Leon, N.D., D.O., *Varicose Veins (New Self-Help Series)*, San Francisco: Thorsons.

////// *Index*